EVOLVING TRENDS IN KIDNEY CANCER

Edited by **Sashi S. Kommu**
and **Inderbir S. Gill**

Evolving Trends in Kidney Cancer
http://dx.doi.org/10.5772/intechopen.70252
Edited by Sashi S. Kommu and Inderbir S. Gill

Contributors

Radu Ion Badea, Lidia Ciobanu, Attila Tama Szora, Alexandru Florin Badea, Mihai Suciu, Xin Ma, Cheng Peng, Liangyou Gu, Xu Zhang, Dan Shen, Songliang Du, Qingbo Huang, Baojun Wang, Luojia Yang, Lingxiang Liu, Yang Wang, Ana Marisa Chudzinski-Tavassi, Katia Luciano Pereira Morais, Roger Chammas, Jean Souza, Le Qu, Cheng Chen, Ding Wu, Camilla Tajzler, Anil Kapoor, Fadil Hassan, Shahid Lambe, Faiz Mumtaz, Menazir Sha, Neelan Das, Keshav Mudgal, Mohammed Kamil Quraishi, Milan Thomas, Ben Eddy, Adrian Simoes, Rakesh Raman, Jennifer Turner, Albert Edwards, Amr Emara, Manar Malki, Hilten Patel, Chris Anderson, Nicholas Mehan, Minna Kankuri-Tammilehto

Notice

First published in London, United Kingdom, 2020 by IntechOpen
IntechOpen is the global imprint of INTECHOPEN LIMITED, registered in England and Wales, registration number: 11086078, 7th floor, 10 Lower Thames Street, London,
EC3R 6AF, United Kingdom
Printed in Croatia

British Library Cataloguing-in-Publication Data
A catalogue record for this book is available from the British Library

Additional hard and PDF copies can be obtained from orders@intechopen.com

Evolving Trends in Kidney Cancer, Edited by Sashi S. Kommu and Inderbir S. Gill
p. cm.
Print ISBN 978-1-83881-959-0
Online ISBN 978-1-83881-960-6
eBook (PDF) ISBN 978-1-83881-964-4

Meet the editors

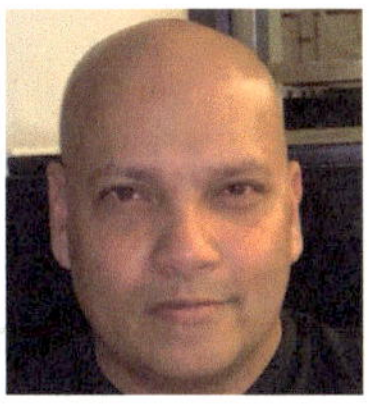

Dr Sashi S. Kommu is an Associate Professor in Uro-oncology and Cancer Biology in The School of Biosciences; The University of Kent, United Kingdom. He is also a Consultant Pelvic Cancer Urological Surgeon with a subspecialty interest in minimally invasive management of urological cancers including laparoscopic and robotic urological surgery at East Kent Hospitals University NHS Foundation Trust. He leads The National Institute for Health Research (NIHR) for all surgical specialties for Kent, Surrey and Sussex in the U.K. His key clinical interests are in the minimally invasive management of urological cancers, surgical robotics and intelligent probes. He has done formal research at The Royal Marsden NHS Foundation Trust and The Institute of Cancer Research with The Translational Cancer Genetics Team where he refined his scientific methodology in advanced laboratory work with an emphasis on cancer genetics and proteomics. He has also gained vast exposure in nanotechnology. He has over 100 peer-reviewed publications in respected scientific and medical journals including The Lancet. He also has over 300 scientific presentations, several book chapters and books. Dr Kommu has over 25 academic awards including The Olympus Award at The 25th World Congress of Endourology in Cleveland U.S.A. 2006. He has nine pending patents including a cost-effective Telerounding Kit for Remote Teleconsultations, which was presented at The House of Commons (Hosted by The British Parliament) in 2006. His ability to blend medical science with engineering and technology has earned him two NASA collaborative scientific commendations. Dr Kommu is reviewer for 15 surgical/urological and 3 basic sciences journals. Several novel concepts described by Dr Kommu include 'suppressor screening in urological cancer screening' and 'the supplementary biomarker approach' for detecting cancers.

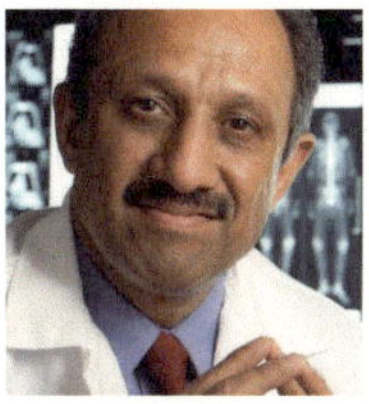

Dr Inderbir Gill is Chairman and Distinguished Professor of the Catherine and Joseph Aresty Department of Urology, Founding Executive Director of the USC Institute of Urology and Associate Dean for clinical innovation. Dr Gill is an internationally recognized leader in the field of robotic and laparoscopic surgery for urologic cancers. An acclaimed innovator, he and his team are the world leaders in robotic urologic cancer surgery for prostate, kidney and bladder cancer, having performed over 15,000 aggregate cases. For his outstanding work, Dr Gill has received numerous prestigious awards, including the Dr B.C. Roy National Award, presented by the President of India for Eminent Medical Person in India. It marked the first time a physician living outside of India was selected for this national award. Dr Gill was also awarded the St. Paul's Medal by the British Association of Urological Surgeons, which is the highest honour bestowed by the organisation. He has published more than 750 peer-reviewed scientific papers, 50 book chapters and eight textbooks. He was elected to the prestigious American Association of Genito-Urinary Surgeons in 2003 and was selected as European Urology's first North American editor. Dr Gill is a distinguished researcher and prolific scholar. He has been listed among the Best Doctors in America for several years.

Contents

Preface

Ours is an exciting time. At no other time in history has there been such an exponential increase in our understanding of disease processes through research and innovation. Kidney cancer is no exception. The recent propulsion and coupling of technological advances and targeted drug therapy in the management of kidney cancer has ushered with it a plethora of significant advances in our current approach. However, kidney cancer continues to impose a significant cancer burden and its incidence continues to rise globally. Mortality in advanced kidney cancer remains high despite oncological, surgical and multimodal optimisation. Genetic associations, heterogeneity and limitations in early diagnosis through lack of optimal biomarkers and early detection tools add to the challenges.

This book is the first in a series that aims to act as a primer and to provide the reader with a comprehensive and up-to-date framework to optimise understanding and stimulate further research and innovation. The chapters were written by a global faculty of leading experts in the respective fields with a multidisciplinary approach. The authorship includes scientists, pathologists, engineers, surgeons, radiologists, oncologists and innovators. The focus of the book is broad and includes genetics, immunology, virtual augmented reality, surgical simulation and robotic surgery. Some chapters explore leading edge concepts while others capture the evolving trends and future concepts.

The Editors would like to acknowledge the respective authors and sponsors for their hard work and support in generating this book.

Dr. Sashi S. Kommu
Associate Professor in Uro-oncology and Cancer Biology
School of Biosciences, University of Kent
Consultant Urological and Minimally Invasive Surgeon
East Kent Hospitals University NHS Foundation Trust
National Institute for Health Research (NIHR) Lead for Surgery in Kent, Surrey and Sussex, UK

Dr. Inderbir S. Gill
Chair and Distinguished Professor of Urology
Shirley and Donald Skinner Chair in Urologic Cancer Surgery
Executive Director, USC Institute of Urology
Associate Dean for Clinical Innovation
University of Southern California (USC)
Los Angeles, California, USA

Section 1

Genetic Susceptibility and Immunotherapy

Chapter 1

Genetic Susceptibility to Kidney Cancer

Minna Kankuri-Tammilehto

Additional information is available at the end of the chapter

http://dx.doi.org/10.5772/intechopen.91933

Abstract

According to the latest knowledge, hereditary kidney cancers may account for 5–8% of all kidney cancers, and it may be more common than previously thought. Hereditary RCC is often characterized by an early age of onset (approximately 45 years), typical histological pattern, and frequently the bilaterality and multicentricity of the primary tumor. Wilms' tumor (nephroblastoma) is the most common kidney tumor of childhood. More than 15 syndromes with inherited susceptibility to kidney cancer are known, and there are over 25 known genes associated with them. Most of these are dominantly inherited in which the offspring of the proband has a 50% chance of inheriting a gene mutation with susceptibility to kidney cancer. The aggressiveness of hereditary RCCs and recommended surgery varies depending on the syndrome and mutation type. Also, systemic therapy may be optional. Multigene next generation sequencing (NGS) panel technology allows genes of interest to be studied quickly and cost-effectively. Sequencing investigations have improved the accuracy of hereditary cancer diagnoses. Diagnostic utility has been hugely increased by multigene NGS panels. It is important to identify hereditary cancer susceptibility, because the risk of cancer in the mutation carriers can be reduced. In this review article, the latest literature on syndromes subjecting to hereditary kidney cancer and recommended follow-up is summarized.

Keywords: von Hippel-Lindau, hereditary papillary RCC, hereditary leiomyomatosis and RCC, Birt-Hogg-Dubé, Wilms' tumor, hereditary kidney cancer syndromes, genetic susceptibility

1. Introduction

Kidney cancer is the 16th most common cancer worldwide with over 400,000 cases in 2018 representing approximately 2.2% of all diagnosed malignancies worldwide [1]. The majority of primary renal malignancies are renal cell carcinomas (RCCs) with most of the remaining comprising upper tract urothelial carcinoma (UTUC). The mean age of onset of RCC is approximately 60–70 years. The most common kidney tumor of childhood is Wilms' tumor (nephroblastoma). In the European Union, the estimated annual number of new kidney cancers is approximately 46,000 [2]. Etiologic risk factors for kidney cancer development are male sex, obesity, and tobacco, in addition to hypertension [3–5], acquired cystic kidney disease [6], and inherited susceptibility. Prognostic factors of different protein and gene expressions in RCC have been studied [7, 8].

According to the latest knowledge, hereditary kidney cancers may account for 5–8% of all kidney cancers [9], and it may be more common than previously thought [10]. In those RCC patients without clear cell RCC (ccRCC) subtype, the amount of germline high-risk mutations is greater, 12% [11]. Susceptibility to kidney cancer may be caused by high-risk, moderate-risk, or low-risk gene mutation [12]. Even the carriership of high-risk gene mutation does not always lead to kidney cancer. The risk for kidney cancer (penetrance) varies in different syndromes. In some cases, the predisposed genetic factor to kidney cancer is chromosomal aberration, for example, as in constitutional chromosomal 3 translocation with 6 or 8 of family (**Table 2**). In hereditary cancer, the impact of environmental factors is small.

More than 15 syndromes with inherited susceptibility to kidney cancer are known, and there are over 25 known genes associated with them. Most of these are dominantly inherited in which the offspring of the proband has a 50% chance of inheriting a gene mutation with susceptibility to kidney cancer.

2. Identifying hereditary kidney cancer

Hereditary kidney cancer syndrome is often characterized by an early age of onset (approximately 45 years) [30], typical histological pattern, and frequently the bilaterality and multicentricity of the primary tumor (**Table 1**). By evaluating the family history of diagnosed cancer cases, benign tumors, and diagnostic gene test results, it is possible to identify families with hereditary kidney cancer (**Tables 2** and **3**).

It is possible that there exists only a single hereditary cancer syndrome case in the family due to de novo mutations (autosomal dominant) which means that the person's parents do not have the same mutation. There are hot spot regions in genes where mutation can easier develop during meiosis of germ cells. In addition to this, the risk of hereditary kidney cancer

Multiple close relatives with benign or malign tumors of the syndrome
Atypically young age of onset for tumors of the syndrome
Relative with two tumors of the syndrome (two examples below)
• RCC and uterine leiomyosarcoma • Colon cancer or endometrial carcinoma in the uterus and upper tract urothelial carcinoma
Typical histological finding (e.g., rare subtype or multiplicity) or clinical picture

Table 1. Factors suggesting inherited cancer syndrome.

	von Hippel-Lindau (VHL)	Hereditary papillary RCC (HPRC)	Hereditary leiomyomatosis and RCC (HLRCC)	Birt-Hogg-Dubé (BHD)	Constitutional chromosomal 3 translocation
RCC subtype	Clear cell carcinoma	Papillary type 1	Papillary type 2, collecting duct	Most often chromophobe ± oncocytoma	Clear cell carcinoma
Risk for RCC	40%	Nearly 100%	20–30%	30%	30%
Gene	*VHL*	*MET*	*FH*	*FLCN(BHD)*	
Typical age of onset for RCC	40 years	50–70 years	Less than 40 years	50 years	
Biology of RCC	Bilaterality, multiple tumors	Bilaterality, multiple tumors, microscopic lesions as much as 1000	Unilaterality, solitarity, aggressive, highly potential to metastasize	Bilaterality, multiple tumors	Bilaterality, multiple tumors
Typical surgery	Minimal invasive	Minimal invasive or radical nephrectomy	Radical nephrectomy	Minimal invasive	
Other signs of the syndrome than RCC	Retinal hemangioma/CNS hemangioblastoma, pheochromocytoma	None	Uterine leiomyomas in almost every patient, uterine leiomyosarcoma, cutaneous leiomyomas	Cutaneous hair follicle benign tumors and pulmonary cysts in almost every patient	Thyroid, bladder, pancreatic and gastric cancer
Reference	[13, 14]	[15, 16]	[17–20]	[21, 22]	[23]

Table 2. Hereditary cancer syndromes in which the kidney cancer risk is high.

is linked to some congenital multisystem syndromes, such as Beckwith-Wiedemann syndrome and tuberous sclerosis (**Table 4**). When such a multisystemic syndrome is detected, appropriate follow-up care is provided as with hereditary kidney cancer families.

It is suspected that hereditary kidney cancer is underdiagnosed. Identifying the families with increased risk for kidney cancer allows clinicians to improve the prognosis of persons with genetic cancer susceptibility. This review discussed the characteristics of inherited kidney cancer and how to improve their prognosis (**Table 5**).

3. Basic cancer genetics

In hereditary and sporadic cancer, the normal genome regulation is impaired [34], and cancer susceptibility is caused by both inherited germline gene mutations and somatic gene mutations in tissue that occurred over time. However, in sporadic cases the inherited gene mutations cause low risk for kidney cancer [35]. Of all clear cell-type RCCs (sporadic or hereditary), 75% have a somatic mutation in the von Hippel-Lindau tumor suppressor gene (VHL) in the short

	Lynch syndrome	Cowden syndrome	Hyperparathyroid jaw tumor syndrome	Hereditary pheochromocytoma and paraganglioma	Li-Fraumeni syndrome	BAP1 tumor predisposition syndrome
Kidney cancer subtype	Upper tract urothelial carcinoma	Clear cell, papillary, chromophobe	Papillary type 1 RCC, adult Wilms' tumor	Clear cell RCC, chromophobe RCC, oncocytoma	RCC and Wilms' tumor	Clear cell RCC
Risk for kidney cancer	Multiple	15%	Uncommon	10%	Low	10%
Gene	*MLH1, MSH2, MSH6, PMS2, EPCAM*	*PTEN*	*CDC73*	*SDHB, SDHC, SDHD*	*p53*	*BAP1*
Other signs of the syndrome than RCC	Bowel cancer, uterine, ovarian cancer	Mucocutaneous papules, hamartomas, macrocephaly, thyroid cancer, uterine cancer, intestinal polyps	Ossifying jaw fibromas, renal cysts, parathyroid adenoma/carcinoma, uterine tumors	Paragangliomas, pheochromocytoma, GIST	Brain tumor, sarcoma, leukemia and other cancer types	Uveal and cutaneous melanoma, mesothelioma
Reference	[24]	[25]	[26]	[27]	[28]	[29]

Table 3. Hereditary cancer syndromes in which the kidney cancer risk is moderate or low.

	Tuberous sclerosis	Beckwith-Wiedemann syndrome	Perlman syndrome
Kidney cancer subtype	Clear cell, papillary, chromophobe	Wilms' tumor	Wilms' tumor
Risk for kidney cancer	Less than 5%	Around 5%	30–60%
Gene	*TSC1, TSC2*	*CDKN1C*	*DIS3L2*
Typical age of onset for kidney cancer	35 years	Primarily in the first 8 years of life	Neonatally
Inheritance	Autosomal dominant	Autosomal dominant, sporadic	Autosomal recessive
Other signs of the syndrome than kidney cancer	Renal angiomyolipomas, hypopigmentation, seizures, learning difficulties, angiofibromas, shagreen patches, oral mucosal lesions, subependymal giant cell astrocytoma	Neonatal hypoglycemia, macrosomia, macroglossia, hemihyperplasia, omphalocele, renal abnormalities	Fetal ascites, macrosomia, visceromegaly, generalized hypotonia
References	[31, 32]	[33]	[33]

Table 4. Congenital multisystem syndromes with susceptibility for the kidney cancer.

The aim is to improve the early detection of cancer
Occurrence can be prevented by removing the precursors identified in the monitoring • In the carriers of Lynch syndrome mutation, removal of colon adenomas decreases the risk of colon cancer
Occurrence can be prevented by surgical procedures • In the carriers of Lynch syndrome mutation, removal of uterus by menopause decreases the risk of endometrial carcinoma in uterus
Sometimes genetic information can guide the choice of medication • In the carriers of p53 mutation, radiation therapy and X-ray imaging will be avoided

Table 5. How to improve prognosis in the carriers of hereditary gene mutation.

arm of chromosome [36]. According to Vogelstein's research group, chance has a major impact in the development of cancer-causing mutations during DNA replication in normal, noncancerous stem cells [37]. Current understanding is that about four to seven mutations in key driver genes is sufficient to cause cancer to develop [38].

Genes associated with cancer predisposition are oncogenes or tumor suppressor genes. Oncogenes act as gain of function. Mutation in the other allele is sufficient to produce the altered protein. An example of this is the *MET* oncogene, in which mutation predisposes to hereditary papillary renal cell carcinoma (HPRC) (**Table 2**). However, typically inherited cancer predisposition is caused by the loss of function of tumor suppressor gene. In nearly all cases, the mutations in tumor suppressor genes function recessively at the cellular level, following Knudson's theory of two hits [39]. Therefore, both alleles must lose function before the carcinogenesis may occur. The first mutation associated with the syndrome, the germline mutation, passes the susceptibility to cancer to the next generation (nearly always) according to the autosomal dominant inheritance and is situated in all the persons' cells. The mutation in the other allele in the same gene occurs during life. The penetrance of the inherited mutation is decreased. Therefore, only part of the mutation carriers will be affected, but the risk of cancer is many times higher than in an average population (**Tables 2** and **3**).

Caretaker genes are responsible for genomic stability by detecting damage to the genome, such as single- or double-stranded DNA breaks [40]. Disruption in these genes leads to genomic instability: an increase in the number of spontaneous mutations that cause new mutations in oncogenes and growth restriction genes. Mutations in the caretaker genes are responsible for a number of cancer susceptibility syndromes. For example, germline mutation in the growth restriction gene *MLH1* exposes for Lynch syndrome, which is associated with a high risk of colon and endometrial carcinoma in the uterus and multiple risk for urothelial carcinoma compared to an average population [24, 41]. Gatekeeper genes control cell growth. Normally, a mutation in a gatekeeper gene activates the caretaker genes to participate in repair [34]. However, if this repair does not work, mutation in the gatekeeper gene will result in tumor formation. For example, *p53* acts as a gatekeeper, and its mutation exposes it to several types of cancers, such as RCC (**Table 3**).

Genetics of cancer is only partially known. Advanced technological methods can detect previously unknown mutations in germline and tumors. Knowledge of the biology of hereditary cancer also increases the understanding of sporadic cancers, as the same disease genes are found in hereditary and non-hereditary cancers: e.g., mutated *MET* is a driver gene in hereditary and sporadic papillary renal carcinomas [42], and mutated *WT1* is observed both in sporadic and hereditary Wilms' tumor. Novel genes and variants may be explored by whole exome (WES) or genome research (WGS), where also noncoding regions are examined, in scientific research projects. Identifying low-risk variants requires data from thousands of patients and controls, which are investigated in genome-wide association studies (GWAS).

4. Genetic counseling and supporting families with hereditary cancer

It is important to identify hereditary cancer susceptibility, because the risk of cancer, morbidity, and mortality in the mutation carriers can be reduced both in cancer patients and healthy relatives in the family. If the family mutation is known, healthy family members with mutation can participate in preventive studies. If the person does not have the known family mutation, there is no need to have follow-up care because the risk of the cancer is the same as for an average population.

Diagnostic gene testing on cancer patients is carried out in the clinical genetic units, but diagnostic genetic testing can also be ordered by a treating oncologist or surgeon for patients with kidney cancer. There are established principles for considering genetic testing in the case of suspected hereditary cancer susceptibility (**Table 6**) [43]. If there is a genetic test that is appropriate for the situation, the American Society of Clinical Oncology (ASCO) recommends access to genetic testing. Before testing the individuals, informed consent should be requested after adequate information and counseling [44]. For genetic testing the patient's peripheral blood, lymphocyte DNA is examined for identifying a possible hereditary mutation.

The investigation for finding the family mutation is always started with the affected person. A medical geneticist will determine who could have mutation with increased kidney cancer risk

Hereditary cancer is suspected
The result of the gene test should be adequately interpreted
Gene testing has one of the following benefits: • Improves diagnosis • Guides to the appropriate medical surveillance for the carriers of gene mutation • Provides information about strategies for prevention in the carriers of gene mutation

The ASCO has provided guidance on when genetic testing for cancer families should be considered [43]. The following three conditions should be met. If the family mutation is found, the access for healthy relatives to genetic counseling should be arranged.

Table 6. ASCO 2010 criteria for genetic testing.

in the family. If there are no surviving cancer patients in the family, with the permission of the relative, from the pathology department, a sample of the deceased person may be requested to have healthy tissue DNA for genetic examination.

The result of the genetic testing gives information about the cancer risk of relatives. Healthy at-risk relatives should have access to genetic counseling and predictive genetic testing after counseling if they decide (Council of Europe's The Convention on Human Rights and Biomedicine in Article 12, 1997). The clinical genetics units offer this service. The geneticist will have the opportunity to provide the laboratory with reliable information about the family mutation and arrange for the laboratory the DNA sample of the family's index patient, which is a control sample, positive control, to obtain a reliable test result. Counseling before predictive genetic testing is nondirective and includes insight of the patient and the family. In counseling, the patient and family receive not only information but also support. Increased anxiety or distress has been documented in both counselors and their families around testing when investigating hereditary VHL susceptibility [45]. The Genetic Information Nondiscrimination Act of the Council of Europe's Convention in Article 11, in 1997, was passed to prevent forms of genetic discrimination by employment and health insurance. The Council of Europe's Convention prohibits the transfer of genetic information to employers in order to prevent employment discrimination. Insurance discrimination is discussed in counseling. In Finland, genetic testing is organized by public health care, which is why very few gene tests are conducted privately.

Participation in predictive genetic testing has been studied in the Finnish Lynch syndrome families, which are at high risk for colorectal cancer and endometrial carcinoma in the uterus. Approximately 80% of the members of the family participated in genetic counseling, and 95% of them performed genetic prediction [46]. The main reasons for participating in predictive genetic testing are the potential for cancer detection in surveillance monitoring, improved treatment options in many Lynch syndrome cancer types, and improved cancer prognosis.

After the genetic testing, the counselor should always receive an interpretation of the significance of the genetic test result [43, 44]. Different mutations in the same disease gene, for example, in the inherited VHL gene, can have varying effects on cancer risk and prognosis [47]. The genetic practitioner will assess the significance of the result for each family separately. It is useful to wait until the age of 18 to allow an offspring to reach an age of consent in those inherited syndromes in which the age of onset is in adulthood. However, the early age of onset in condition like VHL could have devastating complications without early detection and management, and therefore in this syndrome predictive testing is recommended to at-risk children in family.

5. Genotype-phenotype correlation in kidney cancer

VHL is divided to subgroups for academic purposes according to the phenotype based on the likelihood of pheochromocytoma or renal cell carcinoma. In the following some examples are described. For example, a reduced risk for renal cell carcinoma in individuals has been observed with a deletion of *VHL* [13]. A *MET* variant due to a mutation is associated with early-onset HPRC disease [16]. The *WT1* gene mutation may cause hereditary Wilms' tumor without syndrome or with syndrome, like Denys-Drash, Frasier, or nephrotic syndrome type 4. WT1 protein plays an important role in renal and gonadal development, due to which genital abnormalities can be seen in Denys-Drash and Frasier syndrome. In Frasier syndrome patients have progressive nephrotic syndrome, but incidence of Wilms' tumor is rare. Mutations that are responsible for Frasier syndrome are located in intron 9 in *WT1* (an alternative splicing site). In Denys-Drash syndrome, patients' typical symptoms are progressive nephrotic syndrome that early progresses to renal failure less than the age of 4 years. A majority of the Denys-Drash patients have mutations located in exons 8 and 9. The risk of Wilms' tumor is very high (90%).

6. The diagnostic impact of gene testing evolution

Multigene next generation sequencing (NGS) panel technology allows genes of interest to be studied quickly and cost-effectively. By focused massive parallel sequencing, it is possible to examine those exons of the genome's genes that are of interest in diagnosing the cause of inherited kidney cancer. The method can also investigate boundaries between exons and introns. A gene panel for hereditary kidney cancer covers approximately 25 genes and can be ordered from different companies. Clinical picture may sometimes indicate a mutation in particular gene or genes, which can be separately examined. However, often hereditary mutation may be in many different genes according to patient and family history, and then multigene panel-based NGS will be more economical than Sanger or NGS sequencing of several different genes. Sequencing results are obtained in about 4 weeks. The gene content of the panels is regularly updated by laboratories as information on genes associated with kidney cancer is published continuously. A limitation of parallel sequencing is that they cannot recognize large intrinsic deletions or duplicates, and for this another method is required that investigates exome CNVs. A majority of hereditary mutations are located in the exome region. The whole genome NGS is not yet a routine method, but it is used in scientific studies. By the NGS method, the diagnostic utility of hereditary cancers has been hugely improved.

Information on the clinical significance associated with mutations is reviewed in registers (e.g., InSiGHT and ClinVar) [48]. With the development of research techniques, more variants of uncertain significance (VUS) are now observed. Currently, these are also variants of which it is unknown whether they are benign or pathogenic and explain the patient's predisposition to cancer. In some situations, the variant may be classified as likely pathogenic. Prediction programs can be used to evaluate a variant's ability to cause disease (in silico analysis) [49, 50]. For example, the ExAC database can be used to check the prevalence of the variant in the population. As techniques evolve, it is increasingly possible to study the functional change in RNA structure caused by VUS alteration, which would be relevant to the quality of the resulting protein. In order to clarify the nature of the uncertain variants, the geneticist may arrange the so-called segregation analysis in family [49]. Finding the same hereditary variant from several relatives with cancer would strengthen the conclusion that the variant explains the cases in the family. Information is being collected internationally as laboratories collect VUS they observe into databases and doctors publish case reports. However, in already well-known genes such as BRCA and Lynch syndrome genes, VUS alterations are relatively rarely detected.

During counseling, the geneticist will inform what is known about the significance of the identified variant. If the significance of the variant remains open, the geneticist and laboratory experts may reclassify the change after few years. The increased use of multigene NGS panels in patient work expands the knowledge on the different pathogenic variants in the human DNA. The number of VUS changes will therefore decrease in the next few years [50]. It is important that counseling provides reliable information on the examination results and therefore VUS modifications are not used as a basis for prophylactic surgery or to determine the risk of relatives' cancer.

7. Treatment in hereditary kidney cancer

For several RCC syndromes, studies have found that conservative management appears to preserve renal function without increased mortality. In certain syndromes, such as HLRCC, early and aggressive treatment may be preferable [17, 20]. Each subtype of RCC may need to be treated differently by systemic therapy, but no phase III clinical trial data exist from distinct treatments [51, 52]. The prognosis was inferior for papillary metastatic RCC (mRCC) compared to clear cell mRCC when patients were treated with the same evidence-based treatment in a study by Staehler [52]. The understanding of the metabolic and epigenetic abnormalities underlying the symptoms of hereditary kidney cancer-associated genes may lead to the development of novel diagnostic biomarkers and novel treatment modalities for kidney cancer [53].

8. Surveillance in hereditary kidney cancer families

Recommendations for follow-up care should correspond to the level of risk associated with the genetic variant tested [43]. The aim of the monitoring is to improve the early detection of cancer in families with hereditary renal cancer. Monitoring recommendations includes regular kidney imaging: the healthy carrier of a gene mutation predisposing to kidney cancer will usually undergo abdominal MRI scans on a regular basis (**Table 7**). The frequency of follow-up depends on the biological nature of the family syndrome. Several monitoring planes have been proposed for hereditary kidney cancer syndromes, for example, by Freifeld [54] and Carlo [10]. Also, PDQ Cancer Information Summaries [55] has a suggestion for surveillance in certain syndromes predisposing to hereditary renal cancer.

Tracking intervals may be less frequent, for example, for HPRC, and more frequent for others, such as HLRCC in the case of an early onset of 10 years [56] and several reported cases among children. However, the estimated risk of developing RCC before age 20 is estimated to be only around 1–2%, whereas the lifetime risk of RCC among *FH* mutation carriers is approximately 15% [25]. In 2014, consensus guidelines from an international HLRCC symposium recommended annual renal MRI starting at age 8 to 10 years, as also recommended by the HLRCC Family Alliance and the French National Cancer Institute [25]. The starting age is still variable. In HPRC patients, if the tumor smaller than 3 cm is found, imaging should be repeated within the first year to assess the growth rate [55]. Generally, patients with renal

	von Hippel-Lindau (VHL)	Hereditary papillary RCC (HPRC)	Hereditary leiomyomatosis and RCC (HLRCC)	Birt-Hogg-Dubé (BHD)
RCC subtype	Clear cell carcinoma	Papillary type 1	Papillary type 2, collecting duct	Most often chromophobe ± oncocytoma
Risk for RCC	40%	Nearly 100%	20–30%	30%
Gene	*VHL*	*MET*	*FH*	*FLCN(BHD)*
Typical age of onset for RCC	40 years	50–70 years	Less than 40 years	50 years
Abdominal magnetic imaging	Annually starting at the age of 10	Annually starting at the age of 30	Annually starting at the age of 5–20 years	Annually starting at the age of 20 years
Other surveillance	Biannual brain and spine MRI starting at the age of 11 Ophthalmological and audiological exam Plasma-free metanephrines/ urinary metanephrines	None	Dermatological and gynecological exam	Dermatological exam and CT of the chest

Table 7. Follow-up care recommendations in hereditary cancer syndromes in which the kidney cancer risk is high [10, 25, 54].

tumors associated with HPRC are candidates for radiologic surveillance until one or more tumors reach 3 cm. Ultrasound is not sufficient in surveillance of hereditary kidney cancer syndromes [10, 25, 54, 55]. In the near future, more evidence on effective monitoring in different kidney cancer syndromes will be gathered. If the gene mutation has not been identified but the family has a significantly increased risk of kidney cancer, a regular renal imaging examination in the first-degree relative of the patient with renal cancer may be considered on a case-by-case basis. Other surveillance procedures depend on the risks of the specific symptoms in observed gene mutation. In multisystem syndromes, monitoring practices depend on the probability of the kidney cancer, and ultrasound may be used in monitoring.

In Lynch syndrome, which is a high risk for upper tract ureotelic carcinoma, the risk of colorectal cancer can be reduced by removing intestinal adenomas at regular checkups, which results in the same mortality to colorectal cancer in the carriers of Lynch gene mutation as in the general population.

9. Future perspectives

The contents of routine gene panels are based on the knowledge on kidney cancer susceptibility genes. If a patient's DNA sequencing has failed to identify the hereditary mutation, RNA sequencing may identify the specific diagnosis [57]. If there are three patients in the family, trio exome analysis may be a pivotal method. Potentially, tumor tissue-only test would be a useful method to find out novel kidney cancer susceptibility genes and mutations in kidney cancer patients, as the knowledge on hereditary kidney cancer genes is still limited. This investigation is not available currently.

Tumor tissue-only gene tests by next generation sequencing with targeted genes may be soon routinely used for cancer patients' pharmacogenetic genotyping and analyzing their tumor tissue's somatic mutations to tailor their medical treatment [58]. The same method could be also a first step analysis for identifying the hereditary cancer mutation in a gene that is known in literature as a susceptibility gene. An additional test of patient's peripheral lymphocyte should then be used to confirm the susceptive mutation as hereditary mutation.

The growing knowledge on the biology of hereditary kidney cancer produces information about driver genes in kidney cancer tumorigenesis and may develop diagnostics and therapeutic methods for kidney cancer in general [59]. Knowledge on evidence-based medicine in metastatic hereditary kidney cancer [60] is under active study. Analysis of induced pluripotent stem cells (iPSC) from HPRC pointed that drug screening and precision medicine are possible for hereditary kidney cancer [61]. Preventive medicine may be achieved for healthy persons with familial mutation predisposing to kidney cancer [61].

Prospective studies about the method of follow-up in healthy persons with family kidney cancer susceptibility mutation are warranted. The optimal onset to start follow-up in *FH*-related hereditary kidney cancer families should be clarified as currently there is no consensus. It is known that the prognosis in early-stage kidney cancer disease is better than in later stages [62]. Studies about long-term effect of surveillance in healthy carriers in hereditary kidney cancer families are needed. Additionally, further research is needed to understand the actual impact of genetic testing on young family members [63].

10. Conclusion

Knowledge on the clinical significance of mutations helps to improve prognosis in families with hereditary cancer. Understanding of hereditary kidney cancer syndromes on their molecular basis improves the utility of specific diagnosis [64]. In the future, increased knowledge of cancer genetics is likely to enable the development of targeted drug therapies. Today, hereditary mutations are detected by DNA testing of white blood cell lymphocytes. Tumor tissue-only tests to identify the hereditary kidney cancer are not yet available.

Author details

Minna Kankuri-Tammilehto[1,2]*

*Address all correspondence to: mikanku@utu.fi

1 Department of Clinical Genetics, Turku University Hospital, Finland

2 Institute of Biomedicine, University of Turku, Finland

References

[1] Bray F, Ferlay J, Soerjomataram I, Siegel R, Torre L, Jemal A. Global cancer statistics 2018: GLOBOCAN estimates of incidence and mortality worldwide for 36 cancers in 185 countries. CA: A Cancer Journal for Clinicians. 2018;**68**(6):394-426

[2] Ferlay J, Colombet M, Soerjomataram I, Mathers C, Parkin DM, Piñeros M, et al. Estimating the global cancer incidence and mortality in 2018: GLOBOCAN sources and methods. International Journal of Cancer. 2019;**144**(8):1941-1953

[3] Bergström A, Pisani P, Tenet V, Wolk A, Adami HO. Overweight as an avoidable cause of cancer in Europe. International Journal of Cancer. 2001;**91**:421-430. Erratum in: International Journal of Cancer. 2001;**92**:927

[4] Chow WH, Gridley G, Fraumeni JF Jr, Jarvholm B. Obesity, hypertension, and the risk of kidney cancer in men. The New England Journal of Medicine. 2000;**343**:1305-1311

[5] Hunt JD, van der Hel OL, McMillan GP, Boffetta P, Brennan P. Renal cell carcinoma in relation to cigarette smoking: Meta-analysis of 24 studies. International Journal of Cancer. 2005;**114**(1):101-108

[6] Schwarz A, Vatandaslar S, Merkel S, Haller H. Renal cell carcinoma in transplant recipients with acquired cystic kidney disease. Clinical Journal of the American Society of Nephrology. 2007;**2**(4):750-756

[7] Kankuri-Tammilehto MK, Söderström KO, Pelliniemi TT, et al. Prognostic evaluation of COX-2 expression in renal cell carcinoma. Anticancer Research. 2010;**30**(7):3023-3030

[8] Rabjerg M. Identification and validation of novel prognostic markers in renal cell carcinoma. Danish Medical Journal. 2017;**64**(10):B5339

[9] Ball MW, Shuch BM. Inherited kidney cancer syndromes. Current Opinion in Urology. 2019;**29**(4):334-343

[10] Carlo MI, Hakimi AA, Stewart GD, et al. Familial kidney cancer: Implications of new syndromes and molecular insights. European Urology. 2019;**76**(6):754-764

[11] Carlo MI, Mukherjee S, Mandelker D, et al. Prevalence of germline mutations in cancer susceptibility genes in patients with advanced renal cell carcinoma. JAMA Oncology. 2018;**4**(9):1228-1235

[12] Foulkes WD. Inherited susceptibility to common cancers. The New England Journal of Medicine. 2008;**359**:2143-2153

[13] McNeill A, Rattenberry E, Barber R, Killick P, et al. Genotype-phenotype correlations in VHL exon deletions. American Journal of Medical Genetics. Part A. 2009;**149A**(10):2147-2151

[14] Zbar B, Kaelin W, Maher E, Richard S. Third international meeting on von Hippel-Lindau disease. Cancer Research. 1999;**59**(9):2251-2253

[15] Schmidt L, Duh FM, Chen F, et al. Germline and somatic mutations in the tyrosine kinase domain of the MET proto-oncogene in papillary renal carcinomas. Nature Genetics. 1997; **16**(1):68-73

[16] Schmidt LS, Nickerson ML, Angeloni D, et al. Early onset hereditary papillary renal carcinoma: Germline missense mutations in the tyrosine kinase domain of the met proto-oncogene. The Journal of Urology. 2004;**172**(4 Pt 1):1256-1261

[17] Lehtonen HJ, Kiuru M, Ylisaukko-Oja SK, et al. Increased risk of cancer in patients with fumarate hydratase germline mutation. Journal of Medical Genetics. 2006;**43**:523-526

[18] Toro JR, Nickerson ML, Wei MH, et al. Mutations in the fumarate hydratase gene cause hereditary leiomyomatosis and renal cell cancer in families in North America. American Journal of Human Genetics. 2003;**73**:95-106

[19] Vahteristo P, Koski TA, Näätsaari L, et al. No evidence for a genetic modifier for renal cell cancer risk in HLRCC syndrome. Familial Cancer. 2010;**9**(2):245-251

[20] Menko FH, Maher ER, Schmidt LS, Middelton LA, Aittomäki K, Tomlinson I, et al. Hereditary leiomyomatosis and renal cell cancer (HLRCC): Renal cancer risk, surveillance and treatment. Familial Cancer. 2014;**13**(4):637-644

[21] Furuya M, Yao M, Tanaka R, et al. Genetic, epidemiologic and clinicopathologic studies of Japanese Asian patients with Birt-Hogg-Dube syndrome. Clinical Genetics. 2016;**90**: 403-412

[22] Schmidt LS, Warren MB, Nickerson ML, et al. Birt-Hogg-Dubé syndrome, a genodermatosis associated with spontaneous pneumothorax and kidney neoplasia, maps to chromosome 17p11.2. American Journal of Human Genetics. 2001;**69**(4):876-882

[23] Bonné AC, Bodmer D, Schoenmakers EF, van Ravenswaaij CM, Hoogerbrugge N, van Kessel AG. Chromosome 3 translocations and familial renal cell cancer. Current Molecular Medicine. 2004;**4**(8):849-854

[24] Aarnio M, Säily M, Juhola M, et al. Uroepithelial and kidney carcinoma in Lynch syndrome. Familial Cancer. 2012;**11**(3):395-401

[25] Schultz KAP, Rednam SP, Kamihara J, et al. PTEN, DICER1, FH, and their associated tumor susceptibility syndromes: Clinical features, genetics, and surveillance recommendations in childhood. Clinical Cancer Research. 2017;**23**(12):e76-e82

[26] Haven CJ, Wong FK, van Dam EW, van der Juijt R, van Asperen C, Jansen J, et al. A genotypic and histopathological study of a large Dutch kindred with hyperparathyroidism-jaw tumor syndrome. The Journal of Clinical Endocrinology and Metabolism. 2000;**85**(4): 1449-1454

[27] Iwashita H, Okudela K, Matsumura M, et al. Succinate dehydrogenase B-deficient renal cell carcinoma: A case report with novel germline mutation. Pathology International. 2017;**67**(11):585-589

[28] Schlegelberger B, Kreipe H, Lehmann U, et al. A child with Li-Fraumeni syndrome: Modes to inactivate the second allele of TP53 in three different malignancies. Pediatric Blood & Cancer. 2015;**62**(8):1481-1484

[29] Popova T, Herbert L, Jacquemin V, et al. Germline BAP1 mutations predispose to renal cell carcinomas. American Journal of Human Genetics. 2013;**92**:974-980

[30] Stratton KL, Alanee S, Glogowski EA, et al. Outcome of genetic evaluation of kidney cancer patients referred for suspected hereditary cancer syndromes. Urologic Oncology. 2016;**34**(5):238.e1-238.e7

[31] Guo J, Tretiakova MS, Troxell ML, et al. Tuberous sclerosis-associated renal cell carcinoma: A clinicopathologic study of 57 separate carcinomas in 18 patients. The American Journal of Surgical Pathology. 2014;**38**:1457-1467

[32] Peron A, Vignoli A, La Briola F, et al. Do patients with tuberous sclerosis complex have an increased risk for malignancies? American Journal of Medical Genetics. Part A. 2016; **170**(6):1538-1544

[33] Alessandri JL, Cuillier F, Ramful D, et al. Perlman syndrome: Report, prenatal findings and review. American Journal of Medical Genetics - Part A. 2008;**146A**(19):2532-2537. DOI: 10.1002/ajmg.a.32391

[34] Levitt NC, Hickson ID. Caretaker tumour suppressor genes that defend genome integrity. Trends in Molecular Medicine. 2002;**8**(4):179-186

[35] Shu X, Gu J, Huang M, et al. Germline genetic variants in somatically significantly mutated genes in tumors are associated with renal cell carcinoma risk and outcome. Carcinogenesis. 2018;**39**(6):752-757

[36] Maxwell PH, Wiesener MS, Chang GW, Clifford SC, Vaux EC, Cockman ME, et al. The tumor suppressor protein VHL targets hypoxia-inducible factors for oxygen-dependent proteolysis. Nature. 1999;**399**:271-275

[37] Tomasetti C, Vogelstein B. Cancer etiology. Variation in cancer risk among tissues can be explained by the number of stem cell divisions. Science. 2015;**347**(6217):78-81

[38] Haber DA, Settleman J. Cancer: Drivers and passengers. Nature. 2007;**446**:145-146

[39] Knudson AG Jr. Mutation and cancer: Statistical study of retinoblastoma. Proceedings of the National Academy of Sciences of the United States of America. 1971;**68**:820-823

[40] Kinzler KW, Vogelstein B. Cancer-susceptibility genes. Gatekeepers and caretakers. Nature. 1997;**386**:761-763

[41] de Vogel S, Weijenberg MP, Herman JG, et al. MGMT and MLH1 promoter methylation versus APC, KRAS and BRAF gene mutations in colorectal cancer: Indications for distinct pathways and sequence of events. Annals of Oncology. 2009;**20**(7):1216-1222

[42] Tovar EA, Graveel CR. MET in human cancer: Germline and somatic mutations. Annals of Translational Medicine. 2017;**5**(10):205

[43] Robson ME, Storm CD, Weitzel J, et al. American Society of Clinical Oncology policy statement update: Genetic and genomic testing for cancer susceptibility. Journal of Clinical Oncology. 2010;**28**(5):893-901

[44] Robson ME, Bradbury AR, Arun B, et al. American Society of Clinical Oncology policy statement update: Genetic and genomic testing for cancer susceptibility. Journal of Clinical Oncology. 2015;**33**(31):3660-3667

[45] Lammens CR, Bleiker EM, Verhoef S, Ausems MG, Majoor-Krakauer D, Sijmons RH, et al. Distress in partners of individuals diagnosed with or at high risk of developing tumors due to rare hereditary cancer syndromes. Psycho-Oncology. 2011;**20**(6):631-638

[46] Aktan-Collan K, Mecklin JP, Järvinen H. Predictive genetic testing for hereditary non-polyposis colorectal cancer: Uptake and long-term satisfaction. International Journal of Cancer. 2000;**89**(1):44-50

[47] van Leeuwaarde RS, Saya A, Links TP, Giles RH. Von Hippel-Lindau Syndrome. Initial Posting: May 17, 2000; Last Update: September 6, 2018

[48] Balmaña J, Digiovanni L, Gaddam P, et al. Conflicting interpretation of genetic variants and cancer risk by commercial laboratories as assessed by the prospective registry of multiplex testing. Journal of Clinical Oncology. 2016;**34**(34):4071-4078

[49] Richards S, Aziz N, Bale S. Standards and guidelines for the interpretation of sequence variants: A joint consensus recommendation of the American College of Medical Genetics and Genomics and the Association for Molecular Pathology. Genetics in Medicine. 2015; **17**(5):405-424

[50] Shirts BH, Casadei S, Jacobson AL. Improving performance of multigene panels for genomic analysis of cancer predisposition. Genetics in Medicine. 2016;**18**(10):974-981

[51] Choueiri TK, Vaishampayan U, Rosenberg JE, et al. Phase II and biomarker study of the dual MET/VEGFR2 inhibitor foretinib in patients with papillary renal cell carcinoma. Journal of Clinical Oncology. 2013;**31**:181-186

[52] Staehler M, Goebell PJ, Müller L, et al. Rare patients in routine care—Treatment and outcome in advanced papillary renal cell carcinoma in the prospective German clinical RCC-Registry. International Journal of Cancer. 2019;**146**:1307-1315

[53] Hasumi H, Yao M. Hereditary kidney cancer syndromes: Genetic disorders driven by alterations in metabolism and epigenome regulation. Cancer Science. 2018;**109**(3):581-586

[54] Freifeld Y, Ananthakrishnan L, Margulis V. Imaging for screening and surveillance of patients with hereditary forms of renal cell carcinoma. Current Urology Reports. 2018;**19**(10):82

[55] PDQ Cancer Information Summaries. PDQ Cancer Genetics Editorial Board. Genetics of Kidney Cancer (Renal Cell Cancer) Health Professional Version. 2019

[56] Maher ER. Hereditary renal cell carcinoma syndromes: Diagnosis, surveillance and management. World Journal of Urology. 2018;**36**:1891-1898

[57] Gonorazky HD, Naumenko S, Ramani AK, et al. Expanding the boundaries of RNA sequencing as a diagnostic tool for rare Mendelian disease. American Journal of Human Genetics. 2019;**104**(5):1007

[58] Hampel H, Peralman R, et al. Assessment of tumor sequencing as a replacement for lynch syndrome screening and current molecular tests for patients with colorectal cancer. JAMA Oncology. 2018;**4**(6):806-813. DOI: 10.1001/jamaoncol.2018.0104

[59] Hasumi H, Furuya M, Tatsuno K, et al. BHD-associated kidney cancer exhibits unique molecular characteristics and a wide variety of variants in chromatin remodeling genes. Human Molecular Genetics. 2018;**27**(15):2712-2724

[60] Park I, Shim YS, Go H, et al. Long-term response of metastatic hereditary leiomyomatosis and renal cell carcinoma syndrome associated renal cell carcinoma to bevacizumab plus erlotinib after temsirolimus and axitinib treatment failures. BMC Urology. 2019;**19**(1):51

[61] Hwang JW, Desterke C, Féraud O, et al. iPSC-Derived embryoid bodies as models of c-Met-mutated hereditary papillary renal cell carcinoma. International Journal of Molecular Sciences. 2019;**20**(19)

[62] Kankuri M, Pelliniemi TT, Pyrhönen S, et al. Feasibility of prolonged use of interferon-alpha in metastatic kidney carcinoma: A phase II study. Cancer. 2001;**92**(4):761-767

[63] Schultz CL, Alderfer MA, Lindell RB, et al. The influence of adolescence on parents' perspectives of testing and discussing inherited cancer predisposition. Journal of Genetic Counseling. 2018. [published online ahead of print, 2018 Jun 16]. DOI: 10.1007/s10897-018-0267-z

[64] Peng YC, Chen YB. Recognizing hereditary renal cancers through the microscope: A pathology update. Surgical Pathology Clinics. 2018;**11**(4):725-737

Chapter 2

Role of Immune System in Kidney Cancer

Ana Marisa Chudzinski-Tavassi,
Kátia Luciano Pereira Morais,
Jean Gabriel de Souza and Roger Chammas

Additional information is available at the end of the chapter

http://dx.doi.org/10.5772/intechopen.77379

Abstract

Almost all kidney cancers are associated to immune dysfunction. Among these, renal cell carcinoma (RCC) represents approximately 2% of malignancies that affect adults and for 90–95% of all kidney cancers. Recent evidences have collaborated to elucidate the mechanisms involved in the development of this disease. In this view, dysfunctional neutrophil migration, as well as T lymphocyte-DC (dendritic cell) cross talk, DC maturation, immune cell metabolism, and reactivity and abnormal expression of cytokines and chemokines and their receptors have been highlighted in RCC and stroma cells. A rational development of novel therapies to recover antitumor activity of immune system is closely related to the understanding of the complex interactions between immune system and tumor. Some insights have been reached and immunomodulatory molecules, such as interleukin-2 (IL-2) and IFN-α, immune checkpoint inhibitors, and chemokines antagonists have shown clinical efficacy. In this chapter, we overview the essential role of innate and adaptive immune response in RCC and discuss drugs approved or in development for its treatment.

Keywords: renal cell carcinoma, cytokines, chemokines, natural immunity, adaptive immunity

1. Introduction

Basically, the kidney is assigned to the urine production function. Indeed, kidney function overcomes this definition, since it is critical for the regulation of the body's electrolytes, body's fluid balance, body's acid-base balance, and depuration of body waste. Thereby, diseases such as kidney cancer compromise the kidney's ability to perform its functions and bring consequences to the whole organism.

According to the cell type where the tumor starts, kidney cancers are classified as renal cell carcinoma (RCC) subdivided in papillary RCC, chromophobe RCC, rare types of RCC, and unclassified RCC. Also, there are transitional cell carcinoma, Wilms' tumor, which almost always occur in children and renal sarcoma [1–4].

Regardless of the category, kidney tumors have been associated with immune dysfunction [1–3, 5]. RCCs are rich in immune infiltrates consisting of T cells, natural killer (NK), DCs, macrophages among others [6, 7]. Different functions are ascribed to the different subsets of leukocytes. While the function of some of these cells is still elusive, like neutrophils which are essential components of the RCC microenvironment, others have well-defined roles in tumor progression. For example, tumor-associated macrophages (TAMs) are known for their immunosuppressive action, which is associated to the secretion of inhibitory cytokines, the generation of reactive oxygen species, regulatory T cells (Treg) development, and the induction of angiogenesis [6, 8, 9]. Likewise, myeloid-derived suppressor cells (MDSCs) have been reported preventing the formation and execution of an effective antitumor immune response by the inhibition of effector T-cell function and the induction of Tregs maturation [6, 7], besides the inhibition of DC maturation and DC-induced T-cell activation and antitumor cytotoxic T lymphocyte (CTL) [10].

The role of the immune system in RCC is not only observed at the cellular level but also through inflammatory mediators, that is, through the action of cytokines and chemokines which act in tumor and stroma cells [11–13]. These mediators in RCC and stroma cells lead to survival, proliferation, and migration and favor angiogenesis and metastasis [11–13]. Thereby, the modulation of immune system effectors has shown therapeutic potential. In fact, strategies involving immune checkpoint inhibitors, immunotherapy, and antagonists of chemokine receptors have proven clinical efficacy [14, 15].

Herein, we summarize relevant information about the role of natural and adaptive immunity in the development of RCC. Additionally, we describe cytokine and chemokine intracellular signaling pathways and mention how all knowledge has been useful for identification and advancement of therapeutic approaches for RCC.

2. Natural and adaptive immunity in RCC

The tumor microenvironment is a complex structure composed by several mediators that are involved in the cell signaling. The activation profile of extracellular matrix, fibroblasts, immune cells, blood vessels, and endothelial cells is essential to the pathogenesis of cancer, as well as to define therapeutic approaches [16–18]. Resident nontumor cells or infiltrated cells at tumor sites may even suppress the development of RCC. However, tumor cells can avoid the immune response coordinating changes in these cells and stimulating the secretion of immunosuppressive factors for tumorigenesis, pro-inflammatory cytokines including angiogenic factors, thus ensuring the supply of nutrients by newly formed, blood vessels, which further allow for tumor growth [19, 20].

In addition, the profile of soluble factors, such as cytokines and chemokines, present in the tumor microenvironment may undergo dual polarization allowing either tumor growth (leading to progressive disease) or its suppression (leading to regressive disease). Immune cells could interact with tumor cells, especially through immunosuppression, via cell-cell contact, or by the release of factors that maintain a supportive environment for tumor growth. Through some soluble mediators, such as tumor necrosis factor-alpha (TNFα), immune cells can stimulate other cells, such as fibroblasts, to produce proteolytic enzymes for extracellular matrix remodeling and collagen, facilitating the spread of metastases. It may also stimulate the involvement of endothelial cells, which become able to form new vessels [18, 21, 22]. On the other hand, TNFα, which is mainly produced by macrophages, has also an important role in the recruitment of other immune cells to the tumor site where they will be able to assemble a response against the tumor. Thus, the constant interference of mediators may favor/inhibit an adequate environment for tumor maintenance and growth [18, 21].

Indeed, tissue repair promoted by inflammation is self-limited, and the imbalance on this process may be pathogenic, giving inflammatory cells either a beneficial and/or a detrimental role in the pathogenesis of various diseases, including chronic inflammation and neoplasia [23]. The TAMs have at least two well-described states of polarization, according to immunological competences. While M1 (classically activated) macrophages can inhibit tumor growth, M2 (alternatively activated) macrophages stimulate tumor growth [24–26]. The M1 polarization is functionally characterized by the release of pro-inflammatory cytokines (interleukin [IL]-1β, IL-6, and TNFα) and reactive nitrogen/oxygen species (RNI/ROS) acting as microbicidal and tumoricidal [24]. In the tumor context, some authors suggest that macrophages in the initial phase of tumorigenesis can naturally inhibit tumor growth, eradicate tumor cells, and stimulate the immune response. In contrast, M2 macrophages may favor neoplasia by producing anti-inflammatory cytokines that suppress the cellular response, release vascular endothelial growth factors (VEGFs), responsible for angiogenesis, and release transforming growth factors (TGF-beta) [27].

The different subtypes of T lymphocytes are also recruited into the tumor microenvironment and interact with tumor cells, which may induce tumor cell death, becoming anergic or even suppressing the immune response against the tumor [28, 29]. T $CD8^+$ lymphocytes, also known as cytotoxic T cells, play an important role in the adaptive immunity in response to tumor-specific epitopes. Together with NK and Natural killer T (NKT) cells, T $CD8^+$ cells induce tumor cell death by apoptosis through the secretion of cytotoxic factor, such as granzymes and perforins. Besides, when the TCD8 lymphocyte is activated, it secretes IFN-gamma and IL2, activating other TCD8 cells and M1 macrophages, skewing the inflammatory response toward a Th1 profile. However, RCC and some types of tumor-infiltrating immune cells, such as MDSCs, present in the tumor microenvironment can suppress antitumor response T cell mediated by the expression of programmed death ligand-1 (PD-L1, also known as B7-H1 or CD274) [30, 31].

CD4 T lymphocyte is endowed with great plasticity, being able to differentiate into Th1, Th2, Th3, Th17, and Treg subtypes. Treg cells play a critical role in the control of the acute phase of the inflammatory response through immunosuppression. High levels of Treg in the tumor microenvironment are considered as poor prognosis for tumors, for example, in renal and pancreatic tumor, due to the recruitment of other immunosuppressive cells and the stimulation of the angiogenic process [29, 32]. MDSCs are involved in chronic inflammation processes, which are recruited by tumor or Treg, increasing immunosuppression in the tumor microenvironment [33].

A common feature of almost all solid tumors is hypoxia that could lead to the stability of the HIF-1α transcription factor (hypoxia-inducible factor-1α). HIF-1α can bind to a hypoxia-responsive element in the PD-L1 promoter leading to PD-L1 expression, not only on tumor cells but also on MDSCs, macrophages, and DCs within the tumor microenvironment [34].

PD-L1 binds with PD-1 present on the cell surface of activated T cells leading to proliferation blockade, dysfunctional response, and T-cell death. CTLA-4 (CTL -associated antigen 4), a receptor also present in T cells, is the best studied inhibitory molecule, well known for its capacity of blocking T cell-mediated immune responses [35, 36]. CTLA-4 competes with CD28 for CD80 or CD86 binding. When the CTLA-4/CD80 or CD86 interaction occurs, the cell becomes anergic and dies. The overexpression of CTLA-4 is involved in several neoplastic, inflammatory, and autoimmune diseases [37]. The inhibition of T response allows for RCC to avoid effectors of immunologic control and facilitates invasion and metastasis. Accordingly, PD-L1 overexpression is related to worse prognosis for metastatic RCC, and it is therefore an important target for drug discovery [38, 39]. New drugs based on monoclonal antibodies, such as anti-PD-1 and anti-CTLA-4, have been strongly explored in clinical trial and proven to be efficacious to combinatorial treatments [39]. Indeed, immunotherapy is a promising therapeutic strategy for different types of cancers, but it is often not sufficient to control tumor growth [40]. Several therapeutic strategies based on innate, adaptive, humoral, or cytokine immune system responses have been studied in order to combat tumor cells in the host [41–45].

Studies using allogeneic DCs in metastatic Renal Cell Carcinoma (mRCC) and melanoma patients are widespread due to the ability of these cells to mediate the cell signaling between the innate and adaptive immune response. As professional antigen-presenting cells (APCs), these cells phagocytose tumor cell particles, process them, and further present their epitopes to further activate effector lymphocytes [46]. APCs play a crucial role in coordinating the immune response, where the imbalance between populations of macrophages, immature, and mature DCs significantly affects the immune response against solid tumors [47]. Both DCs and macrophages can be activated by some microbial stimulus or cytokines in an inflammatory environment. DCs and macrophages could differentiate from monocytes, according to the tissue environment, where cytokines such as IL4 and macrophage colony-stimulating factor granulocytes (GM-CSF) may induce differentiation, followed by TNFα-induced maturation [47]. In the tumor context, the inflammatory profile present at different stages of disease development may contribute to or eradicate the pathogenesis [47]. The International Society for the Biological Therapy of Cancer (iSBTc), together with the Society for Cancer Immunotherapy (SITC), has been discussing the theme with the purpose of advancing the critical understanding of the involvement of inflammation during pathogenesis and cancer treatment [48, 49]. In fact, the dynamics of tumor progression along with immunoedition has been studied for years, through the realization of which cells, molecules, and pathways of the immune system are engaged at different steps of the evolution of cancers. Nonetheless, an integrative picture of the whole process is still missing [50, 51]. Vesely et al. described several interactions between innate and adaptive immunity in cancer, suggesting a dynamic immuno-delivery model, where cells such as M2 macrophages, MDSC, Th17, Treg, and $TCD8^+$ overexpressing CTLA-4 receptor are present in chronic inflammation and favor the processes related to tumor progression [52]. In contrast, NK, NKT, $TCD8^+$, $TCD4^+$, M1 macrophages, DCs, $T\gamma\delta$ cells and IL12 and IFN-gamma cytokines are important for equilibrium and elimination phases of tumor control [52]. Several cytokines are involved in the differentiation process of immune cells. Interferon-gamma (INF-gamma) belongs to interferon family and is a natural glycoprotein that shows antiviral, antiproliferative, and immunomodulatory properties. INF-gamma plays a key role in the tumor microenvironment, where it aids in tumor eradication. This cytokine is able to recruit and induce the proliferation of T lymphocytes in the tumor microenvironment, to activate innate immunity cells, rendering them cytotoxic, besides polarizing the Th1 response from T CD4

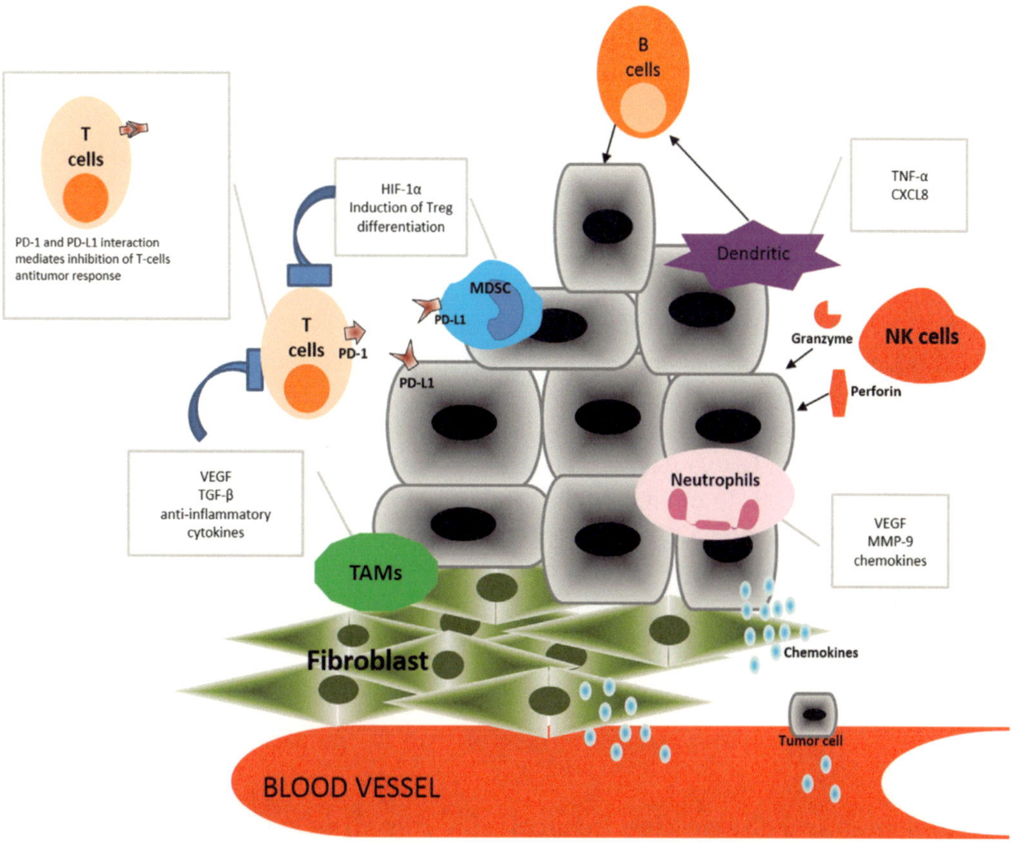

Figure 1. Dual role of natural and adaptive immunity in RCC. Innate immune cells (dendritic cells, macrophages, NK cells, neutrophils, and MDSCs) and adaptive immunity (B and T cells) in the tumor microenvironment may undergo dual polarization allowing either tumor growth (leading to progressive disease) or its suppression (leading to regressive disease). Dendritic cells are primed by tumor antigens, which are then presented to T and B cells for adaptive responses. On the other hand, dendritic cells can directly drive tumor angiogenesis through the release of pro-angiogenic cytokines such as TNFα and CXCL8. Similarly, neutrophils in the tumor microenvironment are able to release pro-angiogenic factors and chemokines that could contribute for cancer progression and metastasis. T CD8+ lymphocytes, also known as cytotoxic T cells, play an important role against tumor cells under response to tumor-specific epitopes. However, the PD-L1/PD-1 interaction on CD8+ T-cell surface induces cellular energy suppressing the effector response, leading CD8 T cell to death. Failure of CD8+ T cells to kill tumor cells involves signals from multiple cells including MDSC, Treg, and TAMs. NK cells are characterized by a high cytolytic capacity against transformed cancer cells by the secretion of granzyme and perforin. Tumor cells and fibroblasts also produce survival/growth-promoting chemokines. Metastatic cancer cells are facilitated by the upregulation of particular chemokine receptors (such as CXCR4) by tumor cells, which enables them to migrate to secondary tissues where the ligands are expressed.

lymphocytes [53, 54]. IL1-beta is one of the major cytokines involved in the pro-inflammatory response, which is synthesized by several immune cells, such as monocytes, macrophages, DCs, B lymphocytes, NK cells, among others. It has similar activities as described for TNFα, favoring tumor invasion and the angiogenic process, as well as favoring vascular permeability and facilitating the recruitment of immune system cells to the tumor microenvironment [55]. However, TNFα is the main mediator of the acute inflammatory response, being secreted primarily by macrophages and T cells. TNFα causes vascular endothelial cells to increase the expression of leukocyte integrins inducing chemotaxis. In addition, TNFα also acts on phagocytic cells, which characterizes an autocrine effect, since macrophages, apart from secreting TNFα, may respond to the stimulus itself, releasing IL1-beta [56, 57]. IL12 is secreted primarily by macrophages, DCs, monocytes, and neutrophils. It has action in the activation of cytotoxic NK cells and TCD8 lymphocytes, but its main function in the antitumor activity is involved in the activation and proliferation of T lymphocytes and NK cells, which induces the production of IFN-gamma. Moreover, IL12 and INF-gamma together are able to differentiate T-helper cells into Th1 cells [58, 59]. IL6 is synthesized by mononuclear phagocytes, such as macrophages and also by some activated T cells and by other cell types that are not part of the immune system in response to microorganisms or IL1-beta and TNFα stimuli [60]. IL10 is a cytokine known to be anti-inflammatory, synthesized in the form of monomers of 18–20 kDa, being functional in the form of homodimers. This cytokine can be produced by Th2 lymphocytes, monocytes, and epithelial cells. Its main action is to suppress the synthesis of several inflammatory cytokines such as IL1-beta, TNFα, IL-6, IL-8, and IL-12, as well as hematopoietic growth factors (GM-CSF, G-CFS) and macrophage colony-stimulating factor (M-CFS). In addition, IL-10 can inhibit the synthesis of nitric oxide, gelatinase, and collagenase, avoiding tissue injury [61]. Although its role in the tumor context remains unclear, IL-17 is a pro-inflammatory cytokine secreted by Th17 lymphocytes, which regulates NFkB and MAPK activities. It is constantly involved in the acute phase of inflammatory diseases, such as autoimmune diseases, and it is associated with poor prognosis in patients with RCC [62, 63].

Taken all these studies together, the dual role of natural and adaptive immunity in RCC is evident (**Figure 1**).

3. Cytokines and chemokine intracellular signaling pathways

Physiologically, inflammation is a mechanism of tissue reaction for elimination, neutralization, and destruction of the cause of aggression, as injurious stimuli such as microbial pathogens, irritants, or toxic cellular components [64]. Cells of the immune system including monocytes, macrophages, neutrophils, basophils, DCs, mast cells, T cells, and B cells play a role in this process [64]. These events are in turn controlled by a host of extracellular molecular regulators, including members of the cytokine and chemokine families that mediate both immune cell recruitment and complex intracellular signaling control mechanisms; as a result, cells assemble and disassemble a complex array of signaling pathways as they move from inactive to dedicated roles within the inflammatory response site. Disruption of these pathways triggers inflammatory disorders that could contribute for the development of some diseases as kidney cancer and other types of cancers [65].

Key pro-inflammatory cytokines in kidney cancer include interleukin-1 beta (IL-1β), IL-6, and TNFα, all of which signal via the type I cytokine receptors that are structurally divergent from other cytokine receptor types [66, 67]. IL-1 signaling starts through its binding to its receptor composed of two subunits, interleukin 1 receptor type I (IL-1RI) and interleukin 1 receptor accessory protein (IL1RAP) [68, 69]. Signaling proceeds with TIR adaptor and MyD88 by recruitment of IL-1R-associated kinases (IRAKs), which promote TNFR-associated factor 6 (TRAF6) polyubiquitination via lysine 63 linkages. Subsequently, TRAF6 interacts with the TAK1/TAB1/TAB2 complex that allows NFκB nuclear translocation (p65/p50) resulting in pro-inflammatory gene expression [69]. Also, TAK1/TAB1/TAB2 complex triggers the activation of the mitogen-activated protein kinases (MAPKs), c-JunN-terminal kinase (JNK), and p38, which induce the expression of pro-inflammatory genes. Similarly, TNFα binding to TNFR1 results in NFκB nuclear translocation, MAPKs, JNK, and p38, but signaling is coordinated by complex I (TRADD/TRAF2/RIP) [67, 70]. Importantly, TNFα signaling following receptor internalization is thought to be pro-apoptotic, via the formation of complex II (TRADD/FADD/Pro-Caspase-8) [67]. On the other hand, IL-6 binds to the FIII domains of the IL-6R chains, unleashing its signal via the gp130 proteins [71, 72]. Consequently, Janus kinases (JAKs) are recruited to the receptor, phosphorylating it and themselves, triggering STAT3 activation and transcription of pro-inflammatory genes and intracellular adhesion molecules [64].

Currently, it is not fully understood how the signaling triggered by these cytokines contributes to tumor progression, but high serum levels of these pro-inflammatory cytokines are associated with advanced disease [73]. Some evidence has arisen, as follows. It is well known that angiogenesis is stimulated by inflammatory mediators in the tumor microenvironment, such as those expressed by TAMs [74]. Interestingly, TAMs isolated from RCC tumors express high levels of IL-1β, TNFa, and IL-6 [75]. In addition, mouse models have demonstrated that the inhibition of IL-1β signaling reduced tumor blood vessel formation [76] and IL-1β mediates metalloproteinase-dependent RCC tumor cell invasion through the activation of cytosine-cytosine-adenosine-adenosine-thymidine (CCAAT) enhancer binding protein b [67]. Regarding TNFα signaling, many studies associated it to chemokine overexpression in tumor and nontumor cells [77, 78]. Moreover, TNFα plays an important role in the progression of RCC by inducing epithelial to mesenchymal transition and CD44 expression, which may be involved in the resistance to the sunitinib treatment [66]. There is no direct correlation between IL-6R and RCC development; however, RCC cells express high levels of IL-6, and its signaling activity seems necessary for carcinogenesis, tumor progression, and tumor evasion of the immune system. STAT3 activation by IL-6 promotes tumorigenesis by preventing apoptosis while enhancing proliferation, angiogenesis, invasiveness, and immune evasion [79]. For example, activated STAT3 induces HIF-1α-mediated VEGF expression in human RCC cell [79].

Besides these pro-inflammatory cytokines, other mediators act as crucial players in RCC. Chemotactic cytokines or chemokines are responsible for the recruitment of cells from both the innate and adaptive immune systems to the site of injury or infection [64]. Chemokines induce integrin expression, such as the β2-integrin lymphocyte function-associated antigen (LFA-1), in target leukocytes, thus acting in the arrest of these cells and favoring diapedesis through the endothelium [71]. Despite this, primary chemotaxis action, chemokines, and their receptors are physiological relevant in many biological process, such as the initiation of adaptive immune responses, immune surveillance and the migration, proliferation, and survival signals in multiple cell types [64]. Chemokine signals are transduced through binding to members of the seven-transmembrane, G-protein-coupled receptor (GPCR) superfamily [80]. GPCRs exist as a heterotrimer containing three subunits: α, β, and γ. In its inactive form, the G protein is complexed in α, β, and γ, with guanosine diphosphate (GDP) fixed to the α subunit. Once stimulated by a receptor activated by its ligand, the α subunit exchanges its GDP for Guanosine-5′-triphosphate (GTP) [81]. This causes the dissociation of α which separate β and γ subunits by interacting with an effector protein or ion channel in order to stimulate or inhibit secondary intracellular messengers [81]. CXCR4 is well known for its role in the homing of progenitor cells into the bone marrow and, recently, associated with poor RCC prognosis, and it is mainly coupled to the Gαi subunit, which, after dissociation of the G$\alpha\beta\gamma$ complex upon CXCR4 stimulation (**Figure 2**), is traditionally been regarded as the major signaling subunit, inhibits adenylyl cyclase activity, and triggers MAPK and phosphatidylinositol-3-kinase (PI3K) pathway activation [82]. The G$\beta\gamma$ subunits, in turn, lead to the activation of phospholipase C (PLC), causing the hydrolysis of the phospholipid membrane phosphatidylinositol 4,5-bisphosphate (PIP2) in inositol 1,4,5-trisphosphate (IP3) and 1,2-diacylglycerol (DAG) [13, 82]. IP3 can bind to channels of the endoplasmic reticulum, inducing the mobilization of Ca^{2+} ions [83, 84]. This could also be considered a downstream effect of Gαi activity, since the inhibition of Gαi activity by its potent inhibitor pertussis toxin has been reported to lead to a decreased Ca^{2+} mobilization from intracellular stores [85]. CXCR4 can also act by interaction with other Gα subunits, that is, Gαq or Gα12, each of which has been associated with different intracellular signaling cascades [86]. Indeed, chemokine receptors also activate signaling pathways independent of G proteins, including p38MAPK and JAK/Stat to regulate cellular processes such as migration and gene transcription [87, 88].

Regarding the signals triggered by pro-inflammatory mediators in RCC, CXCL12 chemokine and its receptors CXCR4 and CXCR7 have gained prominence, since this pathway, which is associated with chronic inflammation, is upregulated in RCC [65, 89, 90]. In RCC cells and in other tumor cells, these chemokines activate the PI3K/Akt pathway; consequently, many downstream elements of the Akt pathway are regulated, leading to tumor cell survival [13, 91, 92]. Frequently, NFκB nuclear translocation is observed following transcription of various apoptosis inhibitors and cell-cycle-promoting genes [93], but can be activated through other pathways, such as PKC [94]. Other downstream targets of Akt include procaspase-9 and the pro-apoptotic Bcl-2 family member, BAD (Bcl-2/Bcl-XL-antagonist, causing cell death), both of which are inhibited upon phosphorylation. Other consequence of Akt activation is the inhibition of members of the FKHR (forkhead in rhabdomyosarcoma) family of transcription factors, which induce the transcription of numerous apoptotic genes [95, 96]. Besides, Akt signaling could induce p53 degradation and inhibition of GSK-3β (glycogen synthase kinase-3β), leading to stabilization of β-catenin, resulting in the downstream inhibition of negative regulators of cell cycle and the activation of cell-cycle-promoting genes [97]. mTOR (mammalian target of rapamycin) activation is also induced by Akt, which leads to p70S6K (p70 S6 kinase) activation and thus enhances protein translation of numerous cell-growth regulators [13]. Furthermore, intracellular events triggered by the activation of chemokines receptors lead to ERK1/2 signaling, following the inhibition of procaspase-9 and BAD [98, 99], the induction of transcription factors involved in cell-cycle regulation, and differentiation, thereby promoting cell proliferation [100]. Other MAPKs, including JNK, have also been implicated in chemokine-induced proliferation signaling [101]. Also, HIF-1α may be

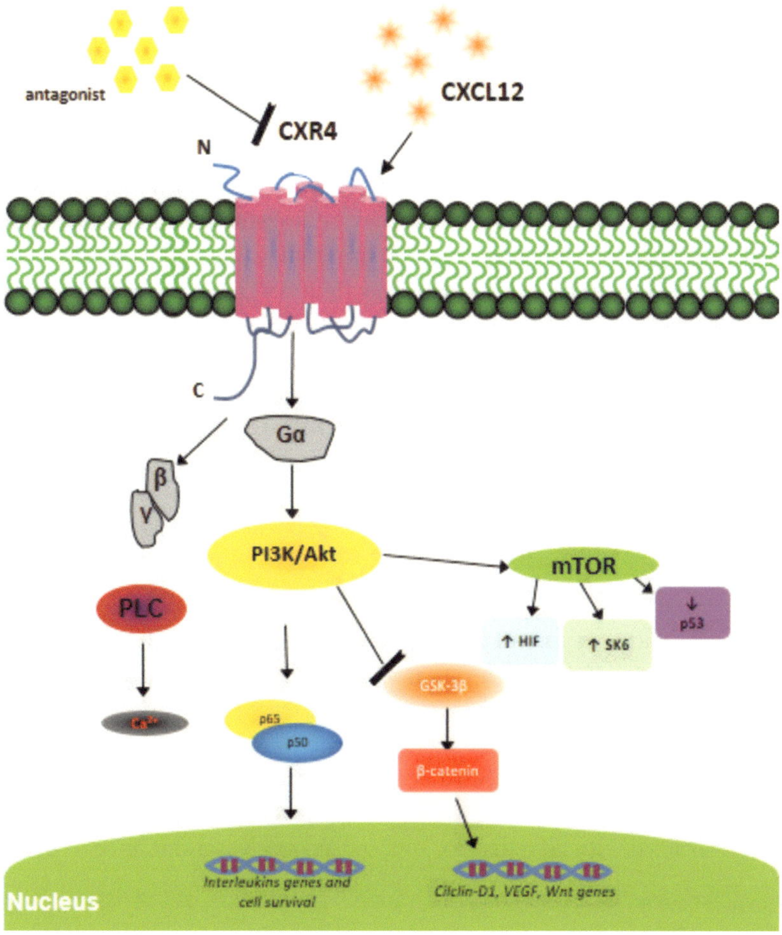

Figure 2. Signaling induced by CXCR4 via G protein. CXCL12 binding causes the dissociation of α which separate β and γ subunits; as a result, βγ PLC is activated leading to calcium mobilization. PI3K/Akt activation by Gα triggers a transduction signal that contributes with cell survival, proliferation, and migration, which is associated with RCC disease. In contrast, the antagonist of CXCR4 blocks CXCR4 intracellular pathway.

induced by chemokines signaling that contributes to VEGF expression, which is known to be the inducer of CXCR4 expression [101]. It is important to mention that not all of these pathways have been studied in detail in RCC cells, but there is strong evidence of their involvement in the development of this disease. For example, Rac1 was not previously reported to be involved in RCC development, but some studies have shown its role in controlling tumor cell growth and chronic kidney disease [102]. In summary, CXCL12, CXCR4, and CXCR7 release result in the activation of transcription factors involved in antiapoptotic mechanisms, cell-cycle regulation, and growth factor production, favoring tumor growth and metastasis.

Also, there are some particularities regarding CXCR7 role in RCC, which are independent of GPCRs. CXCR7 plays a role as a decoy for CXCL12, promoting some CXCL12α accumulation and triggering a differential signaling by CXCR4 [103, 104]. Besides, CXCR7 interacts and signals by β-arrestin in a ligand-dependent manner [83, 104].

Obviously, here we emphasize intracellular events in tumor cells. However, while some processes take place within the tumor cells, others would occur in the stroma: it is the synergism between these responses that contributes to the progression of the disease. RCC and other tumors interact with the surrounding tumor stroma through a variety of cytokines, chemokines, and growth factors [84]. The tumor chemotactic environment recruits inflammatory cells including neutrophils, macrophages, and lymphocytes. Although initially these cells may have a protective antitumoral role, as displayed by neutrophils, which have a higher cytotoxic activity against poorly metastatic cells, secondarily neutrophils could contribute to cancer progression. Leukocytes can produce cytokines, growth factors, and MMPs that enhance growth, proliferation, and angiogenesis, as exemplified by the TAMs, which release growth and angiogenic factors (e.g., VEGF) and basic fibroblast growth factor [105]. Thus, cellular communication by paracrine and autocrine chemokine/cytokine signaling contributes for the survival and growth of metastatic cells. In other words, stroma cells may support tumors at the same time as that tumor cells in turn modulate the microenvironment within which they reside.

4. Immunomodulatory molecules as new therapeutic targets for RCC

Among the standard drugs for metastatic RCC treatment, the most effective regimens include the combination of targeted therapy agents and antiangiogenic agents (tyrosine kinase inhibitors, such as sorafenib, sunitinib, pazopanib, and axitinib), or an antiangiogenic antibody routinely employed in combination with interferon alpha (bevacizumab) [106, 107], and antiproliferative agents (mTOR inhibitors, such as temsirolimus and everolimus) [106, 107]. Despite the effectiveness of these therapies, resistance to antiangiogenic therapy almost always occurs and are associated with high toxicity and, consequently, serious adverse events.

Considering all knowledge previously mentioned in this chapter, it is not surprising that agents altering the immune response in order to prevent tumor growth and metastases have gained space in this scenario [12, 14, 108]. Known as immunomodulators, these molecules have been studied for some time now [109]. Among the first representatives of this class are IL-2 and interferon-alpha (IFN-α). IL-2 is a naturally occurring cytokine, which have antitumor activity by the induction of proliferation of NK cells, lymphokine-activated killer cells (LAKs), and other cytotoxic cells [110, 111]. IFN-α is also a molecule that had its clinical effect for the treatment of RCC demonstrated years ago [109, 112]. It is a pleiotropic cytokine with immunomodulatory activities that is able to induce the differentiation of monocytes into highly activated DCs, which are particularly effective in recognizing complex antigens and inducing T- and B-cell immunity and thus participate in the generation of antitumor T-cell immunity [112]. However, cytokine immunotherapies work effectively only in a minority of RCC patients and currently are not considered for the standard treatment of RCC due to their high toxicity.

In this context, cytokines have been exploited. Combination therapy using an antihuman IL-6R antibody with interferon has been suggested as a novel therapeutic approach for the treatment of RCC. Besides, an IL-6R-neutralizing antibody, tocilizumab, in combination with sorafenib suppressed tumor growth and inhibits angiogenesis *in vivo* more efficiently than sorafenib alone [113, 114]. Similarly, infliximab, an anti-TNFα monoclonal antibody that prevents TNFα binding to its receptors, TNFR1 (p55 receptor) and TNFR2 (p75 receptor) and causes cell death via complement-mediated lysis through interaction with membrane-bound

TNF, has been considered for RCC treatment [115]. However, treatments with anti-TNFα monoclonal antibody showed varying results in independent studies, probably due to reactions given by this cytokine to different conditions, environmental and genetic factors and/or other unknown or unexplained factors [116]. Besides anti-TNFα strategies, targeting IL-1β has also been reported as possible therapy for RCC [117].

Promising candidates for RCC treatment have also been designed to specifically target chemokines and their receptors. One of the most widely studied compounds is AMD3100 which is thought to specifically block CXCR4 signaling [118] and that acts directly in RCC tumor [91] cells as well as local antitumor immune response, by impairing Tregs function [119], know to suppress a whole range of immune cells including B cells, NK cells, NKT cells, CD4+ or CD8+ T cells, monocytes, and DCs [119]. Also, many other chemokine antagonists have also shown potential for clinical application in cancer treatment and could be useful for RCC treatment in the future. For example, anti-CXCR7-12G8 and CCX77, CXCR7 inhibitors or CTCE-9908, which is a peptide analog of CXCL12 and an active inhibitor of the ligand, has shown promising results as well as tolerated drug that stabilized disease in early clinical trials for late-stage cancer patients [12, 120].

Recently, antibodies that inhibit T-cell coinhibitory receptors have emerged as therapeutic promises not only in the treatment of RCC but also in other tumors by inhibiting T-cell regulatory activity and increasing the antitumor immune response [14, 121]. Nivolumab and pembrolizumab (anti-PD-1) [14, 122], avelumab, and durvalumab (anti-PD-L1) are in late-stage clinical development for a number of indications [14, 123], besides the first in its class, ipilimumab (anti-CTLA-4), already approved for use in a number of indications [14, 124].

Finally, the close relationship between cancer and immune system has suggested that current drug therapies used to treat inflammatory diseases or particular types of cancers could function as inhibitors of chemokine signaling and could therefore be redirected toward the treatment of other cancers [12, 116]. This hypothesis needs to be tested by further preclinical and clinical investigation, which elucidates how these drugs would act at molecular and systemic levels.

5. Role of immune system in kidney cancer and the future

The role of immune system in kidney cancer is becoming more clear, whereas new findings that arise from clinical trials and identification of additional predictive biomarkers increase our understanding of the tumor microenvironment. Looking to the future based on the knowledge we have today, the perspective is a better understanding of immune system in tumor stroma as well as in various steps in cancer growth and metastasis.

Regarding RCC therapy, a promising option is the combination therapy based on targeted agents (inhibition of mTOR or VEGF pathways associated with immunotherapies) or immunotherapy + immunotherapy, which would overcome tumor resistance, as well as to restore functional immune system cancer surveillance and response. Currently, there are many clinical trials investigating combination therapy: nivolumab (anti-PD-1) + ipilimumab (anti-CTLA-4) [125], pembrolizumab (anti-PD-1) + ipilimumab (anti-CTLA-4) [126], pidilizumab (anti-PD-1) + vaccine (DC/RCC fusion cell vaccine) [127], atezolizumab (anti-PD-L1) + bevacizumab (anti-VEGF) [127], nivolumab (anti-PD-1) + bevacizumab (anti-VEGF) [128], pembrolizumab (anti-PD-1) + pazopanib (TKI) [129], nivolumab (anti-PD-1) + sunitinib [130].

Also, cell-based therapies have become interesting, which includes adoptive T-cell therapies such as tumor-infiltrating lymphocytes (TILs), T-cell receptor (TCR), and chimeric antigen T-cell (CAR-T) therapy [127].

Other promising alternative of therapy for RCC is vaccine-based immunotherapy. AGS-003 is an autologous DC vaccine that is generated from host DCs in response to tumor mRNA [131], which is also to investigate in combination with sunitinib [132].

All these therapeutic investigations highlighted the importance of immune system in the future study about RCC. Information about immune system may be decisive for clinical decisions.

6. Conclusion

Immune system plays a role in kidney cancer, and this should be considered for both the understanding of the disease and the development of novel therapies.

Acknowledgements

Work in our laboratory is supported by grants provided by the São Paulo Research Foundation (CETICs 2013/07467-1 and 2015/50040-4, São Paulo Research Foundation and GlaxoSmithKline). The authors thank the National Counsel of Technological and Scientific Development (CNPq, INCTTox), Coordination of Improvement of Higher Education Personnel (CAPES), BNDES 13.2.0711.1/2013, and União Química Farmacêutica Nacional for the support.

Conflict of interest

The authors declare they have no conflicts of interest.

Author details

Ana Marisa Chudzinski-Tavassi[1,2]*, Kátia Luciano Pereira Morais[1,2], Jean Gabriel de Souza[1] and Roger Chammas[3]

*Address all correspondence to: ana.chudzinski@butantan.gov.br

1 Laboratory of Molecular Biology, Butantan Institute, SP, Brazil

2 Department of Biochemistry, Federal University of São Paulo, SP, Brazil

3 Experimental Oncology Medical Investigation Laboratory—LIM/24,
University of São Paulo School of Medicine, SP, Brazil

References

[1] Shimodaira S, Hirabayashi K, Yanagisawa R, Higuchi Y, Sano K, Koizumi T. In: van den Heuvel-Eibrink MM, editor. Dendritic Cell-Based Cancer Immunotherapy Targeting Wilms' Tumor 1 for Pediatric Cancer. Brisbane, Australia: Wilms Tumor; 2016

[2] Hanna KS. A review of immune checkpoint inhibitors for the management of locally advanced or metastatic urothelial carcinoma. Pharmacotherapy. 2017;**37**(11):1391-1405. PubMed PMID: 28950037

[3] Alikhan MB, Pease G, Watkin W, Grogan R, Krausz T, Antic T. Primary epithelioid sarcoma of the kidney and adrenal gland: Report of 2 cases with immunohistochemical and molecular cytogenetic studies. Human Pathology. 2017;**61**:158-163. PubMed PMID: 27769872

[4] Kidney Cancer Update. The year in review in kidney cancer. Clinical Advances in Hematology & Oncology: H&O. 2015;**13**(5):327-329. PubMed PMID: 26352778

[5] Florek M, Haase M, Marzesco AM, Freund D, Ehninger G, Huttner WB, et al. Prominin-1/CD133, a neural and hematopoietic stem cell marker, is expressed in adult human differentiated cells and certain types of kidney cancer. Cell and Tissue Research. 2005;**319**(1):15-26. PubMed PMID: 15558321

[6] Santoni M, Berardi R, Amantini C, Burattini L, Santini D, Santoni G, et al. Role of natural and adaptive immunity in renal cell carcinoma response to VEGFR-TKIs and mTOR inhibitor. International Journal of Cancer [Journal International du Cancer]. 2014;**134**(12):2772-2777. PubMed PMID: 24114790

[7] Murphy KA, James BR, Guan Y, Torry DS, Wilber A, Griffith TS. Exploiting natural anti-tumor immunity for metastatic renal cell carcinoma. Human Vaccines & Immunotherapeutics. 2015;**11**(7):1612-1620. PubMed PMID: 25996049. Pubmed Central PMCID: 4514306

[8] Daurkin I, Eruslanov E, Stoffs T, Perrin GQ, Algood C, Gilbert SM, et al. Tumor-associated macrophages mediate immunosuppression in the renal cancer microenvironment by activating the 15-lipoxygenase-2 pathway. Cancer Research. 2011;**71**(20):6400-6409. PubMed PMID: 21900394

[9] Hemmerlein B, Johanns U, Halbfass J, Bottcher T, Heuser M, Radzun HJ, et al. The balance between MMP-2/-9 and TIMP-1/-2 is shifted towards MMP in renal cell carcinomas and can be further disturbed by hydrogen peroxide. International Journal of Oncology. 2004;**24**(5):1069-1076. PubMed PMID: 15067327

[10] Cabillic F, Bouet-Toussaint F, Toutirais O, Rioux-Leclercq N, Fergelot P, de la Pintiere CT, et al. Interleukin-6 and vascular endothelial growth factor release by renal cell carcinoma cells impedes lymphocyte-dendritic cell cross-talk. Clinical and Experimental Immunology. 2006;**146**(3):518-523. PubMed PMID: 17100773. Pubmed Central PMCID: 1810419

[11] O'Hayre M, Salanga CL, Handel TM, Allen SJ. Chemokines and cancer: Migration, intracellular signalling and intercellular communication in the microenvironment. The Biochemical Journal. 2008;**409**(3):635-649. PubMed PMID: 18177271

[12] Hembruff SL, Cheng N. Chemokine signaling in cancer: Implications on the tumor microenvironment and therapeutic targeting. Cancer Therapy. 2009;**7**(A):254-267. PubMed PMID: 20651940. Pubmed Central PMCID: 2907742

[13] Pawig L, Klasen C, Weber C, Bernhagen J, Noels H. Diversity and Inter-connections in the CXCR4 chemokine receptor/ligand family: Molecular perspectives. Frontiers in Immunology. 2015;**6**:429. PubMed PMID: 26347749. Pubmed Central PMCID: 4543903

[14] Ross K, Jones RJ. Immune checkpoint inhibitors in renal cell carcinoma. Clinical Science. 2017;**131**(21):2627-2642. PubMed PMID: 29079639

[15] Chan JY, Choudhury Y, Tan MH. Predictive molecular biomarkers to guide clinical decision making in kidney cancer: Current progress and future challenges. Expert Review of Molecular Diagnostics. 2015;**15**(5):631-646. PubMed PMID: 25837857

[16] Schreiber RD, Old LJ, Smyth MJ. Cancer immunoediting: Integrating immunity's roles in cancer suppression and promotion. Science. 2011;**331**(6024):1565-1570. PubMed PMID: 21436444. Epub 2011/03/26. eng

[17] Balkwill F, Charles KA, Mantovani A. Smoldering and polarized inflammation in the initiation and promotion of malignant disease. Cancer Cell. 2005;**7**(3):211-217

[18] Mantovani A, Allavena P, Sica A, Balkwill F. Cancer-related inflammation. Nature. 2008;**454**(7203):436-444

[19] Ono M. Molecular links between tumor angiogenesis and inflammation: Inflammatory stimuli of macrophages and cancer cells as targets for therapeutic strategy. Cancer Science. 2008;**99**(8):1501-1506. PubMed PMID: 18754859

[20] Hori Y, Stern PJ, Hynes RO, Irvine DJ. Engulfing tumors with synthetic extracellular matrices for cancer immunotherapy. Biomaterials. 2009;**30**(35):6757-6767 PubMed PMID: 19766305. Pubmed Central PMCID: 2788234. Epub 2009/09/22. eng

[21] Mantovani A. Cancer: Inflaming metastasis. Nature. 2009;**457**(7225):36-37

[22] de Visser KE, Coussens LM. The interplay between innate and adaptive immunity regulates cancer development. Cancer Immunology, Immunotherapy. 2005;**54**(11):1143-1152. PubMed PMID: 15889249. Epub 2005/05/13. eng

[23] Coussens LM, Werb Z. Inflammation and cancer. Nature. 2002;**420**(6917):860-867. PubMed PMID: 12490959

[24] Mantovani A, Sozzani S, Locati M, Allavena P, Sica A. Macrophage polarization: Tumor-associated macrophages as a paradigm for polarized M2 mononuclear phagocytes. Trends in Immunology. 2002;**23**(11):549-555. PubMed PMID: 12401408

[25] Sica A, Saccani A, Mantovani A. Tumor-associated macrophages: A molecular perspective. International Immunopharmacology. 2002;**2**(8):1045-1054. PubMed PMID: 12349942

[26] Mantovani A, Bottazzi B, Colotta F, Sozzani S, Ruco L. The origin and function of tumor-associated macrophages. Immunology Today. 1992;**13**(7):265-270. PubMed PMID: 1388654

[27] Gebhard B, Gnant M, Schutz G, Roka S, Weigel G, Kandioler D, et al. Different transendothelial migration behaviour pattern of blood monocytes derived from patients with benign and malignant diseases of the breast. Anticancer Research. 2000;**20**(6B): 4599-4604. PubMed PMID: 11205309

[28] Schlossman SF, Reinherz EL. Human T-cell subsets in health and disease. Springer Seminars in Immunopathology. 1984;**7**(1):9-18

[29] Zikich D, Schachter J, Besser MJ. Predictors of tumor-infiltrating lymphocyte efficacy in melanoma. Immunotherapy. 2016;**8**(1):35-43. PubMed PMID: 26653685. Epub 2015/12/15. Eng

[30] Thompson RH, Kuntz SM, Leibovich BC, Dong H, Lohse CM, Webster WS, et al. Tumor B7-H1 is associated with poor prognosis in renal cell carcinoma patients with long-term follow-up. Cancer Research. 2006;**66**(7):3381-3385. PubMed PMID: 16585157. Epub 2006/04/06. eng

[31] Zhang BY, Thompson RH, Lohse CM, Leibovich BC, Boorjian SA, Cheville JC, et al. A novel prognostic model for patients with sarcomatoid renal cell carcinoma. BJU International. 2015;**115**(3):405-411. PubMed PMID: 24730416. Epub 2014/04/16. eng

[32] Oleinika K, Nibbs RJ, Graham GJ, Fraser AR. Suppression, subversion and escape: The role of regulatory T cells in cancer progression. Clinical and Experimental Immunology. 2013;**171**(1):36-45. PubMed PMID: PMC3530093

[33] Ribas A, Shin DS, Zaretsky J, Frederiksen J, Cornish A, Avramis E, et al. PD-1 blockade expands intratumoral T memory cells. Cancer Immunology Research. 2016;**19**:2016

[34] Noman MZ, Desantis G, Janji B, Hasmim M, Karray S, Dessen P, et al. PD-L1 is a novel direct target of HIF-1α, and its blockade under hypoxia enhanced MDSC-mediated T cell activation. The Journal of Experimental Medicine. 2014;**211**(5):781-790

[35] Figlin RA, Thompson JA, Bukowski RM, Vogelzang NJ, Novick AC, Lange P. Multicenter, randomized, phase III trial of CD8(+) tumor-infiltrating lymphocytes in combination with recombinant interleukin-2 in metastatic renal cell carcinoma. Journal of Clinical Oncology. 1999;**17**(8):2521-2529

[36] Thompson RH, Kwon ED, Allison JP. Inhibitors of B7-CD28 costimulation in urologic malignancies. Immunotherapy. 2009;**1**(1):129-139 PubMed PMID: 20445772. Pubmed Central PMCID: 2864044. Epub 2009/01/01. eng

[37] McCoy KD, Gros G. The role of CTLA-4 in the regulation of T cell immune responses. Immunology and Cell Biology. 1999;**77**(1):1-10

[38] McDermott DF, Sosman JA, Sznol M, Massard C, Gordon MS, Hamid O, et al. Atezolizumab, an anti–programmed death-ligand 1 antibody, in metastatic renal cell carcinoma: Long-term safety, clinical activity, and immune correlates from a phase Ia study. Journal of Clinical Oncology. 2016;**34**(8):833-842. PubMed PMID: 26755520

[39] Philips GK, Atkins MB. New agents and new targets for renal cell carcinoma. American Society of Clinical Oncology Educational Book. 2014:e222-e227 PubMed PMID: 24857106. Epub 2014/05/27. Eng

[40] Pappalardo F, Forero IM, Pennisi M, Palazon A, Melero I, Motta S. SimB16: Modeling induced immune system response against B16-melanoma. PLoS One. 2011;**6**(10):e26523

[41] Dall'Oglio M, Srougi M, Barbuto JA. Complete response of metastatic renal cancer with dendritic cell vaccine. International Brazilian Journal of Urology. 2003;**29**(6):517-519. PubMed PMID: 15748305

[42] Buhtoiarov IN, Neal ZC, Gan J, Buhtoiarova TN, Patankar MS, Gubbels JA, et al. Differential internalization of hu14.18-IL2 immunocytokine by NK and tumor cell: impact on conjugation, cytotoxicity, and targeting. Journal of Leukocyte Biology. 2011; **89**(4):625-638 PubMed PMID: 21248148. Pubmed Central PMCID: 3058817. Epub 2011/01/21. eng

[43] Buhtoiarov IN, Sondel PM, Wigginton JM, Buhtoiarova TN, Yanke EM, Mahvi DA, et al. Anti-tumour synergy of cytotoxic chemotherapy and anti-CD40 plus CpG-ODN immunotherapy through repolarization of tumour-associated macrophages. Immunology. 2011;**132**(2):226-239. PubMed PMID: 21039467. Pubmed Central PMCID: 3050446. Epub 2010/11/03. eng

[44] Gubbels JA, Gadbaw B, Buhtoiarov IN, Horibata S, Kapur AK, Patel D, et al. Ab-IL2 fusion proteins mediate NK cell immune synapse formation by polarizing CD25 to the target cell-effector cell interface. Cancer Immunology, Immunotherapy. 2011;**60**(12): 1789-1800. PubMed PMID: 21792658. Epub 2011/07/28. Eng

[45] Johnson EE, Buhtoiarov IN, Baldeshwiler MJ, Felder MA, Van Rooijen N, Sondel PM, et al. Enhanced T-cell-independent antitumor effect of cyclophosphamide combined with anti-CD40 mAb and CpG in mice. Journal of Immunotherapy. 2011;**34**(1):76-84. PubMed PMID: 21150715. Pubmed Central PMCID: 3031426. Epub 2010/12/15. eng

[46] Barbuto JAM, Ensina LFC, Neves AR, Bergami-Santos PC, Leite KRM, Marques R, et al. Dendritic cell–tumor cell hybrid vaccination for metastatic cancer. Cancer Immunology, Immunotherapy. 2004;**53**(12):1111-1118

[47] Baleeiro RB, Anselmo LB, Soares FA, Pinto CA, Ramos O, Gross JL, et al. High frequency of immature dendritic cells and altered in situ production of interleukin-4 and tumor necrosis factor-alpha in lung cancer. Cancer Immunology, Immunotherapy. 2008;**57**(9):1335-1345. PubMed PMID: 18286287. Epub 2008/02/21. eng

[48] Demaria S, Pikarsky E, Karin M, Coussens LM, Chen YC, El-Omar EM, et al. Cancer and inflammation: Promise for biologic therapy. Journal of Immunotherapy. 2010;**33**(4):335-351. PubMed PMID: 20386472. Pubmed Central PMCID: 2941912. Epub 2010/04/14. eng

[49] Balwit J, Hwu P, Urba W, Marincola F. The iSBTc/SITC primer on tumor immunology and biological therapy of cancer: A summary of the 2010 program. Journal of Translational Medicine. 2011;**9**(1):18. PubMed PMID. DOI: 10.1186/1479-5876-9-18

[50] Reiman JM, Kmieciak M, Manjili MH, Knutson KL. Tumor immunoediting and immunosculpting pathways to cancer progression. Seminars in Cancer Biology. 2007;**17**(4):275-287

[51] Berezhnaya NM. Interaction between tumor and immune system: The role of tumor cell biology. Experimental Oncology. 2010;**32**(3):159-166. PubMed PMID: 21403611. Epub 2011/03/16. eng

[52] Vesely MD, Kershaw MH, Schreiber RD, Smyth MJ. Natural innate and adaptive immunity to Cancer. Annual Review of Immunology. 2011;**29**(1):235-271

[53] Shankaran V, Ikeda H, Bruce AT, White JM, Swanson PE, Old LJ, et al. IFN[gamma] and lymphocytes prevent primary tumour development and shape tumour immunogenicity. Nature. 2001;**410**(6832):1107-1111

[54] Frucht DM, Fukao T, Bogdan C, Schindler H, O'Shea JJ, Koyasu S. IFN-γ production by antigen-presenting cells: Mechanisms emerge. Trends in Immunology. 2001; **22**(10):556-560

[55] Ulloa L, Tracey KJ. The 'cytokine profile': A code for sepsis. Trends in Molecular Medicine. 2005;**11**(2):56-63

[56] Lee H, Baek S, Joe S-J, Pyo S-N. Modulation of IFN-γ production by TNF-α in macrophages from the tumor environment: Significance as an angiogenic switch. International Immunopharmacology. 2006;**6**(1):71-78

[57] Lo SZY, Steer JH, Joyce DA. TNF-[alpha] renders macrophages resistant to a range of cancer chemotherapeutic agents through NF-[kappa]B-mediated antagonism of apoptosis signalling. Cancer Letters. 2011;**307**(1):80-92

[58] Watford WT, Moriguchi M, Morinobu A, O'Shea JJ. The biology of IL-12: Coordinating innate and adaptive immune responses. Cytokine & Growth Factor Reviews. 2003; **14**(5):361-368

[59] Xu M, Mizoguchi I, Morishima N, Chiba Y, Mizuguchi J, Yoshimoto T. Regulation of antitumor immune responses by the IL-12 family cytokines, IL-12, IL-23, and IL-27. Clinical & Developmental Immunology. 2010;**2010**:1-10. PubMed PMID: 20885915. Pubmed Central PMCID: 2946577. Epub 2010/10/05. eng

[60] Heusinkveld M, de Vos van Steenwijk PJ, Goedemans R, Ramwadhdoebe TH, Gorter A, MJP W, et al. M2 macrophages induced by prostaglandin E2 and IL-6 from cervical carcinoma are switched to activated M1 macrophages by CD4+ Th1 cells. The Journal of Immunology. 2011;**187**(3):1157-1165

[61] Ouyang W, Rutz S, Crellin NK, Valdez PA, Hymowitz SG. Regulation and functions of the IL-10 family of cytokines in inflammation and disease. Annual Review of Immunology. 2011;**29**(1):71-109

[62] Dhodapkar KM, Barbuto S, Matthews P, Kukreja A, Mazumder A, Vesole D, et al. Dendritic cells mediate the induction of polyfunctional human IL17-producing cells (Th17-1 cells) enriched in the bone marrow of patients with myeloma. Blood. 2008;**112**(7):2878-2885. PubMed PMID: PMC2556623

[63] Inozume T, K-i H, Wang QJ, Yang JC. IL-17 secreted by tumor reactive T cells induces IL-8 release by human renal cancer cells. Journal of Immunotherapy. 2009;**32**(2):109-117. PubMed PMID: 00002371-200902000-00002

[64] Turner MD, Nedjai B, Hurst T, Pennington DJ. Cytokines and chemokines: At the crossroads of cell signalling and inflammatory disease. Biochimica et Biophysica Acta. 2014;**1843**(11):2563-2582. PubMed PMID: 24892271

[65] Parihar JS, Tunuguntla HS. Role of chemokines in renal cell carcinoma. Reviews in Urology. 2014;**16**(3):118-121. PubMed PMID: 25337041. Pubmed Central PMCID: 4191631

[66] Mikami S, Mizuno R, Kosaka T, Saya H, Oya M, Okada Y. Expression of TNF-alpha and CD44 is implicated in poor prognosis, cancer cell invasion, metastasis and resistance to the sunitinib treatment in clear cell renal cell carcinomas. International Journal of Cancer [Journal International du Cancer]. 2015;**136**(7):1504-1514. PubMed PMID: 25123505

[67] Petrella BL, Vincenti MP. Interleukin-1beta mediates metalloproteinase-dependent renal cell carcinoma tumor cell invasion through the activation of CCAAT enhancer binding protein beta. Cancer Medicine. 2012;**1**(1):17-27. PubMed PMID: 23342250. Pubmed Central PMCID: 3544428

[68] O'Neill LA. The interleukin-1 receptor/toll-like receptor superfamily: 10 years of progress. Immunological Reviews. 2008;**226**:10-18. PubMed PMID: 19161412

[69] Elzinga BM, Twomey C, Powell JC, Harte F, McCarthy JV. Interleukin-1 receptor type 1 is a substrate for gamma-secretase-dependent regulated intramembrane proteolysis. The Journal of Biological Chemistry. 2009;**284**(3):1394-1409. PubMed PMID: 18996842

[70] Baker SJ, Reddy EP. Modulation of life and death by the TNF receptor superfamily. Oncogene. 1998;**17**(25):3261-3270. PubMed PMID: 9916988

[71] Taga T, Kishimoto T. Gp130 and the interleukin-6 family of cytokines. Annual Review of Immunology. 1997;**15**:797-819. PubMed PMID: 9143707

[72] Goette NP, Lev PR, Heller PG, Glembotsky AC, Chazarreta CD, Salim JP, et al. Abnormal regulation of soluble and anchored IL-6 receptor in monocytes from patients with essential thrombocythemia. Experimental Hematology. 2010;**38**(10):868-76 e1. PubMed PMID: 20600579

[73] Yoshida N, Ikemoto S, Narita K, Sugimura K, Wada S, Yasumoto R, et al. Interleukin-6, tumour necrosis factor alpha and interleukin-1beta in patients with renal cell carcinoma. British Journal of Cancer. 2002;**86**(9):1396-1400. PubMed PMID: 11986770. Pubmed Central PMCID: 2375361

[74] Grivennikov SI, Greten FR, Karin M. Immunity, inflammation, and cancer. Cell. 2010; **140**(6):883-899 PubMed PMID: 20303878. Pubmed Central PMCID: 2866629

[75] Ikemoto S, Yoshida N, Narita K, Wada S, Kishimoto T, Sugimura K, et al. Role of tumor-associated macrophages in renal cell carcinoma. Oncology Reports. 2003;**10**(6):1843-1849. PubMed PMID: 14534706

[76] Dinarello CA. Why not treat human cancer with interleukin-1 blockade? Cancer Metastasis Reviews. 2010;**29**(2):317-329. PubMed PMID: 20422276. Pubmed Central PMCID: 2865633

[77] Burns JM, Summers BC, Wang Y, Melikian A, Berahovich R, Miao Z, et al. A novel chemokine receptor for SDF-1 and I-TAC involved in cell survival, cell adhesion, and tumor development. The Journal of Experimental Medicine. 2006;**203**(9):2201-2213. PubMed PMID: 16940167. Pubmed Central PMCID: 2118398

[78] Kulbe H, Hagemann T, Szlosarek PW, Balkwill FR, Wilson JL. The inflammatory cytokine tumor necrosis factor-alpha regulates chemokine receptor expression on ovarian cancer cells. Cancer Research. 2005;**65**(22):10355-10362. PubMed PMID: 16288025

[79] Xin H, Zhang C, Herrmann A, Du Y, Figlin R, Yu H. Sunitinib inhibition of Stat3 induces renal cell carcinoma tumor cell apoptosis and reduces immunosuppressive cells. Cancer Research. 2009;**69**(6):2506-2513. PubMed PMID: 19244102. Pubmed Central PMCID: 2664264

[80] Moser B, Wolf M, Walz A, Loetscher P. Chemokines: Multiple levels of leukocyte migration control. Trends in Immunology. 2004;**25**(2):75-84. PubMed PMID: 15102366

[81] Palczewski K, Kumasaka T, Hori T, Behnke CA, Motoshima H, Fox BA, et al. Crystal structure of rhodopsin: A G protein-coupled receptor. Science. 2000;**289**(5480):739-745. PubMed PMID: 10926528

[82] Teicher BA, Fricker SP. CXCL12 (SDF-1)/CXCR4 pathway in cancer. Clinical Cancer Research: An Official Journal of the American Association for Cancer Research. 2010;**16**(11):2927-2931. PubMed PMID: 20484021

[83] Kalatskaya I, Berchiche YA, Gravel S, Limberg BJ, Rosenbaum JS, Heveker N. AMD3100 is a CXCR7 ligand with allosteric agonist properties. Molecular Pharmacology. 2009;**75**(5):1240-1247. PubMed PMID: 19255243

[84] McAllister SS, Weinberg RA. Tumor-host interactions: A far-reaching relationship. Journal of Clinical Oncology: Official Journal of the American Society of Clinical Oncology. 2010;**28**(26):4022-4028. PubMed PMID: 20644094

[85] Putney JW , Broad LM, Braun FJ, Lievremont JP, Bird GS. Mechanisms of capacitative calcium entry. Journal of Cell Science. 2001;**114**(Pt 12):2223-2229. PubMed PMID: 11493662

[86] Mukherjee D, Zhao J. The role of chemokine receptor CXCR4 in breast cancer metastasis. American Journal of Cancer Research. 2013;**3**(1):46-57. PubMed PMID: 23359227. Pubmed Central PMCID: 3555200

[87] Goda S, Inoue H, Umehara H, Miyaji M, Nagano Y, Harakawa N, et al. Matrix metalloproteinase-1 produced by human CXCL12-stimulated natural killer cells. The American Journal of Pathology. 2006;**169**(2):445-458. PubMed PMID: 16877347. Pubmed Central PMCID: 1698790

[88] Vila-Coro AJ, Rodriguez-Frade JM, Martin De Ana A, Moreno-Ortiz MC, Martinez AC, Mellado M. The chemokine SDF-1alpha triggers CXCR4 receptor dimerization and activates the JAK/STAT pathway. FASEB Journal: Official Publication of the Federation of American Societies for Experimental Biology. 1999;**13**(13):1699-1710. PubMed PMID: 10506573

[89] Sun X, Cheng G, Hao M, Zheng J, Zhou X, Zhang J, et al. CXCL12/CXCR4/CXCR7 chemokine axis and cancer progression. Cancer Metastasis Reviews. 2010;**29**(4):709-722. PubMed PMID: 20839032. Pubmed Central PMCID: 3175097

[90] Schrader AJ, Lechner O, Templin M, Dittmar KE, Machtens S, Mengel M, et al. CXCR4/CXCL12 expression and signalling in kidney cancer. British Journal of Cancer. 2002; **86**(8):1250-1256. PubMed PMID: 11953881. Pubmed Central PMCID: 2375348

[91] Ierano C, Santagata S, Napolitano M, Guardia F, Grimaldi A, Antignani E, et al. CXCR4 and CXCR7 transduce through mTOR in human renal cancer cells. Cell Death & Disease. 2014;**5**:e1310. PubMed PMID: 24991762. Pubmed Central PMCID: 4123065

[92] Curnock AP, Logan MK, Ward SG. Chemokine signalling: Pivoting around multiple phosphoinositide 3-kinases. Immunology. 2002;**105**(2):125-136. PubMed PMID: 11872087. Pubmed Central PMCID: 1782650

[93] Karin M. Nuclear factor-kappaB in cancer development and progression. Nature. 2006; **441**(7092):431-436. PubMed PMID: 16724054

[94] Ye RD. Regulation of nuclear factor kappaB activation by G-protein-coupled receptors. Journal of Leukocyte Biology. 2001;**70**(6):839-848. PubMed PMID: 11739545

[95] Lee BC, Lee TH, Avraham S, Avraham HK. Involvement of the chemokine receptor CXCR4 and its ligand stromal cell-derived factor 1alpha in breast cancer cell migration through human brain microvascular endothelial cells. Molecular Cancer Research: MCR. 2004;**2**(6):327-338. PubMed PMID: 15235108

[96] Johnson-Holiday C, Singh R, Johnson EL, Grizzle WE, Lillard JW Jr, Singh S. CCR9-CCL25 interactions promote cisplatin resistance in breast cancer cell through Akt activation in a PI3K-dependent and FAK-independent fashion. World Journal of Surgical Oncology. 2011;**9**:46. PubMed PMID: 21539750. Pubmed Central PMCID: 3110128

[97] Diehl JA, Cheng M, Roussel MF, Sherr CJ. Glycogen synthase kinase-3beta regulates cyclin D1 proteolysis and subcellular localization. Genes & Development. 1998;**12**(22): 3499-3511. PubMed PMID: 9832503. Pubmed Central PMCID: 317244

[98] Allan LA, Morrice N, Brady S, Magee G, Pathak S, Clarke PR. Inhibition of caspase-9 through phosphorylation at Thr 125 by ERK MAPK. Nature Cell Biology. 2003;**5**(7): 647-654. PubMed PMID: 12792650

[99] Bonni A, Brunet A, West AE, Datta SR, Takasu MA, Greenberg ME. Cell survival promoted by the Ras-MAPK signaling pathway by transcription-dependent and -independent mechanisms. Science. 1999;**286**(5443):1358-1362. PubMed PMID: 10558990

[100] Kyriakis JM. MAP kinases and the regulation of nuclear receptors. Science's STKE: Signal Transduction Knowledge Environment. 2000;**2000**(48):pe1. PubMed PMID: 11752606

[101] Zagzag D, Lukyanov Y, Lan L, Ali MA, Esencay M, Mendez O, et al. Hypoxia-inducible factor 1 and VEGF upregulate CXCR4 in glioblastoma: Implications for angiogenesis and glioma cell invasion. Laboratory Investigation; A Journal of Technical Methods and Pathology. 2006;**86**(12):1221-1232. PubMed PMID: 17075581

[102] van Golen KL, Ying C, Sequeira L, Dubyk CW, Reisenberger T, Chinnaiyan AM, et al. CCL2 induces prostate cancer transendothelial cell migration via activation of the small GTPase Rac. Journal of Cellular Biochemistry. 2008;**104**(5):1587-1597. PubMed PMID: 18646053

[103] Boldajipour B, Mahabaleshwar H, Kardash E, Reichman-Fried M, Blaser H, Minina S, et al. Control of chemokine-guided cell migration by ligand sequestration. Cell. 2008;**132**(3):463-473. PubMed PMID: 18267076

[104] Rajagopal S, Kim J, Ahn S, Craig S, Lam CM, Gerard NP, et al. Beta-arrestin-but not G protein-mediated signaling by the "decoy" receptor CXCR7. Proceedings of the National Academy of Sciences of the United States of America. 2010;**107**(2):628-632. PubMed PMID: 20018651. Pubmed Central PMCID: 2818968

[105] Kovaleva OV, Samoilova DV, Shitova MS, Gratchev A. Tumor associated macrophages in kidney Cancer. Analytical Cellular Pathology. 2016;**2016**:9307549. PubMed PMID: 27807511. Pubmed Central PMCID: 5078639

[106] Banumathy G, Cairns P. Signaling pathways in renal cell carcinoma. Cancer Biology & Therapy. 2010;**10**(7):658-664. PubMed PMID: 20814228. Pubmed Central PMCID: 3093809

[107] Ghidini M, Petrelli F, Ghidini A, Tomasello G, Hahne JC, Passalacqua R, et al. Clinical development of mTor inhibitors for renal cancer. Expert Opinion on Investigational Drugs. 2017;**26**(11):1229-1237. PubMed PMID: 28952411

[108] Song M. Recent developments in small molecule therapies for renal cell carcinoma. European Journal of Medicinal Chemistry. 2017;**142**:383-392. PubMed PMID: 28844802

[109] Minasian LM, Motzer RJ, Gluck L, Mazumdar M, Vlamis V, Krown SE. Interferon alfa-2a in advanced renal cell carcinoma: Treatment results and survival in 159 patients with long-term follow-up. Journal of Clinical Oncology: Official Journal of the American Society of Clinical Oncology. 1993;**11**(7):1368-1375. PubMed PMID: 8315435

[110] Yagoda A, Bander NH. Failure of cytotoxic chemotherapy, 1983-1988, and the emerging role of monoclonal antibodies for renal cancer. Urologia Internationalis. 1989;**44**(6): 338-345. PubMed PMID: 2696193

[111] Iguchi M, Matsumoto M, Hojo K, Wada T, Matsuo Y, Arimura A, et al. Antitumor efficacy of recombinant human interleukin-2 combined with sorafenib against mouse renal

cell carcinoma. Japanese Journal of Clinical Oncology. 2009;**39**(5):303-309. PubMed PMID: 19336449

[112] Rizza P, Moretti F, Belardelli F. Recent advances on the immunomodulatory effects of IFN-alpha: Implications for cancer immunotherapy and autoimmunity. Autoimmunity. 2010;**43**(3):204-209. PubMed PMID: 20187707

[113] Ishibashi K, Haber T, Breuksch I, Gebhard S, Sugino T, Kubo H, et al. Overriding TKI resistance of renal cell carcinoma by combination therapy with IL-6 receptor blockade. Oncotarget. 2017;**8**(33):55230-55245. PubMed PMID: 28903416. Pubmed Central PMCID: 5589655

[114] Oguro T, Ishibashi K, Sugino T, Hashimoto K, Tomita S, Takahashi N, et al. Humanised antihuman IL-6R antibody with interferon inhibits renal cell carcinoma cell growth in vitro and in vivo through suppressed SOCS3 expression. European Journal of Cancer. 2013;**49**(7):1715-1724. PubMed PMID: 23274199

[115] Harrison ML, Obermueller E, Maisey NR, Hoare S, Edmonds K, Li NF, et al. Tumor necrosis factor alpha as a new target for renal cell carcinoma: Two sequential phase II trials of infliximab at standard and high dose. Journal of Clinical Oncology: Official Journal of the American Society of Clinical Oncology. 2007;**25**(29):4542-4549. PubMed PMID: 17925549

[116] Kobak S, Karaarslan A, Aktakka Y. Renal cell carcinoma in a patient with rheumatoid arthritis treated with adalimumab. Current Drug Safety. 2014;**9**(1):69-72. PubMed PMID: 24191905

[117] Triozzi PL, Kim JA, Martin EW, Young DC, Benzies T, Villasmil PM. Phase I trial of escalating doses of interleukin-1 beta in combination with a fixed dose of interleukin-2. Journal of Clinical Oncology: Official Journal of the American Society of Clinical Oncology. 1995;**13**(2):482-489. PubMed PMID: 7844609

[118] Burger JA, Burger M, Kipps TJ. Chronic lymphocytic leukemia B cells express functional CXCR4 chemokine receptors that mediate spontaneous migration beneath bone marrow stromal cells. Blood. 1999;**94**(11):3658-3667. PubMed PMID: 10572077

[119] Santagata S, Napolitano M, D'Alterio C, Desicato S, Maro SD, Marinelli L, et al. Targeting CXCR4 reverts the suppressive activity of T-regulatory cells in renal cancer. Oncotarget. 2017;**8**(44):77110-77120. PubMed PMID: 29100374. Pubmed Central PMCID: 5652768

[120] Kavsak PA, Henderson M, Moretto P, Hirte H, Evans K, Wong D, et al. Biochip arrays for the discovery of a biomarker surrogate in a phase I/II study assessing a novel antimetastasis agent. Clinical Biochemistry. 2009;**42**(10-11):1162-1165. PubMed PMID: 19389390

[121] Atkins MB, Clark JI, Quinn DI. Immune checkpoint inhibitors in advanced renal cell carcinoma: Experience to date and future directions. Annals of Oncology : Official Journal of the European Society for Medical Oncology. 2017;**28**(7):1484-1494. PubMed PMID: 28383639

[122] McDermott DF, Drake CG, Sznol M, Choueiri TK, Powderly JD, Smith DC, et al. Survival, durable response, and long-term safety in patients with previously treated

advanced renal cell carcinoma receiving Nivolumab. Journal of Clinical Oncology: Official Journal of the American Society of Clinical Oncology. 2015;**33**(18):2013-2020. PubMed PMID: 25800770. Pubmed Central PMCID: 4517051

[123] Swaika A, Hammond WA, Joseph RW. Current state of anti-PD-L1 and anti-PD-1 agents in cancer therapy. Molecular Immunology. 2015;**67**(2 Pt A):4-17. PubMed PMID: 25749122

[124] Nivolumab Plus Ipilimumab Has Antitumor Activity in Metastatic RCC. Cancer Discovery. 2017;**7**(9):OF7. PubMed PMID: 28710099

[125] Hao C, Tian J, Liu H, Li F, Niu H, Zhu B. Efficacy and safety of anti-PD-1 and anti-PD-1 combined with anti-CTLA-4 immunotherapy to advanced melanoma: A systematic review and meta-analysis of randomized controlled trials. Medicine. 2017;**96**(26):e7325. PubMed PMID: 28658143. Pubmed Central PMCID: 5500065

[126] Alsaab HO, Sau S, Alzhrani R, Tatiparti K, Bhise K, Kashaw SK, et al. PD-1 and PD-L1 checkpoint signaling inhibition for cancer immunotherapy: Mechanism, combinations, and clinical outcome. Frontiers in Pharmacology. 2017;**8**:561. PubMed PMID: 28878676. Pubmed Central PMCID: 5572324

[127] Weinstock M, McDermott D. Targeting PD-1/PD-L1 in the treatment of metastatic renal cell carcinoma. Therapeutic Advances in Urology. 2015;**7**(6):365-377. PubMed PMID: 26622321. Pubmed Central PMCID: 4647139

[128] Mazza C, Escudier B, Albiges L. Nivolumab in renal cell carcinoma: Latest evidence and clinical potential. Therapeutic Advances in Medical Oncology. 2017;**9**(3):171-181. PubMed PMID: 28344662. Pubmed Central PMCID: 5349425

[129] Rodriguez-Vida A, Hutson TE, Bellmunt J, Strijbos MH. New treatment options for metastatic renal cell carcinoma. ESMO Open. 2017;**2**(2):e000185 PubMed PMID: 28761748. Pubmed Central PMCID: 5519813

[130] Wallin JJ, Bendell JC, Funke R, Sznol M, Korski K, Jones S, et al. Atezolizumab in combination with bevacizumab enhances antigen-specific T-cell migration in metastatic renal cell carcinoma. Nature Communications. 2016;**7**:12624. PubMed PMID: 27571927. Pubmed Central PMCID: 5013615 provided the study drug. Some of the authors of this manuscript are employees of Genentech/Roche. The remaining authors declare no competing financial interests

[131] Gill DM, Hahn AW, Hale P, Maughan BL. Overview of current and future first-line systemic therapy for metastatic clear cell renal cell carcinoma. Current Treatment Options in Oncology. 2018;**19**(1):6. PubMed PMID: 29368125

[132] Amin A, Dudek AZ, Logan TF, Lance RS, Holzbeierlein JM, Knox JJ, et al. Survival with AGS-003, an autologous dendritic cell-based immunotherapy, in combination with sunitinib in unfavorable risk patients with advanced renal cell carcinoma (RCC): Phase 2 study results. Journal for Immunotherapy of Cancer. 2015;**3**:14. PubMed PMID: 25901286. Pubmed Central PMCID: 4404644

Chapter 3

Immunotherapy for Renal Cell Carcinoma

Le Qu, Ding Wu, Haowei He, Xiaofeng Xu and
Cheng Chen

Additional information is available at the end of the chapter

http://dx.doi.org/10.5772/intechopen.77377

Abstract

Despite the rapid development of therapeutic modalities for advanced or metastatic renal cell carcinoma (mRCC) over the past decade to include traditional immunotherapy, such as high-dose interleukin-2 and interferon-α, as well as a number of targeted anti-angiogenic therapies, mRCC continues to be associated with poor prognosis. Currently, immunotherapy has seen tremendous development in the form of immune checkpoint inhibition and vaccines at a dizzying pace, which are being studied in mRCC and are showing promise as important steps in the management of this disease. With so many drugs available to clinicians and patients, properly integrating immunotherapy especially immune checkpoint blockade (ICB) into the treatment paradigm is challenging. Emerging research with additional ICB agents and novel combination strategies is likely to further impact clinical decision-making. The further development of biomarkers for predicting a response is required to achieve optimal efficacy with these therapeutic interventions. This chapter summarizes the current landscape of standard and emerging immune therapeutics and other modalities for mRCC.

Keywords: immunotherapy, renal cell carcinoma, immune checkpoint inhibitors

1. Introduction

Renal cell carcinoma (RCC) is the most prevalent kidney cancer, with nearly 63,990 cases diagnosed and 14,400 deaths in 2017 [1]. Approximately 25–30% of cases are metastatic at diagnosis [2] and 20–30% of patients who undergo surgical management for local RCC show metastases [3]. Recently, the enhanced comprehension of RCC pathogenesis led to the development of von Hippel-Lindau/ hypoxia-inducible factor (VHL/HIF) targeted therapy as the mainstay of therapeutic options for advanced RCC patients, improving the survival rates of patients [4].

However, the current 3-year overall survival rate is yet no more than 40% and a majority of patients will die because of the progressed disease [5]. As a consequence, new targets and therapies are needed to improve patient outcomes. The rapidly evolving field of immuno-oncology yields several novel immunotherapeutic agents. Currently, cancer vaccines, adoptive T-cell therapy, and immune checkpoint inhibitors (ICIs) are being investigated in advanced RCC and are producing durable responses and noteworthy overall survival improvement. This chapter mainly introduces the treatment landscape of immune therapeutics for RCC.

2. Immunotherapy

The immune system interacts intimately with tumors over the entire disease process. The complex crosstalk between the immune system and cancer cells determines the eventual outcome, either inhibiting or enhancing tumor development [6]. First, antigen-presenting cells (APCs), primarily dendritic cells (DCs), must encounter tumor-associated antigen (TAA), which can emerge via the altered protein structure caused by somatic mutations or differentially expressed proteins. The antigen expression pattern needs to be different from that on normal cells to avoid immune tolerance. APCs process TAA into peptide fragments, which then form a complex with major histocompatibility complex (MHC) class I and II molecules. The initial step of T-cell activation is the recognition of antigen presented on the MHC molecule of APCs by T-cell receptor (TCR). Full T-cell activation also requires a co-stimulatory signal by the binding of CD28 on T cell to B7 ligands (CD80 and CD86) on APCs [7].

Multiple feedback mechanisms exert stimulatory or inhibitory effects on T cells, regulating immune function and preventing an excessive immune response. These mechanisms include immune checkpoint molecules on the surface of T cells and other immune cells such as regulatory T (T_{reg}) cells and myeloid-derived suppressor cells (MDSCs) [8]. Tumor cells can take advantage of these mechanisms to prevent a potential anticancer immune response. RCC usually presents prominent immune cell infiltration, including T cells, natural killer (NK) cells, DCs, and macrophages. During early stages, malignant cells can be poor stimulators and become resistant to the innate immune response. Later, progressively growing tumors impair the adaptive immune response by blocking T-cell signal transduction and function [9]. An increased understanding of these processes has enabled the development of immunotherapy for cancer management.

Immunotherapy is defined as excluding cancer by activating the autoimmune response against the tumor rather than by attacking the tumor directly. Immunotherapy can induce long-lasting anticancer responses owing to the generation of antigen-specific immune memory, either through memory T-cells or antibodies. Several crucial steps are needed to mount an initial effective immune response against tumors [10]. Immune checkpoint blockade disrupts negative immune regulations to enhance immune system activity and boost antitumor immune response. Other immunomodulatory therapies such as cytokine therapy and vaccines potentiate co-stimulatory pathways or stimulate the innate immunity or interact with the immune suppressive tumor microenvironment. The past decade has witnessed the emergence of immunotherapy as an exciting treatment option for different malignancies, including RCC. The following sections discuss these in more detail (**Figure 1**).

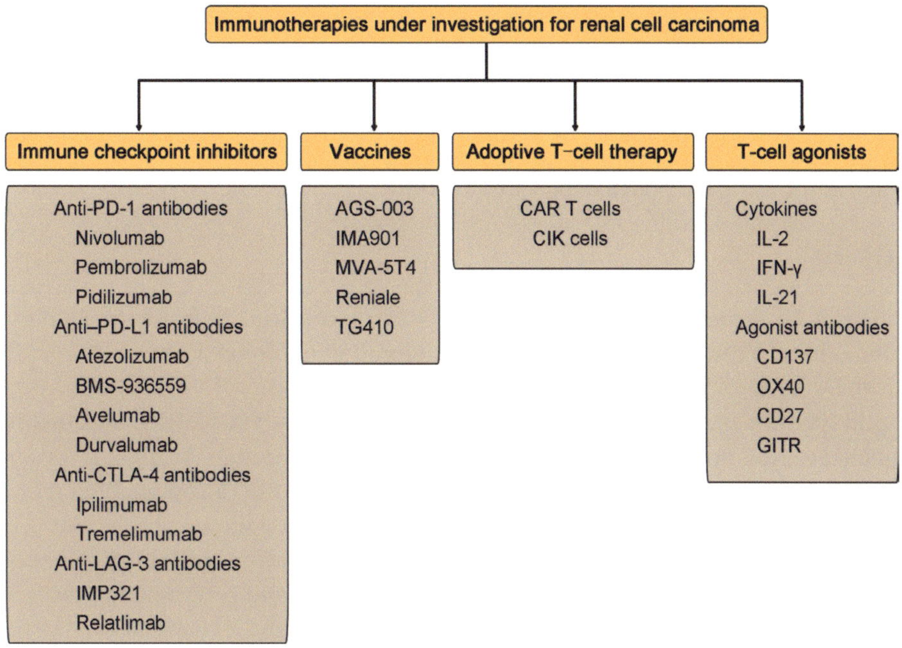

Figure 1. Immunotherapies under investigation for renal cell carcinoma.

3. Traditional immunotherapy for mRCC

Cytokine therapy, involving IFN-α and IL-2, was the main treatment for mRCC before the approval of targeted therapies. IFN-α has antiangiogenic effects, promoting antigen presentation and dendritic cell maturation. The efficacy of IFN-α for mRCC patients was first reported in 1989, and it was confirmed that IFN-α is active [11]. The response rate of IFN-α was 15%, with 3–7 months increase in overall survival [12]. However, most responses to IFN-α were not long-lasting and rare patients showed complete responses. In addition, side effects such as flu-like symptoms and liver toxicity disenabled the long-term use of IFN-α. IL-2 is a potent stimulator of T-cell proliferation and differentiation. High dose IL-2 (HD IL-2) was approved in 1992 for treatment of mRCC based on an objective response rate (ORR) between 10 and 20%; many of the responses were durable and continued for a long time [13]. Despite HD IL-2 having become the preferred treatment, there is a limitation of severe toxicity that can prove in various organ systems, most significantly the heart, lungs, kidney, and central nervous system. The treatment of cytokine alone has gradually fallen out of favor from the first-line setting in the current era of targeted therapy and immunotherapy.

4. Vaccines

Studies on vaccine therapies in mRCC are still ongoing. They mainly focus on the treatment of primary tumors rather than prevention. Tumor vaccines have been designed to enhance the ability of the immune system to recognize tumor antigens, improve immune microenvironment, and trigger strong specific antitumor cell immunity. Currently, clinical trials evaluating various vaccines have been conducted, although none has demonstrated an improvement in survival thus far. In the future, vaccination approaches will probably be further tailored to the patient's mutanome and tumor-associated antigen profile, with the goal of individualizing treatments and, thus, maximizing the potential benefits [14–16].

4.1. AGS-003

AGS-003 is a dendritic cell immunotherapeutic vaccine constructed from autologous blood dendritic cells and generated through the electroporation of tumor-derived RNA and CD40 ligands (CD40L) RNA into host immune cells [17–19]. The tumor RNA-loaded mature dendritic cells present patient tumor-specific antigens in T-cells via MHC I. Meanwhile, the upregulated CD40L promotes the recruitment of $CD8^+$ T-cell through the regional production of IL-12. A phase II study on 21 mRCC patients were treated by a combination therapy of AGS-003 with 1 cycle of sunitinib (4 weeks on, 2 weeks off), followed by AGS-003 immunotherapy until tumor progression or the end of the study. The median progression-free survival (PFS) and overall survival (OS) were 11.2 months and 30.2 months, respectively. Remarkably, OS was more than 5 years in 5 patients (24%), with 2 patients achieving durable responses for more than 5 years. Of 21 patients, 13 (62%) achieved a clinical benefit (9 with a partial response and 4 with stable disease). Treatment with AGS-003 was well tolerated, with injection site reactions as the primary adverse event (AE). Based on these promising results, a randomized multicenter phase III ADAPT trial is currently under way, to determine whether there is an overall survival benefit between AGS-003 and sunitinib in comparison to sunitinib alone in mRCC patients undergoing de-bulking nephrectomy (NCT01582672).

4.2. IMA901

IMA901 is a therapeutic vaccine consisting of nine different HLA class I-binding tumor-associated peptides and one HLA class II-binding tumor-associated peptide. A phase II trial investigating the addition of cyclophosphamide (which reduces the T regulatory cells) to IMA901 showed that pretreatment with cyclophosphamide prolonged the survival of RCC patients compared with IMA901 therapy alone [20]. The majority of adverse events reported were local injection site reactions. A phase III trial comparing sunitinib with or without this vaccine for mRCC was recently completed. Unfortunately, the OS did not differ significantly between the 2 groups [21].

4.3. Modified vaccinia Ankara (MVA-5 T4; TroVax)

MVA-5 T4 was created to stimulate the immune system to destroy cells expressing 5 T4 antigen. The 5 T4 oncofetal antigen is rarely detected in normal adult tissues but is over-expressed in kidney cancer [22–24]. A randomized, double-blind phase III study (TRIST trial) assessed OS and safety in patients with mRCC [25]. Patients were randomized to MVA-5 T4 (n = 365) or placebo (n = 368) in combination with IL-2, IFN-α, or sunitinib. Unfortunately, MVA-5 T4 in combination with IFN-α, IL-2, or sunitinib as a first-line mRCC therapy did not lead to a significant difference in OS when compared to the arm without MVA-5 T4 (median 20.1 months MVA-5 T4 versus 19.2 months placebo, p = 0.55). The adverse events' profile was also similar between the treatment arms.

4.4. Autologous tumor cell lysate (Reniale)

Principally, autologous tumor cell lysate vaccine active APCs, such as dendritic cells, which stimulate a cytotoxic T lymphocyte response toward tumor-associated antigens, leading to tumor cell destruction [26–28]. Adjuvant treatment with autologous vaccination Reniale (Liponova AG, Hannover, Germany) improved OS in pT3 RCC patients (10-year OS rates: 53.6% in vaccine group versus 36.2% in control group; p = 0.022) in a phase III study [29]. Additional current studies on nonprotein antigens have been limited. There are other ongoing trials involving the DC-based vaccines. Some of the promising ones involve the transduction of a fusion gene construct of GM-CSF and carbonic anhydrase IX into autologous DCs (NCT01826877), DC/RCC fusion cells in combination with pidilizumab (a PD-1 antibody) (NCT01441765), and DCs in combination with cytokine-induced killer cells (NCT00862303).

5. Immune checkpoint inhibitors

Peptides derived from tumor-associated antigens are presented via MHC I and II epitopes to stimulate $CD8^+$ and $CD4^+$ T cells, respectively [30]. The binding of the T-cell receptor (TCR) to the peptide presented by MHC requires further co-stimulatory signals, resulting in the activation of downstream pathways and secretion of cytotoxic molecules, such as granzyme and perforin [31]. Regulatory mechanisms exist to weaken or inhibit immune response, avoiding excessive autoimmune response. These breaks in the immune system are often referred to as "immune checkpoints," including PD-1/PD-L1, CTLA4/CD80, and so on. Immune checkpoint proteins on CTLs cut off co-stimulatory signals after ligand binding and give rise to T-cell anergy and immune suppression. However, immune checkpoint proteins may become dysregulated under tumor settings, typically via an overexpression of inhibitory ligands and receptors [32]. Blocking these immune checkpoint proteins could improve the capability of CTL to mount and maintain an effective T-cell response [32–34].

Over the past decade, immune checkpoint inhibition (ICI) has become a major focus of research given its durable response rates and promising survival benefits in various malignancies. Current ICIs include the cytotoxic T-lymphocyte associated antigen 4 (CTLA-4) antibodies (ipilimumab and tremelimumab), the programmed cell death protein 1 (PD-1) antibodies (nivolumab, pembrolizumab, and pidilizumab), and the programmed cell death protein ligand 1 (PD-L1) antibodies (atezolizumab, BMS-936559, durvalumab, and avelumab) [35] (**Figure 2**). Multiple clinical trials studying the efficacy of these agents on mRCC are being conducted (**Table 1**), among which nivolumab is the only agent approved for the treatment of mRCC by USFDA in 2015 [36].

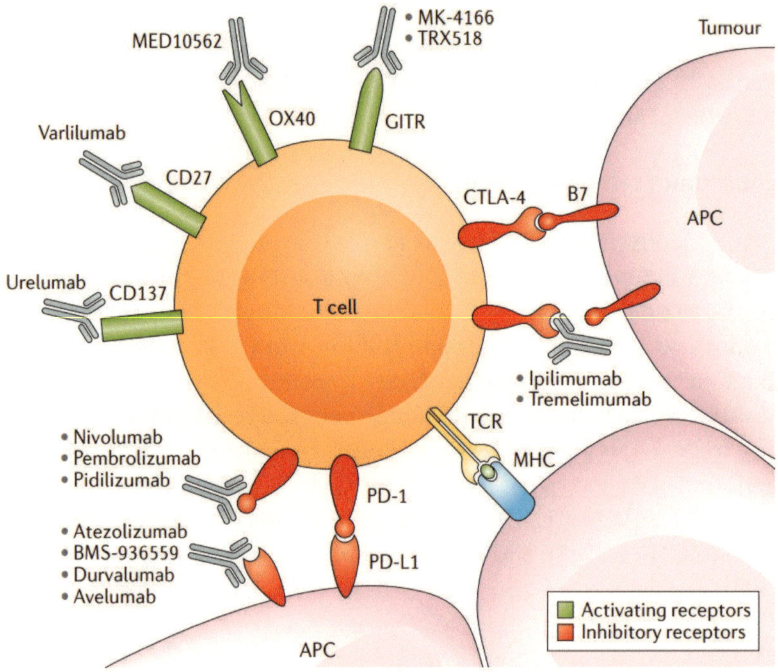

Figure 2. Immune checkpoint inhibitors and agonists being tested in renal cell carcinoma.

Checkpoint inhibitors cause immune-associated adverse events due to hyper-activated T-cell response in healthy tissues. The most common adverse reactions include skin rash, fatigue, and colitis. The incidence and grade of toxicities caused by CTLA-4 antibodies are greater than PD-1/PD-L1-directed monotherapy. Asymptomatic hepatitis and endocrinopathies are also occasionally encountered. Other rare, affected organs include eyes, lungs, kidneys, pancreas, and the hematologic system [37].

T-cell activation is regulated by various co-stimulatory and inhibitory checkpoints. Both agonistic antibodies to activating receptors and blocking antibodies to inhibitory receptors can stimulate T-cell activity and are being tested in advanced renal cell carcinoma and other solid tumors. Activation of T-cells first requires an antigen-presenting cell (APC), such as a dendritic cell, to present an antigen. Here, an APC presents a tumor antigen complexed to major histocompatibility complex (MHC) class I to the T-cell via the T-cell receptor (TCR). Co-stimulatory signals are also needed at this time. At this point, B7 on an APC can bind to cytotoxic T-lymphocyte-associated antigen 4 (CTLA-4) creating an inhibitory signal, but ipilimumab or tremelimumab—CTLA-4 antibodies—can inhibit the inhibitory signal by binding to CTLA-4 and promote T-cell activation. Once the activated T-cell is in the tumor environment it can recognize the antigen presented by an APC cell in the tumor. At this time, the programmed cell death protein 1 (PD-1) receptor can also send an inhibitory signal to the T-cell when the receptor binds to programmed cell death 1 ligand 1 (PD-L1), which is often expressed on tumor cells. Inhibition of PD-L1 or PD-1 could block that signal. Several PD-1 inhibitors are under investigation for RCC, including pembrolizumab and pidilizumab, and

Agent and trial	Phase	Population	Line	Design	*n*	Response	Toxicities	Comments	Refs
Nivolumab (CheckMate 025/ NCT01668784)	III	Advanced and metastatic RCC Prior systemic therapies: antiangiogenic therapy MSKCC risk group: • favorable: 36% • intermedi-ate: 49% • poor: 15%	Second	Open-label, 1:1 randomized trial Arm A: nivolumab 3 mg/kg every 2 weeks Arm B: everolimus 10 mg every 2 weeks	821	OS (months) • nivolumab: 25 • everolimus: 19 ORR • nivolumab: 25% • everolimus: 5% PFS (months) • nivolumab: 4.6 • everolimus: 4.4	Grade 3–4 treatment-related AEs: • nivolumab: 19% • everolimus: 37%	Hazard ratio for death with nivolumab = 0.73 ($P = 0.002$)	[36]
NCT01354431	II	Metastatic RCC Prior systemic therapies: Antiangiogenic therapy	Second	Blinded, 1:1 randomized trial Arm A: nivolumab 0.3 mg/kg every 3 weeks Arm B: nivolumab 2 mg/kg every 3 weeks Arm C: nivolumab 10 mg/kg every 3 weeks	168	OS (months) • Arm A: 18.2 • Arm B: 25.5 • Arm C: 24.7 ORR • Arm A: 20% • Arm B: 22% • Arm C: 20% PFS (months) • Arm A: 2.7 • Arm B: 4.0 • Arm C: 4.2	Grade 3–4 treatment-related AEs: • Arm A: 5% • Arm B: 17% • Arm C: 13%	No dose-response relationship was detected as measured by PFS	[46]

Agent and trial	Phase	Population	Line	Design	*n*	Response	Toxicities	Comments	Refs
NCT01358721	Ib	Metastatic RCC Prior systemic therapies: not specified	First, second	Arm A: previously treated group Nivolumab 0.3 mg/kg every 3 weeks Arm B: previously treated group Nivolumab 2 mg/kg every 3 weeks Arm C: previously treated group Nivolumab 10 mg/kg every 3 weeks Arm D: treatment-naive group Nivolumab 10 mg/kg every 3 weeks	91	OS (months) • Arm A: 16.4 • Arm B: NR • Arm C: 25.2 • Arm D: NR ORR • Arm A: 9% • Arm B: 18% • Arm C: 22% • Arm D: 13%	Grade 3–4 treatment-related AEs: • Arm A: 68% • Arm B: 36% • Arm C: 57% • Arm D: 50%	This is the first prospective translational study involving analysis of both baseline and on-treatment biopsies in RCC	Clin Cancer Res 2016;22:5461–71.
Nivolumab and ipilimumab	I	• Previously treated or treatment-naive • All MSKCC risk groups permitted	First, second	Randomized trial of three dosing cohorts: • Arm A: nivolumab 3 mg/kg plus ipilimumab 1 mg/kg every 3 weeks × 4 • Arm B: nivolumab 1 mg/kg plus ipilimumab 3 mg/kg every 3 weeks × 4 • Arm C: nivolumab 3 mg/kg ipilimumab 3 mg/kg every 3 weeks × 4 All followed by nivolumab 3 mg/kg every 2 weeks until substantial disease progression or toxicity	100	ORR: • ArmA:38% • ArmB:40% PFS at 24 weeks: • ArmA:54% • ArmB:68% Median duration of response: • ArmA: 67 weeks • ArmB: 81 weeks	Treatment in Arm C stopped owing to toxicity Grade 3–4 treatment related AEs: • ArmA:34% • ArmB:64% • ArmC:83%	Median OS not reached with median follow-up duration ranging from 46 to 90 weeks	J. Clin. Oncol. 32:5s (Suppl.), 4504 (2014).

Table 1. Results of immune checkpoint inhibitors in patients with renal cell carcinoma.

nivolumab was recently FDA approved for patients with RCC who have failed prior antiangiogenic therapy. PD-L1 inhibitors under investigation include atezolizumab, BMS-936559, durvalumab, and avelumab. In addition to inhibitory receptors, several activating receptors exist that stimulate T-cell activity, including CD137, CD27, OX40, and GITR. Similarly, several agonist antibodies target these receptors which are under investigation for RCC. These include urelumab targeting CD137, varlilumab targeting CD27, MEDI10562 targeting OX40, and MK-4166 and TRX518 targeting GITR.

5.1. Anti-PD-1 antibodies

PD-1 (CD279) is a cell surface receptor that is expressed on $CD4^+$ and $CD8^+$ T cells as well as NK cells and B cells. The expression of PD-1 is increased by several cytokines, such as IL-2, IL-7, IL-15, and IL-21. PD-1 belongs to the CD28/CTLA-4 superfamily and has an immunoreceptor tyrosine-based inhibitory motif (ITIM) and an immunoreceptor tyrosine-based switch motif (ITSM) which is able to recruit tyrosine phosphatases, anti-SRC homology phosphatase (SHP)-1 and SHP-2, to modulate inhibitory signaling [38, 39]. When interacting with its ligands, PD-1 suppresses signaling pathways that are involved in T-cell activity [32, 40]. Blockade of PD-1 was evaluated and the initial clinical trial demonstrated impressive antitumor response in several refractory cancer types, including RCC [41]. Thompson and his colleagues examined the expression of PD-1 and PD-L1 in a large number of renal tumors and found PD-1 being expressed in 56% of patient tumors with mononuclear cell infiltration. In addition, PD-1 expression was correlated with advanced tumor stage and worse survival in RCC patients [42–44].

5.1.1. Nivolumab

Nivolumab is a fully human immunoglobulin (Ig) G4 anti-PD-1 monoclonal antibody that selectively inhibits the interaction between PD-1 and its ligands PD-L1 and PD-L2. Several clinical trials of nivolumab have been performed for RCC (**Table 1**). In a phase I study that enrolled 33 patients with mRCC, nivolumab demonstrated an objective response rate of 27% and a manageable safety profile; responses were durable [45]. A phase II study enrolled 168 patients with mRCC who had received previous treatment targeting the vascular endothelial growth factor (VEGF) pathway. Nivolumab was dosed at 0.3, 2, or 10 mg/kg every 3 weeks and showed antitumor activity with no dose-response relationship observed. There was no association between nivolumab dosage and the number of adverse events (AEs), which suggested that the incidence of immune-related AEs was limited [46]. Moreover, a randomized phase III study (Check Mate 025) evaluating nivolumab (3 mg/kg every 2 weeks) versus second-line everolimus (10 mg orally every day, pretreated with antiangiogenic therapy) represented a 5.4-month improvement in median OS (25 months and 19.6 months, respectively). Although the ORR was significantly higher in the nivolumab group than in the everolimus group (25% versus 5%, odds ratio: 5.98 [95% CI, 3.68–9.72], $p < 0.001$), PFS was similar (4.6 versus 4.4 months, HR 0.88 [95% CI, 0.75–1.03], $p = 0.11$). This is the first time that an immune checkpoint inhibitor has demonstrated an OS benefit when compared with patients treated with TKIs for mRCC. The exact mechanism behind the discrepancy between PFS and OS is still unknown, and the authors hypothesized that there might be a potential delayed benefit in PFS with nivolumab. Nivolumab was very well tolerated, and a lower proportion of patients developed grade 3 or 4 treatment-related AEs (19 and 37%, respectively), including fatigue, nausea, and diarrhea, which suggested that the safety profile of nivolumab was favorable [36]. Nivolumab was approved by the FDA for pretreated advanced clear-cell RCC in November 2015 [36, 41, 46, 47] and is still under investigation as pre- and postoperative therapy in mRCC (ADAPTeR) (NCT02446860) and is also being studied in combination with other drugs (NCT01472081, NCT02231749, NCT02210117, NCT02335918, and NCT02614456).

5.1.2. Pembrolizumab

Pembrolizumab (formerly known as MK3475 or lambrolizumab), a highly selective humanized IgG4 monoclonal antibody against PD-1, has been approved for metastatic melanoma, head and neck cancer, and non-small cell lung cancer (NSCLC) mainly as combinational therapy. Pembrolizumab is currently being investigated in two randomized phase II trials of mRCC patients [48]. A phase I/II study (KEYNOTE-029) involving pembrolizumab plus ipilimumab or pegylated interferon alfa-2b (PEGIFN) in patients with advanced melanoma and RCC reported an acceptable safety profile [49]. Nowadays, several trials evaluating pembrolizumab in combination with various agents with different mechanisms are ongoing (NCT02014636, NCT02133742, NCT02348008, NCT02089685, NCT02501096, NCT02619253, NCT02298959, NCT02646748, NCT02178722, and NCT02475213). The most common adverse events were fatigue, pruritus, and dyspnea. Antitumor activity was observed [50].

5.1.3. Pidilizumab

Pidilizumab (CT-011), another humanized IgG1 kappa monoclonal antibody targeting PD-1, is already under evaluation in several hematologic malignancies, including acute myeloid leukemia (AML), multiple myeloma, Hodgkin lymphoma, non-Hodgkin lymphoma, and chronic lymphocytic leukemia [51]. There are several efforts under way to assess the agent in several solid tumors. As for mRCC, a study is currently under way to assess the combination of pidilizumab with a novel dendritic cell (DC) fusion cell vaccine (NCT01441765). The first group will receive pidilizumab at a dose of 3 mg/kg every 2 weeks intravenously, for a total of 4 cycles. The second group will receive infusions of an autologous DC vaccine during 2–4 cycles of pidilizumab therapy. The noted trial of pidilizumab with an autologous DC vaccine is of substantial interest, especially with emerging vaccine-based therapies, such as AGS-003 and IMA901 [52–54].

5.2. Anti-PD-L1 antibodies

The encouraging results of PD-1 antibodies in cancer management inspired interest in the inhibition of the PD-1 ligands, namely PD-L1. PD-L1 is expressed on a variety of cells, including cancer cells, APCs, T-cells, B cells, and myeloid cells. PD-L1 inhibits T-cell proliferation and adhesion, as well as cytokine production [17, 55, 56]. PD-L1 expression was detected by immune staining in the RCC tissue, and PD-L1 expression by tumor cells (>10%), on infiltrating lymphocytes (>50%), or the composite of both makers was strongly associated with poor prognosis [42, 57].

5.2.1. Atezolizumab

Atezolizumab (MPDL3280A), a fully humanized monoclonal IgG1 antibody against PD-L1, is being evaluated in different cancers, including RCC. It has showed promising results in a multicenter phase I trial involving 17 mRCC patients. The ORR was 12% with responses that lasted for 4–17 months. Seven patients (41%) had stable disease for more than 24 weeks [55]. In another phase Ia study, of the 63 patients with clear-cell RCC that were evaluable, median PFS was 5.6 months and median OS was 28.9 months. The ORR was 15% (18% in patients with >1 and 9% in those with <1% PD-L1 expression) [58].

5.2.2. BMS-936559

BMS-936559 (MDX-1105) is a fully human monoclonal antibody with high affinity to PD-L1 and blocks the binding of PD-L1 to both PD-1 and B7.1. In a phase I trial of evaluating BMS-936559 in 207 patients with different advanced cancer types, 17 patients had mRCC. The study showed that 2 of 17 RCC patients had an objective response with response durations for 4 and 17 months, respectively [59].

5.2.3. Avelumab

Avelumab (MSB0010718C) is a fully human IgG1 monoclonal antibody against PD-L1 and inhibits PD-1-PD-L1 interactions. It also has a native Fc region that could induce antibody-dependent cell-mediated cytotoxicity (ADCC). In a phase Ib, open-label expansion study, avelumab was used in patients with advanced solid tumors and showed an acceptable safety profile [60]. Two ongoing trials evaluate avelumab in combination with axitinib (NCT02493751, NCT02684006).

5.2.4. Durvalumab

Durvalumab (MEDI4736) is another human anti-PD-L1 IgG1 monoclonal antibody. It blocks PD-L1 binding to PD-1 and CD80, with no binding to PD-L2. ADCC and complement-dependent cytotoxicities are removed by an engineered triple mutation in the Fc domain. A Phase 1/2, multicenter, open-label study which evaluated the safety and clinical activity of the drug in patients with multiple solid tumor types such as non-small cell lung cancer noted a very manageable safety profile [61]. There are ongoing trials evaluating durvalumab in combination with other drugs, including tremelimumab (NCT01975831) and MEDI0680 (AMP-514) (a humanized IgG4 monoclonal antibody against PD-1) (NCT02118337) for patients with advanced malignancies including RCC.

5.3. Anti-CTLA-4 antibodies

In addition to the PD-1/PD-L1 checkpoint, CTLA-4, an immune checkpoint on the surface of cytotoxic T-cells, counteracts the action of the co-stimulatory receptor CD28 and plays a key role in the immune response. Both CTLA-4 and CD28 bind identical ligands CD80 and CD86 (called B7-1 and B7-2), but CTLA4 has a higher affinity for both ligands than CD28. Therefore, CTLA4 can antagonize CD28-ligand interactions by competing for ligand binding. In addition, the interaction of CTLA4 with CD80 or CD86 can lead to the endocytosis of these ligands from the APC surface into a CTLA4-expressing T-cell (a process called trans-endocytosis). The ligand removal impairs the stimulatory capacity of APCs by limiting CD28 signaling and thus inhibits T-cell responses [32, 62]. CTLA-4 antibodies were initially tested on colon adenocarcinoma and sarcoma in mouse models with noted tumor shrinkage [63]. These encouraging results led to the subsequent development of CTLA-4 antibodies, including ipilimumab and tremelimumab.

5.3.1. *Ipilimumab*

Ipilimumab, an anti-CTLA-4 IgG1 monoclonal antibody, received US FDA approval for the treatment of melanoma in 2011 [64, 65]. It has been investigated as monotherapy plus nivolumab in metastatic melanoma, with the combination treatment being more effective albeit accompanied with significantly more toxicity [66]. Currently, ipilimumab is being investigated in mRCC with the combination of nivolumab. In a phase II study of ipilimumab in patients with mRCC, 1 of 21 patients had a partial response in the lower dose group (3 mg/kg followed by 1 mg/kg every 3 weeks). A total of 5 of 40 patients had partial responses at the higher dose (3 mg/kg every 3 weeks). AEs were highly significant and associated with tumor regression [67]. Ipilimumab has also been investigated in another phase II trial in mRCC; however, just 12% of patients achieved a partial response, with a substantial amount of toxicities [67]. Further phase III trials investigating ipilimumab alone (NCT00057889) and in combination with other drugs have not yet been studied (NCT02231749, NCT02381314).

5.3.2. *Tremelimumab*

Tremelimumab is another anti-CTLA-4 antibody that is actively being investigated in mRCC. Unlike ipilimumab, it is an IgG2 antibody. It is currently being evaluated with durvalumab in the treatment of patients with mRCC (NCT01975831).

5.4. Anti-LAG-3 antibodies

Lymphocyte activation gene 3 (LAG-3) is expressed on activated T cells and T_{reg}-cells [68]. Upon binding to the MHC class II on APCs, LAG-3 induces an inhibitory signal in T-cells [69], whereas LAG-3 enhances the suppressive function of T_{reg}-cells [70, 71]. Co-expression of LAG-3 and PD-1 is a marker of exhausted T cells and, therefore, the blockade of both receptors confers additive therapeutic activity in preclinical models of chronic infection and cancer [72–74]. In a phase I study, a soluble LAG-3-Ig fusion protein (IMP321), which was designed to stimulate MHC class II-driven DC activation, has been evaluated in patients with advanced RCC. IMP321 induced CD8 T-cell activation in patients and disease stabilization with the absence of toxicity [75]. Currently, a blocking mAb targeting LAG-3 is being tested in the clinic (NCT01968109).

6. Combined therapy

Preclinical studies point out that the dual blockade of PD-1 and CTLA-4 reduced regulatory T_{reg} cell infiltration and increased effector T-cell infiltration and interferon-γ production, achieving a heightened antitumor effect [76]. This approach has demonstrated clinically effective synergy from nivolumab plus ipilimumab treatment in patients with advanced melanoma [77]. Several studies are ongoing in patients with mRCC on the combinations of ICIs with different targets, for example, anti-PD-1 or PD-L1 and anti-CTLA-4 antibodies [78, 79], allowing dual/multifaceted manipulation of immunosuppression. A combination of nivolumab and ipilimumab has acquired success in patients with treatment naïve or previously treated RCC (CheckMate 016 study) with an ORR of about 40% [80] these provided the rationale for a phase III trial comparing this combination with sunitinib in treatment-naïve patients (CheckMate 214, NCT02231749).

Emerging evidence suggests that antiangiogenic therapies may have immune-modulatory effects such as the enhancement of cytotoxic T-cell trafficking and infiltration in addition to their known direct antiangiogenic effects, possibly potentiating the effectiveness of checkpoint inhibitors when administered concurrently [81]. Based on this rationale, several clinical studies are ongoing in patients with mRCC under the combinations of ICIs and VEGF pathway inhibitors (**Table 2**) [78, 79]. While a few of these combinations have produced unacceptable hepatic toxicity [82, 83], the use of the combinations of PD-1 pathway inhibitors with more selective inhibitors of the VEGF pathway (e.g., atezolizumab with bevacizumab, pembrolizumab with axitinib, or avelumab with axitinib) has proven to be more tolerable [55, 84–87]. Preliminary results from studies combining immune checkpoints and VEGF pathway inhibitors have shown encouraging clinical activity in terms of PFS and ORR [83–86]. In an ongoing phase Ib study of 52 treatment-naïve patients, pembrolizumab plus axitinib resulted in an ORR of 67%, including 2 complete responses and 33 PR; median PFS is not yet mature, with 7 patients of 11 enrolled in the dose-finding phase remaining progression-free at 11 months [84]. Smaller phase I studies evaluating avelumab plus axitinib and pembrolizumab plus pazopanib combination therapy reported ORRs of 83% (5 PRs of 6 treated patients) and 60% (6 of 10 patients; pazopanib 800 mg cohort), respectively [47, 85]. Atezolizumab plus bevacizumab combination therapy in 10 previously untreated patients with mRCC also resulted in clinical benefits (4 patients with PRs and 4 with stable disease) [86]. Confirmatory randomized phase III trials comparing sunitinib versus either atezolizumab with bevacizumab (NCT02420821), avelumab with axitinib (NCT02684006), or pembrolizumab with axitinib (NCT02853331) are ongoing. Preclinical data from an RCC mouse model showed that radiation enhanced the therapeutic effect of IL-2 immunotherapy on pulmonary metastases [88]. One explanation is that DCs are recruited to the irradiated site when radiotherapy is applied in few-fraction and high-dose manners [89]. Currently, a clinical trial evaluating the combination of radiation therapy with pembrolizumab for patients with recurrent or mRCC is ongoing (NCT02318771).

Therefore, a number of combination strategies, such as PD-1/PD-L1 blockade, PD-1 antibody with other immunotherapeutic agents, PD-1 antibody with antiangiogenesis agents, and combination with radiotherapy, are currently in clinical trial research to determine whether there is a most favorable sequence of treatment and if combination strategy benefits mRCC patients. Results from recent clinical trials with immunotherapeutic agents suggest that immunotherapy in combination with other agents is capable of producing durable responses and significant overall survival improvement. Thus, in the future, immunotherapy, together with other treatments, will likely cause a paradigm shift in the clinical management of mRCC patients. However, the combination of immunotherapeutic agents does have considerable

Checkpoint inhibitor	Targeted therapy	Phase	Population	Identifier
Nivolumab	Sunitinib Pazopanib	I	Advanced RCC, prior cytokine therapy allowed	NCT01472081 (CheckMate 016)
Atezolizumab	Bevacizumab	Ib	Untreated, advanced clear cell RCC	NCT01633970
Nivolumab	Bevacizumab	Neoadjuvant pilot	Metastatic clear cell RCC, prior therapy allowed	NCT02210117
Nivolumab	Temsirolimus	Ib/II	Metastatic RCC, prior therapy allowed	NCT02423954
Pembrolizumab	Pazopanib	I/II	Untreated, advanced clear cell RCC	NCT02014636
Pembrolizumab	Axitinib	Ib	Untreated, advanced clear cell RCC	NCT02133742
Pembrolizumab	Bevacizumab	Ib/II	Metastatic clear cell RCC treated with failure of at least one prior therapy	NCT02348008
Pembrolizumab	Aflibercept	I	Metastatic RCC treated with at least one prior VEGF TKI	NCT02298959
Avelumab	Axitinib	Ib	Untreated, advanced clear cell RCC	NCT02493751
Atezolizumab	Bevacizumab	III	Untreated, advanced clear cell RCC	NCT02420821
Avelumab	Axitinib	III	Untreated, advanced clear cell RCC	NCT02684006
Pembrolizumab	Axitinib	III	Untreated, advanced clear cell RCC	NCT02853331 (MK-3475-426/ KEYNOTE-426)

RCC, renal cell carcinoma; TKI, tyrosine kinase inhibitor; VEGF, vascular endothelial growth factor.

Table 2. Ongoing immune checkpoint inhibitor and targeted therapy combinational trials in RCC.

toxicities such as gastrointestinal and hepatic toxicities, and careful patient selection must be guaranteed [90, 91]. Therefore, much more studies must be taken to define the role of combination treatment with immunotherapy agents in mRCC. Moreover, further studies are warranted to identify biomarkers that reliably predict the treatment benefit from these new therapies.

7. Adjuvant and neoadjuvant immunotherapy

With the promising outcome of immunotherapy in mRCC, it is reasonable to explore whether immunotherapy works in the non-metastatic adjuvant setting. Noteworthy, spontaneous antitumor immune infiltration was shown to be higher in primary tumors with respect to matched metastases [92], suggesting that the administration of immunotherapy in the early setting might be more effective than in the advanced setting. However, trials of adjuvant therapy involving tumor cell vaccination, IFN-α, or HD IL-2 have not shown survival benefits [93]. Trials studying the role of checkpoint inhibition (anti PD-1/PD-L1 agents) are proceeding, and the results are eagerly awaited. Studies are also under way to determine the feasibility of ICIs as neoadjuvant (nivolumab, NCT02575222, NCT02595918; durvalumab with or without tremelimumab, NCT02762006) or adjuvant therapy (nivolumab; NCT02595944, NCT02388906, NCT02743494, NCT02632409; pembrolizumab, NCT02362594, NCT02504372; atezolizumab, NCT02450331, NCT02927301, NCT02912559, NCT02486718). We believe that a big movement in RCC management will occur if we can find a way to increase survival rates in the adjuvant or neoadjuvant setting of surgically managed patients.

8. Non-clear cell RCC (nccRCC)

Non-clear cell histology constitutes 20–25% of RCCs [94, 95]. However, this group is heterogeneous, and individually each subtype is relatively rare and thus difficult to study in large prospective trials. nccRCC includes papillary, chromophobe, sarcomatoid, collecting duct, medullary, and various hereditary forms, among which papillary is the most common subtype [94]. Patients with metastatic nccRCC have generally proven to be less responsiveness to the drugs shown to be active in ccRCC [96]. Although some patients with nccRCC may obtain some benefit from VEGF-targeting TKIs, retrospective studies have generally suggested that these agents have inferior efficacy compared with what would be expected in patients with ccRCC [97]. This was also true in the previous era of immunotherapy HD IL-2. Although included in some of the large trials of HD IL-2, patients with nccRCC rarely experienced clinical benefits [95, 98, 99]. Treatment with IFN-α has also showed limited efficacy in patients with non-clear cell histology [95]. No prospective data currently exist to characterize the response of patients with nccRCC to ICIs, though several case reports have been published identifying single responses across various histologies [100–102]. Several ongoing studies are evaluating ICIs as a single agent or in combination in patients with nccRCC.

9. Therapy response and predictive biomarkers

The use of immunotherapies for RCC provides evidence that immune-based treatments can drastically improve survival or antitumor effects for patients with advanced RCC. However, only certain patients obtain clinic benefit as a durable response, so we need to identify reliable predictive biomarkers of treatment response to optimize patient selection.

The evaluation of responses to immunotherapeutic agents represents a challenge in the clinic. Specific tumor response patterns with ICI treatment sometimes differ from those with chemotherapeutic and targeted agents. Due to immune-mediated mechanisms, tumor flare, which shows enlarged size of baseline lesions or increased total tumor burden, may occur before cellular immune responses have a chance to affect the actual tumor size [103]. Additionally, transient immune cell infiltration at the tumor site may boost the appearance of tumor growth [103, 104]. Therefore, tumor flare can confuse tumor response interpretation by appearing as disease progression, hence the term pseudoprogression, and may result in inappropriately switching therapy before ongoing clinical benefits manifest on imaging [105]. While pseudoprogression is relatively uncommon (occurring in <10% of patients) versus true progression, it sometimes presents a challenge for patients and for clinicians in determining when to stop and/or switch therapy [105]. Recently updated guidelines for the use of modified RECIST (iRECIST) in trials of immunotherapies were published in an effort to standardize and validate these criteria and harmonize the interpretation of the results [106].

Response to ICI has been associated with specific intrinsic and extrinsic properties of tumors or of the host that have been recently classified as the elements of the cancer-immune set point [107]. Intrinsic properties reflect the degree of tumor foreignness [108], linked to the mutational burden and the presence of neoantigens that can be recognized by the immune system, as shown in NSCLC and melanoma [109, 110]. Foreignness of RCC might vary by molecular subtype and a higher number of mutations [111]. In addition, the general individual immune status, mirrored by the levels of circulating lymphocytes and the neutrophil to lymphocyte ratio (NLR), the increase of the C reactive protein, the erythrocyte sedimentation rate PD-L1 expression (although controversial), and LDH were shown to influence the response to ICI.

In addition to the intrinsic properties of the tumors, extrinsic factors, such as exposure to sunlight and to cigarette smoke, the presence of viral infections, and the composition of the gut microbiota, were classified as elements of the cancer-immune set point [107]. The exposure to sunlight and cigarette smoke was relevant for melanoma and NSCLC, respectively, while the presence of viral infections might impact the response to ICI in human papilloma virus positive tumors and Epstein-Barr virus related tumors. Preclinical evidence showed that several bacteroides and bifidobacterium species influenced the efficacy of ICI with anti-CTLA-4 and anti-PD-L1 mAb in mice [112–114]. The role of the gut microbiota in patients with renal cancer treated with ICB requires further investigations.

Taken together, these data suggest that multiple parameters should be taken into account to identify ideal candidates for immunotherapy in RCC. The genomic landscape likely has a role in determining the putative immunogenicity of the tumor [115]; TIL, PD-L1 expression, and immune gene signatures could detect tumors with an inflamed phenotype, which have higher chances of response to ICB [107, 116].

10. Perspective

The advent of immunotherapy has brought about a paradigm shift in the treatment of advanced RCC. Properly integrating immunotherapy into the present treatment is challenging.

Preclinical research has demonstrated the role of VEGF in suppressing tumor immune responses—an attractive strategy to combine with ICIs [117–119]. This successful synergy has been confirmed in phase 1 and 2 studies with axitinib-pembrolizumab [84], axitinib-avelumab [120], lenvatinib-pembrolizumab [121], and bevacizumab-atezolizumab [122, 123]. The ORR ranged between 32% and 67%, and AEs were manageable in all these studies, in contrast to studies in other combinations as TKIs (pazopanib/sunitinib) plus immunotherapy, which did not move forward because of unacceptable toxicity [83, 124, 125]. Although preliminary, the abovementioned results are encouraging and have led to larger, confirmatory, phase 3 trials, which are now actively accruing patients.

In addition, different novel immunotherapies beyond ICIs are being investigated, including adoptive T-cell therapy and T-cell agonists.

Adoptive T-cell transfer therapy refers to the autologous or allogeneic infusion of T-cells. One such therapy involves the generation and infusion of chimeric antigen receptor (CAR) T-cells—T cells that have been genetically modified to express a receptor specific to tumor epitopes independent of HLA. The promising efficacy of anti-CD19 CAR T cells in hematological malignancies has inspired further investigations in solid tumors [126]. One of the key aspects of designing effective CAR T cells is finding a tumor-associated antigen that is uniformly expressed in tumor cells but not in the normal tissue. Carbonic anhydrase 9 (CAIX) is an enzyme that is overexpressed in clear-cell RCC but minimally expressed in normal tissue [127]. Early efforts in using CAIX as a tumor-associated antigen for CAR resulted in liver enzyme elevations that limited its use, likely owing to the therapy also targeting CAIX expressed in the liver bile duct epithelium [128]. Cor H.J. Lamers and his colleagues gave patients a CAIX monoclonal antibody before infusion of CAR T cells to reduce this off-target toxicity [129]. However, in the study, no clinical responses were observed, and the efficacy of CAIX CAR T cells is yet to be proven.

Another form of adoptive immune cell therapy tested in RCC is autologous cytokine-induced killer (CIK) cell immunotherapy. CIK cells are created in vitro by harvesting peripheral mononuclear cells in the blood using an anti-CD3 antibody. The resulting phenotype by IL-1, IFNγ, and IL-2 shares features of effector T-cells and natural killer cells [130]. A phase II trial randomly assigned 148 patients with mRCC to CIK cell immunotherapy or IL-2 combined with IFNα [131]. PFS and OS at 3 years in the CIK cell therapy arm were 18% and 61%, respectively, compared with 12% and 23% in the IL-2 plus IFNα arm ($p = 0.031$ and $p < 0.001$, respectively). This therapy is being further investigated in conjunction with DC vaccines and early results show that therapy is well tolerated and might have activity against RCC [132].

Stimulatory molecules expressed on immune cells can also be targeted with agonist antibodies. CD137 is a co-stimulatory molecule for T-cells that increases T-cell effector activity and survival. Its use in combination with anti-DR5 and anti-CD40 antibodies in mouse models of RCC has shown to improve survival compared with control mice ($p < 0.001$) [133]. The CD137 agonist PF-05082566 is currently being tested in combination with pembrolizumab in a phase I trial of advanced solid tumors, including RCC (NCT02179918). Varlilumab is an agonist antibody targeting CD27, another co-stimulatory molecule for T-cell activation. In a phase I trial in solid tumors, including 11 patients with RCC, of the six evaluable RCC patients, two had stable diseases [134]. This antibody is currently being studied in combination with sunitinib and in combination with atezolizumab in phase I/II trials in RCC (NCT02386111).

In addition to CD137 and CD27, other co-stimulatory molecules such as OX40 and GITR are also promising therapeutic targets. Trials of monotherapy with the OX40 agonist MEDI0562, and with the GITR agonists MK-4166 and TRX518, are under way in solid tumor malignancies (NCT02318394, NCT02132754, and NCT02628574). Like combination checkpoint blockade strategies, much enthusiasm exists for combined treatment strategies with other immunomodulatory agents [135, 136].

Owing to the unique antitumor mechanisms elicited by immunotherapy, patients treated with these agents can have tumor response patterns that are different from conventional tumor-response criteria, such as the WHO criteria [137, 138]. A subset of patients receiving ICI therapy develop pseudoprogression, in which tumor burden decreases after an initial increase or during or after the appearance of new lesions. The evaluation of pseudoprogression provides new challenges in treatment monitoring and therapeutic decision-making because it cannot be evaluated with the existing response-evaluation criteria. The establishment of a standardized strategy to evaluate immune-related responses in patients receiving ICIs is extremely important. However, advances in the knowledge of immune-related responses have been challenged by the fact that only a few clinical trials have used the immune-related response criteria (irRC) [103] or immune-related response evaluation criteria in solid tumors (irRECIST) [139] as the primary criteria to define their end points [77, 104, 140].

In addition, the development of robust biomarkers to assist prediction of response and clinical benefits of immunotherapy is essential to further advance the field as precision immuno-oncology. Despite the remarkable success of clinical applications of immunotherapy reported in the past decade, the effectiveness of these therapies varies greatly across individual patients and among different tumor types. A substantial unmet need is the development of biomarkers of response to immunotherapeutic agents, in order to identify, before the initiation of treatment, which patients are likely to experience clinical benefit from such treatments. This aspect is particularly important in the management of tumors with low response rates, such as NSCLC (response rate ≤ 20%), RCC, and urothelial carcinoma (UCC) [141]. The growing knowledge of molecular subtypes of RCC with next-generation sequencing is the first step toward developing RCC-specific genomic signatures and guiding therapy selection, thereby moving toward precision medicine [142].

Taken together, the therapeutic activity of immunotherapy is the result of a complex interplay between multiple factors in the tumor, tumor microenvironment, and immune system, requiring a collaborative approach to translate the emerging knowledge into the clinical context.

11. Conclusions

Novel immune therapies are emerging as an important addition to targeted therapies in the treatment of RCC. Many questions regarding their use remain to be optimized including dose, schedule, AEs, and adjuvant or neoadjuvant application. An investigation of the rational combination of different treatment modalities is also critical in maximizing the potential of immunotherapy. Additional investigations into predictive biomarkers or resistance mechanisms are needed to optimize patient selection. To date, nivolumab has been approved in the second-line setting, and randomized phase III trials with novel immunotherapy combinations are challenging the first-line standard of care in RCC—in the near future, immunotherapy will likely be a new standard therapy.

Author details

Le Qu[1*†], Ding Wu[1†], Haowei He[1†], Xiaofeng Xu[1†] and Cheng Chen[2]

*Address all correspondence to: septsoul@hotmail.com

1 Department of Urology, Jinling Hospital, Clinical School of Medical College, Nanjing University, Nanjing, China

2 Department of Medical Oncology, Jinling Hospital, Clinical School of Medical College, Nanjing University, Nanjing, China

† These authors contributed equally to this paper.

References

[1] Siegel RL, Miller KD, Jemal A. Cancer statistics, 2017. CA: A Cancer Journal for Clinicians. 2017;**67**(1):7-30

[2] Ljungberg B, Campbell SC, Choi HY, et al. Corrigendum to "the epidemiology of renal cell carcinoma" [Eur Urol 2011;60:615-21]. European Urology. 2011;**60**(6):1317

[3] Athar U, Gentile TC. Treatment options for metastatic renal cell carcinoma: A review. The Canadian Journal of Urology. 2008;**15**(2):3954-3966

[4] Iacovelli R, Sternberg CN, Porta C, et al. Inhibition of the VEGF/VEGFR pathway improves survival in advanced kidney cancer: A systematic review and meta-analysis. Current Drug Targets. 2015;**16**(2):164-170

[5] Heng DY, Xie W, Regan MM, et al. Prognostic factors for overall survival in patients with metastatic renal cell carcinoma treated with vascular endothelial growth factor-targeted agents: Results from a large, multicenter study. Journal of Clinical Oncology. 2009;**27**(34):5794-5799

[6] Hanahan D, Weinberg RA. Hallmarks of cancer: The next generation. Cell. 2011;**144**(5): 646-674

[7] Chen L. Co-inhibitory molecules of the B7–CD28 family in the control of T-cell immunity. Nature Reviews Immunology. 2004;**4**(5):336-347

[8] Gabrilovich DI, Nagaraj S. Myeloid-derived suppressor cells as regulators of the immune system. Nature Reviews Immunology. 2009;**9**(3):162-174

[9] Campoli M, Ferrone S, Zea AH, et al. Mechanisms of tumor evasion. Cancer Treatment and Research. 2005;**123**:61-88

[10] Mellman I, Coukos G, Dranoff G. Cancer immunotherapy comes of age. Nature. 2011; **480**(7378):480-489

[11] Oliver RT, Nethersell AB, Bottomley JM. Unexplained spontaneous regression and alpha-interferon as treatment for metastatic renal carcinoma. British Journal of Urology. 1989; **63**(2):128-131

[12] Fossa SD. Interferon in metastatic renal cell carcinoma. Seminars in Oncology. 2000;**27**(2): 187-193

[13] Floros T, Tarhini AA. Anticancer cytokines: Biology and clinical effects of interferon-alpha2, interleukin (IL)-2, IL-15, IL-21, and IL-12. Seminars in Oncology. 2015;**42**(4):539-548

[14] Ophir E, Bobisse S, Coukos G, et al. Personalized approaches to active immunotherapy in cancer. Biochimica et Biophysica Acta. 2016;**1865**(1):72-82

[15] Keenan BP, Jaffee EM. Whole cell vaccines—Past progress and future strategies. Seminars in Oncology. 2012;**39**(3):276-286

[16] Fritsch EF, Hacohen N, Wu CJ. Personal neoantigen cancer vaccines: The momentum builds. Oncoimmunology. 2014;**3**:e29311

[17] Combe P, De Guillebon E, Thibault C, et al. Trial watch: Therapeutic vaccines in metastatic renal cell carcinoma. Oncoimmunology. 2015;**4**(5):e1001236

[18] Figlin RA. Personalized immunotherapy (AGS-003) when combined with sunitinib for the treatment of metastatic renal cell carcinoma. Expert Opinion on Biological Therapy. 2015;**15**(8):1241-1248

[19] Amin A, Dudek AZ, Logan TF, et al. Survival with AGS-003, an autologous dendritic-cell-based immunotherapy, in combination with sunitinib in unfavorable risk patients with advanced renal cell carcinoma (RCC): Phase 2 study results. Journal for Immuno Therapy of Cancer. 2015;**3**:14

[20] Walter S, Weinschenk T, Stenzl A, et al. Multipeptide immune response to cancer vaccine IMA901 after single-dose cyclophosphamide associates with longer patient survival. Nature Medicine. 2012;**18**(8):1254-1261

[21] Rini BI, Stenzl A, Zdrojowy R, et al. IMA901, a multipeptide cancer vaccine, plus sunitinib versus sunitinib alone, as first-line therapy for advanced or metastatic renal cell carcinoma (IMPRINT): A multicentre, open-label, randomised, controlled, phase 3 trial. The Lancet Oncology. 2016;**17**(11):1599-1611

[22] Kaufman H, Taback B, Sherman W, et al. Phase II trial of Modified Vaccinia Ankara (MVA) virus expressing 5T4 and high dose Interleukin-2 (IL-2) in patients with metastatic renal cell carcinoma. Journal of Translational Medicine. 2009;**7**:2

[23] Amato RJ. 5T4-modified vaccinia Ankara: Progress in tumor-associated antigen-based immunotherapy. Expert Opinion on Biological Therapy. 2010;**10**(2):281-287

[24] Amato RJ, Shingler W, Goonewardena M, et al. Vaccination of renal cell cancer patients with modified vaccinia Ankara delivering the tumor antigen 5T4 (TroVax) alone or administered in combination with interferon-alpha (IFN-alpha): A phase 2 trial. Journal of Immunotherapy. 2009;**32**(7):765-772

[25] Amato RJ, Hawkins RE, Kaufman HL, et al. Vaccination of metastatic renal cancer patients with MVA-5T4: A randomized, double-blind, placebo-controlled phase III study. Clinical Cancer Research. 2010;**16**(22):5539-5547

[26] Wittke S, Baxmann S, Fahlenkamp D, et al. Tumor heterogeneity as a rationale for a multi-epitope approach in an autologous renal cell cancer tumor vaccine. OncoTargets and Therapy. 2016;**9**:523-537

[27] Matsushita H, Enomoto Y, Kume H, et al. A pilot study of autologous tumor lysate-loaded dendritic cell vaccination combined with sunitinib for metastatic renal cell carcinoma. Journal for ImmunoTherapy of Cancer. 2014;**2**:30

[28] Wang H, Feng F, Zhu M, et al. Therapeutic efficacy of dendritic cells pulsed by autologous tumor cell lysate in combination with CIK cells on advanced renal cell carcinoma. Xi Bao Yu Fen Zi Mian Yi Xue Za Zhi. 2015;**31**(1):67-71

[29] May M, Kendel F, Hoschke B, et al. Adjuvant autologous tumour cell vaccination in patients with renal cell carcinoma. Overall survival analysis with a follow-up period in excess of more than 10 years. Urologe A. 2009;**48**(9):1075-1083

[30] Kirkwood JM, Butterfield LH, Tarhini AA, et al. Immunotherapy of cancer in 2012. CA: A Cancer Journal for Clinicians. 2012;**62**(5):309-335

[31] Schwartz RH. A cell culture model for T lymphocyte clonal anergy. Science. 1990; **248**(4961):1349-1356

[32] Pardoll DM. The blockade of immune checkpoints in cancer immunotherapy. Nature Reviews. Cancer. 2012;**12**(4):252-264

[33] Webster RM. The immune checkpoint inhibitors: Where are we now? Nature Reviews. Drug Discovery. 2014;**13**(12):883-884

[34] Byun DJ, Wolchok JD, Rosenberg LM, et al. Cancer immunotherapy—Immune checkpoint blockade and associated endocrinopathies. Nature Reviews. Endocrinology. 2017;**13**(4):195-207

[35] Ghatalia P, Zibelman M, Geynisman DM, et al. Checkpoint inhibitors for the treatment of renal cell carcinoma. Current Treatment Options in Oncology. 2017;**18**(1):7

[36] Motzer RJ, Escudier B, Mcdermott DF, et al. Nivolumab versus Everolimus in advanced renal-cell carcinoma. The New England Journal of Medicine. 2015;**373**(19):1803-1813

[37] Postow MA. Managing immune checkpoint-blocking antibody side effects. American Society of Clinical Oncology Educational Book. 2015;**35**(76):76-83

[38] Nirschl CJ, Drake CG. Molecular pathways: Coexpression of immune checkpoint molecules: Signaling pathways and implications for cancer immunotherapy. Clinical Cancer Research. 2013;**19**(18):4917-4924

[39] Macfarlane AWT, Jillab M, Plimack ER, et al. PD-1 expression on peripheral blood cells increases with stage in renal cell carcinoma patients and is rapidly reduced after surgical tumor resection. Cancer Immunology Research. 2014;**2**(4):320-331

[40] Amarnath S, Mangus CW, Wang JC, et al. The PDL1-PD1 axis converts human TH1 cells into regulatory T cells. Science Translational Medicine. 2011;**3**(111):111ra120

[41] Brahmer JR, Drake CG, Wollner I, et al. Phase I study of single-agent anti-programmed death-1 (MDX-1106) in refractory solid tumors: Safety, clinical activity, pharmacodynamics, and immunologic correlates. Journal of Clinical Oncology. 2010;**28**(19):3167-3175

[42] Tykodi SS. PD-1 as an emerging therapeutic target in renal cell carcinoma: Current evidence. OncoTargets and Therapy. 2014;**7**:1349-1359

[43] Thompson RH, Kuntz SM, Leibovich BC, et al. Tumor B7-H1 is associated with poor prognosis in renal cell carcinoma patients with long-term follow-up. Cancer Research. 2006;**66**(7):3381-3385

[44] Thompson RH, Dong H, Kwon ED. Implications of B7-H1 expression in clear cell carcinoma of the kidney for prognostication and therapy. Clinical Cancer Research. 2007;**13** (2 Pt 2):709s-715s

[45] Topalian SL, Hodi FS, Brahmer JR, et al. Safety, activity, and immune correlates of anti-PD-1 antibody in cancer. The New England Journal of Medicine. 2012;**366**(26):2443-2454

[46] Motzer RJ, Rini BI, Mcdermott DF, et al. Nivolumab for metastatic renal cell carcinoma: Results of a randomized phase II trial. Journal of Clinical Oncology. 2015;**33**(13):1430-1437

[47] Mcdermott DF, Drake CG, Sznol M, et al. Survival, durable response, and long-term safety in patients with previously treated advanced renal cell carcinoma receiving Nivolumab. Journal of Clinical Oncology. 2015;**33**(18):2013-2020

[48] Godwin JL, Zibelman M, Plimack ER, et al. Immune checkpoint blockade as a novel immunotherapeutic strategy for renal cell carcinoma: A review of clinical trials. Discovery Medicine. 2014;**18**(101):341-350

[49] Atkins MB, Choueiri TK, Hodi FS, et al. Pembrolizumab (MK-3475) plus low-dose ipilimumab (IPI) in patients (pts) with advanced melanoma (MEL) or renal cell carcinoma (RCC): Data from the KEYNOTE-029 phase 1 study. Journal of Clinical Oncology. 2015;**33**(15_suppl):3009-3009

[50] Patnaik A, Kang SP, Rasco D, et al. Phase I study of pembrolizumab (MK-3475; anti-PD-1 monoclonal antibody) in patients with advanced solid tumors. Clinical Cancer Research. 2015;**21**(19):4286-4293

[51] Berger R, Rotem-Yehudar R, Slama G, et al. Phase I safety and pharmacokinetic study of CT-011, a humanized antibody interacting with PD-1, in patients with advanced hematologic malignancies. Clinical Cancer Research. 2008;**14**(10):3044-3051

[52] Reinhardt C, Zdrojowy R, Szczylik C, et al. Results of a randomized phase II study investigating multipeptide vaccination with IMA901 in advanced renal cell carcinoma (RCC). Journal of Clinical Oncology. 2010;**28**(15_suppl):4529-4529

[53] Figlin RA, Nicolette CA, Amin A, et al. Monitoring T-cell responses in a phase II study of AGS-003, an autologous dendritic cell-based therapy in patients with newly diagnosed advanced stage renal cell carcinoma in combination with sunitinib. Journal of Clinical Oncology. 2011;**29**(15_suppl):2532-2532

[54] Amin A, Dudek A, Logan T, et al. A phase II study testing the safety and activity of AGS-003 as an immunotherapeutic in subjects with newly diagnosed advanced stage renal cell carcinoma (RCC) in combination with sunitinib. Journal of Clinical Oncology. 2010;**28**(15_suppl):4588-4588

[55] Weinstock M, Mcdermott D. Targeting PD-1/PD-L1 in the treatment of metastatic renal cell carcinoma. Therapeutic Advances in Urology. 2015;**7**(6):365-377

[56] Gunturi A, Mcdermott DF. Potential of new therapies like anti-PD1 in kidney cancer. Current Treatment Options in Oncology. 2014;**15**(1):137-146

[57] Thompson RH, Gillett MD, Cheville JC, et al. Costimulatory B7-H1 in renal cell carcinoma patients: Indicator of tumor aggressiveness and potential therapeutic target. Proceedings of the National Academy of Sciences of the United States of America. 2004;**101**(49):17174-17179

[58] Mcdermott DF, Sosman JA, Sznol M, et al. Atezolizumab, an anti-programmed death-ligand 1 antibody, in metastatic renal cell carcinoma: Long-term safety, clinical activity, and immune correlates from a phase Ia study. Journal of Clinical Oncology. 2016;**34**(8):833-842

[59] Brahmer JR, Tykodi SS, Chow LQ, et al. Safety and activity of anti-PD-L1 antibody in patients with advanced cancer. The New England Journal of Medicine. 2012;**366**(26): 2455-2465

[60] Kelly K, Patel MR, Infante JR, et al. Avelumab (MSB0010718C), an anti-PD-L1 antibody, in patients with metastatic or locally advanced solid tumors: Assessment of safety and tolerability in a phase I, open-label expansion study. Journal of Clinical Oncology. 2015;**33**(15_suppl):3044-3044

[61] Rizvi NA, Brahmer JR, Ou S-HI, et al. Safety and clinical activity of MEDI4736, an anti-programmed cell death-ligand 1 (PD-L1) antibody, in patients with non-small cell lung cancer (NSCLC). Journal of Clinical Oncology. 2015;**33**(15_suppl):8032-8032

[62] Walker LS, Sansom DM. The emerging role of CTLA4 as a cell-extrinsic regulator of T cell responses. Nature Reviews. Immunology. 2011;**11**(12):852-863

[63] Leach DR, Krummel MF, Allison JP. Enhancement of antitumor immunity by CTLA-4 blockade. Science. 1996;**271**(5256):1734-1736

[64] Lipson EJ, Drake CG. Ipilimumab: An anti-CTLA-4 antibody for metastatic melanoma. Clinical Cancer Research. 2011;**17**(22):6958-6962

[65] Hodi FS, O'day SJ, Mcdermott DF, et al. Improved survival with ipilimumab in patients with metastatic melanoma. The New England Journal of Medicine. 2010;**363**(8):711-723

[66] Larkin J, Hodi FS, Wolchok JD. Combined nivolumab and ipilimumab or monotherapy in untreated melanoma. The New England Journal of Medicine. 2015;**373**(13):1270-1271

[67] Yang JC, Hughes M, Kammula U, et al. Ipilimumab (anti-CTLA4 antibody) causes regression of metastatic renal cell cancer associated with enteritis and hypophysitis. Journal of Immunotherapy. 2007;**30**(8):825-830

[68] Huard B, Gaulard P, Faure F, et al. Cellular expression and tissue distribution of the human LAG-3-encoded protein, an MHC class II ligand. Immunogenetics. 1994;**39**(3):213-217

[69] Huard B, Prigent P, Tournier M, et al. CD4/major histocompatibility complex class II interaction analyzed with CD4- and lymphocyte activation gene-3 (LAG-3)-Ig fusion proteins. European Journal of Immunology. 1995;**25**(9):2718-2721

[70] Huang CT, Workman CJ, Flies D, et al. Role of LAG-3 in regulatory T cells. Immunity. 2004;**21**(4):503-513

[71] Okamura T, Fujio K, Shibuya M, et al. CD4+CD25-LAG3+ regulatory T cells controlled by the transcription factor Egr-2. Proceedings of the National Academy of Sciences of the United States of America. 2009;**106**(33):13974-13979

[72] Blackburn SD, Shin H, Haining WN, et al. Coregulation of CD8+ T cell exhaustion by multiple inhibitory receptors during chronic viral infection. Nature Immunology. 2009;**10**(1):29-37

[73] Butler NS, Moebius J, Pewe LL, et al. Therapeutic blockade of PD-L1 and LAG-3 rapidly clears established blood-stage Plasmodium infection. Nature Immunology. 2011; **13**(2):188-195

[74] Woo SR, Turnis ME, Goldberg MV, et al. Immune inhibitory molecules LAG-3 and PD-1 synergistically regulate T-cell function to promote tumoral immune escape. Cancer Research. 2012;**72**(4):917-927

[75] Brignone C, Escudier B, Grygar C, et al. A phase I pharmacokinetic and biological correlative study of IMP321, a novel MHC class II agonist, in patients with advanced renal cell carcinoma. Clinical Cancer Research. 2009;**15**(19):6225-6231

[76] Curran MA, Montalvo W, Yagita H, et al. PD-1 and CTLA-4 combination blockade expands infiltrating T cells and reduces regulatory T and myeloid cells within B16 melanoma tumors. Proceedings of the National Academy of Sciences of the United States of America. 2010;**107**(9):4275-4280

[77] Wolchok JD, Kluger H, Callahan MK, et al. Nivolumab plus ipilimumab in advanced melanoma. New England Journal of Medicine. 2013;**369**(2):122-133

[78] Parekh H, Rini BI. Emerging therapeutic approaches in renal cell carcinoma. Expert Review of Anticancer Therapy. 2015;**15**(11):1305-1314

[79] Aoun F, Kourie HR, Sideris S, et al. Checkpoint inhibitors in bladder and renal cancers: Results and perspectives. Immunotherapy. 2015;**7**(12):1259-1271

[80] Hammers HJ, Plimack ER, Infante JR, et al. Safety and efficacy of nivolumab in combination with ipilimumab in metastatic renal cell carcinoma: The CheckMate 016 study. Journal of Clinical Oncology. 2017;**35**(34):3851-3858

[81] Hughes PE, Caenepeel S, Wu LC. Targeted therapy and checkpoint immunotherapy combinations for the treatment of cancer. Trends in Immunology. 2016;**37**(7):462-476

[82] Amin A, Plimack ER, Infante JR, et al. Nivolumab (anti-PD-1; BMS-936558, ONO-4538) in combination with sunitinib or pazopanib in patients (pts) with metastatic renal cell carcinoma (mRCC). American Society of Clinical Oncology. 2014:5010

[83] Mcdermott D, Infante J, Chowdhury S, et al. 2622 A phase I/II study to assess the safety and efficacy of pazopanib (paz) and pembrolizumab (pembro) in patients (pts) with advanced renal cell carcinoma (aRCC). European Journal of Cancer. 2015;**51**:S519-S520

[84] Atkins M, Plimack E, Puzanov I, et al. Axitinib in combination with pembrolizumab in patients (pts) with advanced renal cell carcinoma (aRCC): Preliminary safety and efficacy results. European Society for Medical Oncology. 2016

[85] Larkin J, Rini B, Nathan P, et al. Phase 1b dose-finding study of avelumab (anti-PD-L1)+ axitinib in treatment-naïve patients with advanced renal cell carcinoma. European Society for Medical Oncology. 2016:775PD

[86] Wallin JJ, Bendell JC, Funke R, et al. Atezolizumab in combination with bevacizumab enhances antigen-specific T-cell migration in metastatic renal cell carcinoma. Nature Communications. 2016;**7**:12624

[87] Atkins MB, Gupta S, Choueiri TK, et al. Phase Ib dose-finding study of axitinib plus pembrolizumab in treatment-naïve patients with advanced renal cell carcinoma. Journal for Immunotherapy of Cancer. 2015;**3**(S2):P353

[88] Chakrabarty A, Hillman GG, Maughan RL, et al. Radiation therapy enhances the therapeutic effect of immunotherapy on pulmonary metastases in a murine renal adenocarcinoma model. In Vivo. 1994;**8**(1):25-31

[89] De Meerleer G, Khoo V, Escudier B, et al. Radiotherapy for renal-cell carcinoma. The Lancet Oncology. 2014;**15**(4):e170-e177

[90] Pal SK, Vogelzang NJ. Sequential treatment strategies and combination therapy regimens in metastatic renal cell carcinoma. Clinical Advances in Hematology & Oncology. 2013;**11**(3):146-155

[91] Buonerba C, Di Lorenzo G, Sonpavde G. Combination therapy for metastatic renal cell carcinoma. Annals of Translational Medicine. 2016;**4**(5):100

[92] Remark R, Alifano M, Cremer I, et al. Characteristics and clinical impacts of the immune environments in colorectal and renal cell carcinoma lung metastases: Influence of tumor origin. Clinical Cancer Research. 2013;**19**(15):4079-4091

[93] Smaldone MC, Fung C, Uzzo RG, et al. Adjuvant and neoadjuvant therapies in high-risk renal cell carcinoma. Hematology/Oncology Clinics of North America. 2011;**25**(4):765-791

[94] Valenca LB, Hirsch MS, Choueiri TK, et al. Non-clear cell renal cell carcinoma, part 1: Histology. Clinical Advances in Hematology & Oncology. 2015;**13**(5):308-313

[95] Motzer RJ, Bacik J, Mariani T, et al. Treatment outcome and survival associated with metastatic renal cell carcinoma of non-clear-cell histology. Journal of Clinical Oncology. 2002;**20**(9):2376-2381

[96] Zibelman M, Plimack ER. Integrating immunotherapy into the management of renal cell carcinoma. Journal of the National Comprehensive Cancer Network. 2017;**15**(6):841-847

[97] Kroeger N, Xie W, Lee JL, et al. Metastatic non-clear cell renal cell carcinoma treated with targeted therapy agents: Characterization of survival outcome and application of the international mRCC database consortium criteria. Cancer. 2013;**119**(16):2999-3006

[98] Mcdermott DF, Cheng SC, Signoretti S, et al. The high-dose aldesleukin "select" trial: A trial to prospectively validate predictive models of response to treatment in patients with metastatic renal cell carcinoma. Clinical Cancer Research. 2015;**21**(3):561-568

[99] Mcdermott DF, Regan MM, Clark JI, et al. Randomized phase III trial of high-dose interleukin-2 versus subcutaneous interleukin-2 and interferon in patients with metastatic renal cell carcinoma. Journal of Clinical Oncology. 2005;**23**(1):133-141

[100] Adra N, Cheng L, Pili R. Unclassified renal cell carcinoma with significant response to nivolumab. Clinical Genitourinary Cancer. 2017;**15**(3):e517-e519

[101] Beckermann KE, Jolly PC, Kim JY, et al. Clinical and immunologic correlates of response to PD-1 blockade in a patient with metastatic renal medullary carcinoma. Journal for ImmunoTherapy of Cancer. 2017;**5**:1

[102] Geynisman DM. Anti-programmed cell death protein 1 (PD-1) antibody Nivolumab leads to a dramatic and rapid response in papillary renal cell carcinoma with Sarcomatoid and Rhabdoid features. European Urology. 2015;**68**(5):912-914

[103] Wolchok JD, Hoos A, O'day S, et al. Guidelines for the evaluation of immune therapy activity in solid tumors: Immune-related response criteria. Clinical Cancer Research. 2009;**15**(23):7412-7420

[104] Chiou VL, Burotto M. Pseudoprogression and immune-related response in solid tumors. Journal of Clinical Oncology. 2015;**33**(31):3541-3543

[105] Adams S, Diamond JR, Hamilton EP, et al. Phase Ib trial of atezolizumab in combination with nab-paclitaxel in patients with metastatic triple-negative breast cancer (mTNBC). American Society of Clinical Oncology. 2016:1009

[106] Seymour L, Bogaerts J, Perrone A, et al. iRECIST: Guidelines for response criteria for use in trials testing immunotherapeutics. The Lancet Oncology. 2017;**18**(3):e143-e152

[107] Chen DS, Mellman I. Elements of cancer immunity and the cancer-immune set point. Nature. 2017;**541**(7637):321-330

[108] Blank CU, Haanen JB, Ribas A, et al. Cancer immunology. The "cancer immunogram". Science. 2016;**352**(6286):658-660

[109] Chan TA, Wolchok JD, Snyder A. Genetic basis for clinical response to CTLA-4 blockade in melanoma. The New England Journal of Medicine. 2015;**373**(20):1984

[110] Rizvi NA, Hellmann MD, Snyder A, et al. Cancer immunology. Mutational landscape determines sensitivity to PD-1 blockade in non-small cell lung cancer. Science. 2015;**348**(6230):124-128

[111] Pena-Llopis S, Vega-Rubin-De-Celis S, Liao A, et al. BAP1 loss defines a new class of renal cell carcinoma. Nature Genetics. 2012;**44**(7):751-759

[112] Vetizou M, Pitt JM, Daillere R, et al. Anticancer immunotherapy by CTLA-4 blockade relies on the gut microbiota. Science. 2015;**350**(6264):1079-1084

[113] Sivan A, Corrales L, Hubert N, et al. Commensal Bifidobacterium promotes antitumor immunity and facilitates anti-PD-L1 efficacy. Science. 2015;**350**(6264):1084-1089

[114] Pitt JM, Vetizou M, Gomperts Boneca I, et al. Enhancing the clinical coverage and anticancer efficacy of immune checkpoint blockade through manipulation of the gut microbiota. Oncoimmunology. 2017;**6**(1):e1132137

[115] Luen S, Virassamy B, Savas P, et al. The genomic landscape of breast cancer and its interaction with host immunity. Breast. 2016;**29**:241-250

[116] Hegde PS, Karanikas V, Evers S. The where, the when, and the how of immune monitoring for cancer immunotherapies in the era of checkpoint inhibition. Clinical Cancer Research. 2016;**22**(8):1865-1874

[117] Ott PA, Hodi FS, Buchbinder EI. Inhibition of immune checkpoints and vascular endothelial growth factor as combination therapy for metastatic melanoma: An overview of rationale, preclinical evidence, and initial clinical data. Frontiers in Oncology. 2015;**5**:202

[118] Alfaro C, Suarez N, Gonzalez A, et al. Influence of bevacizumab, sunitinib and sorafenib as single agents or in combination on the inhibitory effects of VEGF on human dendritic cell differentiation from monocytes. British Journal of Cancer. 2009;**100**(7):1111-1119

[119] Vanneman M, Dranoff G. Combining immunotherapy and targeted therapies in cancer treatment. Nature Reviews. Cancer. 2012;**12**(4):237-251

[120] Choueiri TK, Larkin JM, Oya M, et al. First-line avelumab+ axitinib therapy in patients (pts) with advanced renal cell carcinoma (aRCC): Results from a phase Ib trial. American Society of Clinical Oncology. 2017:4504

[121] Taylor M, Dutcus C, Schmidt E, et al. A phase 1b trial of lenvatinib (LEN) plus pembrolizumab (PEM) in patients with selected solid tumors. Annals of Oncology. 2016;**27**(suppl_6):776

[122] Mcdermott DF, Atkins MB, Motzer RJ, et al. A phase II study of atezolizumab (atezo) with or without bevacizumab (bev) versus sunitinib (sun) in untreated metastatic renal cell carcinoma (mRCC) patients (pts). American Society of Clinical Oncology. 2017:431

[123] Sznol M, Mcdermott DF, Jones SF, et al. Phase Ib evaluation of MPDL3280A (anti-PDL1) in combination with bevacizumab (bev) in patients (pts) with metastatic renal cell carcinoma (mRCC). American Society of Clinical Oncology. 2015

[124] Rini BI, Vogelzang NJ. Future challenges for drug development in renal cell carcinoma. American Society of Clinical Oncology. 2016

[125] Rini BI, Stein M, Shannon P, et al. Phase 1 dose-escalation trial of tremelimumab plus sunitinib in patients with metastatic renal cell carcinoma. Cancer. 2011;**117**(4):758-767

[126] Kakarla S, Gottschalk S. CAR T cells for solid tumors: Armed and ready to go? Cancer Journal (Sudbury, Mass.). 2014;**20**(2):151

[127] Bui MH, Seligson D, Han K-R, et al. Carbonic anhydrase IX is an independent predictor of survival in advanced renal clear cell carcinoma. Clinical Cancer Research. 2003; **9**(2):802-811

[128] Lamers CH, Sleijfer S, Vulto AG, et al. Treatment of metastatic renal cell carcinoma with autologous T-lymphocytes genetically retargeted against carbonic anhydrase IX: First clinical experience. Journal of Clinical Oncology. 2006;**24**(13):e20-e22

[129] Lamers CH, Sleijfer S, Van Steenbergen S, et al. Treatment of metastatic renal cell carcinoma with CAIX CAR-engineered T cells: Clinical evaluation and management of on-target toxicity. Molecular Therapy. 2013;**21**(4):904-912

[130] Kim JS, Chung IS, Lim SH, et al. Preclinical and clinical studies on cytokine-induced killer cells for the treatment of renal cell carcinoma. Archives of Pharmacal Research. 2014;**37**(5):559-566

[131] Liu L, Zhang W, Qi X, et al. Randomized study of autologous cytokine-induced killer cell immunotherapy in metastatic renal carcinoma. Clinical Cancer Research. 2012;**18**(6): 1751-1759

[132] Wang D, Zhang B, Gao H, et al. Clinical research of genetically modified dendritic cells in combination with cytokine-induced killer cell treatment in advanced renal cancer. BMC Cancer. 2014;**14**(1):251

[133] Westwood JA, Darcy PK, Guru PM, et al. Three agonist antibodies in combination with high-dose IL-2 eradicate orthotopic kidney cancer in mice. Journal of Translational Medicine. 2010;**8**(1):42

[134] Infante JR, Burris HA, Ansell SM, et al. Immunologic activity of an activating anti-CD27 antibody (CDX-1127) in patients (pts) with solid tumors. American Society of Clinical Oncology. 2014:3027

[135] Sanmamed MF, Pastor F, Rodriguez A, et al. Agonists of co-stimulation in cancer immunotherapy directed against CD137, OX40, GITR, CD27, CD28, and ICOS[C]. Seminars in Oncology. 2015:640-655

[136] Peggs K, Quezada S, Allison J. Cancer immunotherapy: Co-stimulatory agonists and co-inhibitory antagonists. Clinical & Experimental Immunology. 2009;**157**(1):9-19

[137] Miller A, Hoogstraten B, Staquet M, et al. Reporting results of cancer treatment. Cancer. 1981;**47**(1):207-214

[138] Eisenhauer E, Therasse P, Bogaerts J, et al. New response evaluation criteria in solid tumours: Revised RECIST guideline (version 1.1). European Journal of Cancer. 2009;**45**(2):228-247

[139] Nishino M, Giobbie-Hurder A, Gargano M, et al. Developing a common language for tumor response to immunotherapy: Immune-related response criteria using unidimensional measurements. Clinical Cancer Research. 2013;**19**(14):3936-3943

[140] Lynch TJ, Bondarenko I, Luft A, et al. Ipilimumab in combination with paclitaxel and carboplatin as first-line treatment in stage IIIB/IV non–small-cell lung cancer: Results from a randomized, double-blind, multicenter phase II study. Journal of Clinical Oncology. 2012;**30**(17):2046-2054

[141] Nishino M, Ramaiya NH, Hatabu H, et al. Monitoring immune-checkpoint blockade: Response evaluation and biomarker development. Nature Reviews Clinical Oncology. 2017;**14**(11):655

[142] Posadas EM, Limvorasak S, Figlin RA. Targeted therapies for renal cell carcinoma. Nature Reviews Nephrology. 2017;**13**(8):496-511

Section 2

Current Concepts in Kidney Cancer

Chapter 4

Simulation and Training in Kidney Cancer Surgery

Nicholas Mehan, Nicholas Simson and
Ben Challacombe

Additional information is available at the end of the chapter

http://dx.doi.org/10.5772/intechopen.85683

Abstract

The rise of robotic surgery coupled with the increased detection of small renal masses has led to a marked increase in renal cancer surgery and, in particular, robotic partial nephrectomy. Given the associated learning curves of these procedures and added external pressures such as work-time directives, training programmes have had to adapt and move away from the traditional apprenticeship model. Simulation in surgery has greatly expanded over the past 20 years to fill this divide and is now commonplace for surgical training and fellowship programmes. This chapter explores the different modalities of simulation available in renal cancer surgery including the latest procedural-specific simulation platforms for both radical and partial nephrectomy. Exciting new developments such as 3D printing and patient-specific modelling are addressed as well as the emerging role of artificial intelligence. Finally, the integration of simulation into a comprehensive surgical training programme is explored.

Keywords: renal cancer, simulation, partial nephrectomy, radical nephrectomy, surgical training, robotic surgery, surgical curriculum

1. Introduction

The traditional apprenticeship style of surgical training is evolving due to a multitude of challenges. The old Halstedian mantra of 'do one, see one, teach one' [1] has become less acceptable as societal and professional expectations change. Current trainees are now expected to achieve a similar level of competency to their mentors despite mounting restrictions on available training opportunities [2]. Initiatives such as the European Work Time Directive (EWTD) [3] have resulted in reduced working hours, and financial restrictions on healthcare budgets have led to increased focus on operating room efficiency. The concurrent emergence of minimally invasive surgical techniques, such as laparoscopy and robotic-assisted surgery, and their associated learning curves has further compounded the issue. As a result, the development of quality surgical training opportunities in the non-clinical setting has long been on the agenda of the profession, and today, surgical simulation has ascended to occupy a central role in the modern surgical curriculum [4, 5]. For *trainees*, simulation allows the opportunity to develop surgical skills in an environment free of risk to the patient. It overcomes the limitations of operating room exposure and affords flexibility in an often chaotic work schedule. For *trainers,* the controlled nature of simulation allows objective appraisal of performance and progression, as well as a tailored approach to meet individual learning needs.

2. Development and validation of simulators

The ideal simulator should have a significant educational impact, improve subsequent performance in the operating room, shorten the procedural learning curve and subsequently increase patient safety. For novices, it should offer a realistic introduction to basic technical skills, allowing part-task training, while becoming increasingly procedure-specific and patient-specific for the more experienced operator [6].

Simulators must be rigorously evaluated across a number of parameters before they can be used for training and assessment. Validity is a measure of the extent a simulator succeeds in teaching the skill for which it was designed [7]. An ideal simulator would perform well in all of the following aspects of validity [8];

- Face validity: the extent to which the simulator is realistic.
- Content validity: the extent to which the simulator's content is representative of the skill required to be learnt.
- Construct validity: the extent to which experienced and novice operators can be differentiated.
- Concurrent validity: the extent to which the simulation correlates with the current gold standard test used to measure the skill.
- Predictive validity: the extent to which future performance can be predicted by simulator performance.

With the increased pressure on healthcare expenditure and efficiency, the importance of independent and robust validation is critical to ensure that resources are invested in simulator platforms that provide the highest levels of educational impact [9].

3. Different modalities of simulation

Simulators can broadly be divided into two categories: physical and 'virtual reality' simulators. Physical (or mechanical) simulators use physical objects as substitutes for patients and include bench-top models, animal tissue, live animals and human cadavers. Virtual reality simulators use a computer-based platform with artificially generated virtual environments to interact [9]. This group includes the recent introduction of 'augmented reality' platforms, which integrate real-life patient data into a virtual reality environment. The range of different modalities, as well as their perceived advantages and disadvantages is summarised in **Table 1**.

Simulation modality	Description/ examples	Advantages	Disadvantages	Use in kidney cancer surgery
Bench-top model	Synthetic, dry-lab models; e.g. box trainers	Re-usable, portable, use of real instruments	Low fidelity: unrealistic Unable to teach entire procedure High fidelity: Cost	Basic laparoscopic skills Partial Nephrectomy dry-lab models [11, 12] 3D printing allows tumours to be incorporated into models [13, 14]
Animal tissue	Ex-vivo animal tissue; e.g. porcine urinary tract	Tissue handling Cost-effective	Single-use Storage facilities No blood flow Anatomical differences	Partial nephrectomy with porcine kidney and various tumour-mimics (e.g. polystyrene ball, injection of liquid plastic) [15, 16]
Live animals	Live, anaesthetised animals; e.g. pigs, sheep, rabbits	Tissue handling Ability to perform entire procedures Realistic Blood flow	Ethical concerns Need for storage facilities and trained veterinary personnel Single-use Cost Anatomical differences	Live rabbits for laparoscopic nephrectomy [17] Anaesthetised pigs for nephrectomy and partial nephrectomy [18]
Cadaveric material	Fresh frozen or thiel-embalmed cadaveric material	Ability to perform entire procedures Highest face validity	Cost Availability Single use No blood flow	Full procedure training (Nephrectomy and partial nephrectomy) [19]
Virtual-reality	Interaction with computer-generated environment (e.g. RoSS, SEP, dvSS)	Objective evaluation Data capture Repetitive use	Cost/maintenance No availability when robot in use Poor 3D vision	Familiarisation with robotic equipment and basic technical skills [20] Procedure-specific simulation allows for procedures to be performed in their entirety [21, 22]
Augmented reality	Integration of real patient data into virtual reality simulation (e.g. HoST, Maestro AR)	Patient-specific information Data capture Repetitive use	Cost	Patient-specific tumours incorporated into simulation [23] Patient imaging or 3D surgical video incorporated [22, 24]

dvSS, da Vinci skills simulator; RoSS, robotic surgical simulator; HoST, Hands-On Surgical Simulator; SEP, SimSurgery Educational Platform; 3D, three-dimensional.

Table 1. Available simulation modalities (adapted from Aydin et al. [10]).

3.1. Physical simulators (mechanical)

3.1.1. Bench-top/'dry-lab' models

Bench-top models are synthetic models that can vary from simple (i.e. peg-transfer) to more complex tasks (i.e. suturing and knot-tying) in order to acquire surgical skills. These are often incorporated into different surgical platforms via a box-trainer allowing the utilisation of actual surgical instruments and giving the trainee an opportunity to familiarise with the controls and limitations of that platform [12]. Higher-fidelity synthetic models can be utilised for more advanced skills and part-procedural simulation. With the advent of 3D printing, several authors have described high-fidelity partial-nephrectomy models whereby tumour excision and renorrhaphy can be rehearsed [13, 14, 25]. Patient-specific models have even been utilised by expert surgeons to pre-operatively rehearse RAPN in order to determine feasibility of PN and predict warm-ischaemia times [26].

3.1.2. Ex-vivo animal tissue/'wet-lab' models

Inanimate animal tissue has been used to simulate a range of endourological, laparoscopic and robotic-assisted procedures ex-vivo [10]. These models utilise the actual surgical instruments or console similar to dry-lab models and subsequently have similar advantages with regard to developing familiarity with the surgical platform. Porcine kidneys in particular have been utilised successfully for procedural simulation in renal cancer surgery and offer advantages in terms of higher-fidelity tissue handling and even the ability to be artificially perfused, allowing simulation of vascular control and haemostasis [16, 27]. These advantages need to be weighed against the special facilities required for storage and subsequent increased costs, which can be a limiting factor in some institutions.

3.1.3. Live animal tissue

Live animal models facilitate the closest simulation to live surgical cases and also provide an opportunity for whole procedural simulation. Whole-procedural simulation has the significant advantage, allowing development in dissection technique, energy control, vascular control and haemostasis techniques. Several groups have even described the creation of artificial tumours in live porcine models, subsequently allowing specific procedural simulation for robotic-assisted partial nephrectomy (RAPN) [15, 16]. Despite these benefits, however, the higher costs, ethical issues and local legislative restrictions can significantly impact the availability. Subsequently, access to live animal simulation is often limited to a few programmes.

3.1.4. Cadaveric tissue

Human cadaveric material has long been used in surgical training, and it is generally accepted that cadaveric simulation has the highest face validity of all simulation modalities [19, 28]. Simulation using fresh frozen cadavers (FFCs) or thiel-embalmed cadavers (TECs) has shown face, content and construct validity in a range of endourological and laparoscopic procedures [10]. Despite utilisation in various training programmes, validation of the effectiveness of cadaveric training in robotic-assisted procedures remains limited [28], and further research in this area is needed.

3.1.5. *Virtual reality (VR) and augmented reality (AR) simulators*

Robotic surgery in particular lends itself to VR simulation, and as such, there has been a significant development in this modality in recent times. At present, there exist a number of commercially available products as outlined in **Table 2**.

In recent years, the introduction of augmented reality (AR) simulators has provided increasingly realistic and procedure-specific platforms for simulation. The two AR systems in common use are the Hands-On Surgical Training (HoST) and the Maestro AR system. HoST

Simulation model	Manufacturer	Focus	Advantages	Disadvantages
dV-Trainer	Mimic Technologies, USA	Basic skills	Standalone Availability Extensively validated [20, 29–31]	Mechanically different hand controls
dvSS	Intuitive Surgical, USA	Basic skills	Fixed to console Uses actual console Extensively validated [32–34]	Can only be used when da Vinci robot not in use
RoSS/HoST	Simulated Surgical Systems, USA	Basic skills, procedural specific simulation (RARP, cystectomy, lymph node dissection)	Standalone Availability Extensively validated [35–37] Augmented reality procedural tasks (HoST)	Mechanically different hand controls Cost Limited availability outside USA
RobotiX mentor	Simbionix, USA	Basic skills Procedural simulation	Standalone Availability Laparoscopic assistant module [38]	Mechanically different hand controls No urological procedural tasks
SEP robot	SimSurgery, Norway	Basic skills	Standalone Availability	2D vision Mechanically different hand controls Less robust validity [39]
Pro-MIS	CAE Healthcare, Canada	Basic skills	Standalone VR and use with box trainers	2D vision Originally designed for laparoscopy Limited robotic validation [40] Mechanically different hand controls
Maestro AR	Mimic Technologies, USA	Augmented Reality Procedural simulation (RAPN, RARP) [22]	Standalone Availability Procedural simulation	Unable to manipulate surgical field

dV-Trainer, da Vinci trainer; dvSS, da Vinci skills simulator; RoSS, robotic surgical simulator; HoST, Hands-On Surgical Simulator; SEP, SimSurgery Educational Platform; 3D, three-dimensional; 2D, two-dimensional; RARP, robotic-assisted radical prostatectomy; RAPN, robotic-assisted partial nephrectomy.

Table 2. Available VR simulation platforms.

(Simulated Surgical Systems, USA) incorporates a real surgical procedure into the virtual reality framework and guides the user through an enhanced version of the operation, with audio-visual illustration, haptic cues and guided movements [24]. The HoST system currently does not offer procedural simulation for nephrectomy or partial nephrectomy. Maestro AR (Mimic Technologies, USA) provides procedure-specific 3D video and interaction via virtual reality robotic instruments. This includes a module on partial nephrectomy that demonstrates face, content, construct and concurrent validity [22].

4. Procedural simulation for renal cancer

Competently performing a whole procedure requires knowledge of surgical anatomy, procedural steps and the ability to perform each surgical component. Whole procedure simulation is challenging and at present time in renal surgery, it is largely limited to cadaveric and animal models. As a result of these limitations part-procedural simulation, where a particular procedural step is simulated (i.e. tumour excision or renorraphy), has advanced significantly over the last decade. The majority of these models are bench-top, either wet or dry, and have the advantage of being able to be utilised for open, laparoscopic and robotic platforms. The following section aims to explore the models available for radical and partial nephrectomy.

4.1. Radical nephrectomy

Radical nephrectomy remains the most utilised treatment approach for renal malignancy [41, 42]. Traditionally performed as an open procedure, laparoscopic radical nephrectomy has become widespread due to the benefits of shorter convalescence and less procedural morbidity [42]. The initial experience with laparoscopy was technically challenging, and the learning curve and associated complication rates for novice surgeons were a significant barrier to uptake [43]. Developments in training and simulation subsequently followed in an attempt to provide an adjunct for skill development outside of the operating theatre [44, 45]. At present there are a vast array of simulators available for acquiring laparoscopic skills with extensive validation ranging from box trainers to develop basic skills, to whole procedural simulation on live animals and VR platforms.

4.1.1. Physical simulation

The first clinical laparoscopic radical nephrectomy (LRN) was performed in 1990 by Clayman and colleagues [46] after extensive experimentation on porcine models. The benefits of animal models for teaching dissection, tissue handling, haemostasis and vascular control are significant, and subsequently this simulation modality remains central to the development and dissemination of minimally invasive surgical techniques [47].

Molinas and colleagues [17] demonstrated the validity of live simulation in LRN using a rabbit model. Ten gynaecologists and 10 medical students each performed 20 laparoscopic nephrectomies over a 20-day training course. The overall time required to perform the LRN decreased from 44 ± 18 to 11 ± 2 minutes for the first and the last procedure, respectively, and complication rates similarly decreased. Despite the rabbit's smaller size compared to pigs for example, pneumoperitoneum was able to be established, and conventional instruments were used for all procedures. Reduction in acquisition and handling costs associated with the rabbits allowed the authors to provide a more prolonged period of training demonstrating the impact of repetition on learning curves and complication rates.

Cruz and colleagues [48] assessed the impact of repeated LRN in the porcine model on overall surgical performance among established surgeons. Six urologists with limited laparoscopic experience were recruited to perform a live porcine LRN weekly for 10 weeks. Surgical performance was judged quantitatively including total operative time and estimated blood loss. Qualitative measures were also assessed using the Global Operative Assessment of Laparoscopic Skills (GOALS) including depth perception, dexterity, efficiency, tissue handling and autonomy. Over the course of the study, blood loss, depth perception and dexterity showed statistically significant improvements. The remaining domains including operative time showed no statistical improvement.

4.1.2. *Virtual reality*

Despite the obvious benefits of high-fidelity animal models, the costs and associated ethical issues restrict access which is often limited to several day courses. A high-fidelity virtual reality LRN simulation platform has obvious advantages in overcoming some of these barriers. The LAP Mentor (Simbionix, USA) and LapSim (Surgical Sciences, Sweden) are two commercially available laparoscopic simulators, which provide VR laparoscopic training including a full nephrectomy module. While both simulators have been validated in terms of basic laparoscopic skills [49, 50], the nephrectomy modules remain to be formally scientifically assessed. Despite this, these simulators provide full procedure simulation that is reproducible and able to provide feedback on performance metrics such as economy of motion, procedure time and error rates. These metrics have potential utility in assessing progression and setting benchmarks for training curriculums.

4.2. Partial nephrectomy

With the advent of widespread cross-sectional imaging, there has been a surge in incidental detection of small renal masses. This has subsequently led to increased utilisation of partial nephrectomy (PN) in order to preserve normal renal parenchyma in these otherwise well patients [51]. PN is a technically challenging operation with a significant learning curve and variability unrivalled by almost any other frequently performed kidney procedure [52]. Perhaps, most challenging, however, is the *time-critical* nature of PN. The vast blood supply to the kidney means bleeding is a significant intraoperative risk and efficient excision, and renorrhaphy is therefore crucial. Furthermore, prolonged warm ischaemia is deleterious to healthy renal tissue and can impact post-operative renal function [53, 54]. Finally, each tumour is highly variable in size, location and relation to critical structures, making oncological excision a persistent challenge even for experienced surgeons. For these reasons, training in PN is subsequently fraught with complexity, and mentors must try and negotiate sometimes the discordant goals of training with patient safety. Simulation for PN has rapidly progressed in response to this dilemma, and the availability of PN models is becoming more widespread.

4.2.1. *Physical simulation*

Tumour-mimic models for PN rose to prominence in the initial laparoscopic era in response to the technically challenging nature of the procedure and associated learning curve. Taylor and colleagues [55] described one of the earliest models in 2004, whereby a pigmented mixture was injected into a series of ex-vivo and in-vivo porcine kidneys. The authors were able to create a variety of lesions both endo- and exophytic with a mean size of 10 mm. This model was not formally assessed as part of a training programme but established the feasibility of artificial tumour creation. Hidalgo et al. [15] similarly described the creation of an in-vivo porcine PN model through the percutaneous injection of a liquefied plastic solution into the subscapular renal space to create exophytic lesions. This model was evaluated as part of a laparoscopic training programme and found to enhance the learning experience in 96% of participants. While advantageous for the novice, the inability of these techniques to create large endophytic or central lesions may limit the utility to more advanced surgeons.

Yang et al. [27] described an ex-vivo porcine model, whereby the kidney was secured to a specifically designed box for use with a laparoscopic trainer. The renal vessels were preserved, and simulated vascular perfusion was achieved through infusion of red-dyed water through the artery. Urology trainees were requested to excise a 2 cm spherical piece of renal parenchyma and then complete renorrhaphy. The model was validated by five urology trainees, each of whom completed 10 attempts at the LPN model over a 20-day period. Trainees demonstrated a decrease in the total operative and renorrhaphy times with progressive attempts, as well as increase in the quality of the PN as assessed by two blinded experts. Trainees also reported an improvement in their confidence to perform a LPN, particularly with respect to tissue manipulation, intra-corporeal suturing and knot tying.

The proliferation of robotic-assisted surgery has helped overcome many of the barriers associated with LPN, resulting in shorter learning curves and subsequent growth in this area [56]. Eun and colleagues [57] described a novel technique for creating renal tumour mimics for RAPN in addition to a renal vein/inferior vena cava (IVC) tumour model for tumour thrombectomy. A tumour-mimic mixture was percutaneously injected into eight live pigs and one human cadaver in order to create 33 renal pseudotumours. A renal vein thrombus model was also created by injecting the material into the renal vein while clamped and allowing this to solidify. In addition, a renal-vein thrombus with extension into the IVC was created through partial clamping of the IVC with a long, curved bulldog clamp. Subsequent robotic radical nephrectomy with excision of the involved IVC cuff and IVC reconstruction was performed. This model was not validated by the authors but was the first demonstration of the feasibility of artificial renal vein and IVC tumour thrombus creation. While all procedures in this paper were performed robotically, such a model could be beneficial in both laparoscopic and open surgery.

Hung and colleagues [16] devised a novel robotic specific model for RAPN using an ex-vivo porcine kidney embedded with a 3.8 cm Styrofoam ball to mimic an exophytic renal tumour. The model task included tumour excision with a parenchymal margin but did not incorporate renorrhaphy. Forty-six participants were classified into 3 groups for validation, 24 novices (no robotic cases), 9 intermediates (1–100 robotic cases), and 13 experts (>100 robotic cases). Among expert surgeons, the model demonstrated excellent face and content validity. Experts rated the applicability for advanced surgeons as lower, however, which likely reflects the lack of renorrhaphy and haemostasis component associated with the simulation.

The recent advent of rapid prototyping (3D-printing) has allowed the formation of synthetic surgical renal tumour models. Several groups have already demonstrated that high-fidelity 3D printed renal models can be created using specialised software to import diagnostic cross-sectional imaging [26, 58]. Monda and colleagues [14] recently developed and validated a silicone tumour model from a 3D printed cast of a kidney with a tumour. A medium complexity tumour was selected from a patient who had previously undergone RAPN at the authors' institution, and a 3D printed negative-volume mould was created. Following this, tumour models could be repeatedly cast with silicone using this mould. The model was validated by surgeons of different training levels and demonstrated face, construct, and content validity. Through the use of a 3D printed mould, the authors were able to subsequently reproduce multiple models reliably with minimal cost.

Von Rundstedt et al. [26] used advanced 3D printing to create a high-fidelity, patient-specific, synthetic renal tumour model for the purposes of surgical rehearsal prior to actual RAPN. Surgical models were created for 10 patients and the same surgeon performed all rehearsals and actual RAPNs. The resection times and resection volumes were compared between rehearsal and live procedure and found to be predictive. Being able to predict, excision time has significant implications and could be utilised in assessing the feasibility of more complex masses for PN within an acceptable warm-ischaemia time. Furthermore, the authors reported altering their actual surgical approach in several patients based on difficulties encountered with tumour excision in the simulated rehearsal.

Maddox and colleagues [13] used a slightly different process to construct patient-specific tumour models by 3D printing an outer polymer 'shell' which was subsequently filled with an agarose gel solution to resemble normal renal parenchyma. The renal mass of interest, as well as critical structures such as renal vasculature and collecting system, was able to be pigmented to distinguish them from the normal parenchyma. It is very conceivable that 3D-printed bench models may ultimately decrease the learning curve and potentially improve surgical outcomes; however, further studies are needed to fully elucidate this effect. Current limitations include the lack of 'real-life' confounders such as perinephric fat and an active blood supply; however, it is very possible that these could be overcome in the future.

4.2.2. *Virtual reality*

No PN specific whole procedure VR simulation is commercially available at present. In an attempt to bridge the gap, Hung and colleagues [22] developed and validated an augmented reality platform now commercially available as Maestro AR (Mimic Technologies, USA). In this 'hybrid' model, augmented reality and virtual reality were combined to create a procedural specific platform that aimed to teach surgical anatomy, procedural steps and operative skills. High-definition actual surgical video of a full length RAPN was embedded with interactive VR exercises and virtual instruments in five modules: colon mobilisation, kocherisation of duodenum, hilar dissection, kidney mobilisation, tumour resection and renorrhaphy. In the final module, an embedded VR exercise was developed, whereby a mobile sponge could be manipulated around a central pivot point (renal hilum) and sutured. This platform was internally validated throughout development, and concurrent validity was assessed by comparison to an in-vivo porcine model. Expert surgeons rated the platform a useful tool for training residents and fellows particularly with respect to teaching the steps of the procedure and surgical anatomy. Performance in the VR renorrhaphy task correlated with that of the in-vivo porcine model in the intermediate and expert groups. While this platform is a significant progression towards procedure-specific VR simulation, further advances are needed before this could feasibly replace wet lab training. Allowing the user to alter the surgical view and perform embedded tasks for each step of the procedure would likely increase validity.

5. Training in renal cancer surgery

With substantial progress having being made in surgical simulation, the next challenge is formally integrating this into surgical training programmes. At present, access to simulation is often limited and certainly is not routinely incorporated into trainee assessment and technical skill development [59]. The learning curves for minimally invasive renal cancer surgery and in particular partial nephrectomy are well documented, and subsequently complications early in the surgical experience are more likely [43]. Progressing training surgeons along the learning curve in the safety of the simulation environment has obvious benefits to patient outcomes. Simulators can also be utilised at the convenience of the trainee accommodating theatre and on-call commitments and local work-time directives. Furthermore, multiple studies have demonstrated the positive attitude of trainees towards simulation with benefits reported in learning anatomy, procedural steps, skill acquisition and confidence for subsequent performance in the operating theatre [19].

An ideal training programme needs to match the trainee with appropriate levels of simulation and operating theatre exposure [60]. Initially, trainees should acquire basic skills on lower fidelity VR simulators, with higher fidelity bench models and whole procedure simulation on live animals or human cadavers introduced with subsequent progression [10]. Advancement through simulation platforms should be coupled with, or followed by, a modular training programme for live operative cases. Modular training involves the breakdown of a procedure into sequential steps of increasing difficulty. Novice trainees begin with a period of observation and assistance and subsequently progress through each graded step of the procedure [61]. Under this structure, a whole procedure shall only be attempted once a trainee has individually mastered all steps of the procedure.

The European Association of Urology (EAU) Robotic Urology Section (ERUS) training curriculum has been endorsed by British Association of Urological Surgeons (BAUS) and incorporates such an approach (**Figure 1**) [62]. This programme has already been validated for robotic-assisted radical prostatectomy [63].

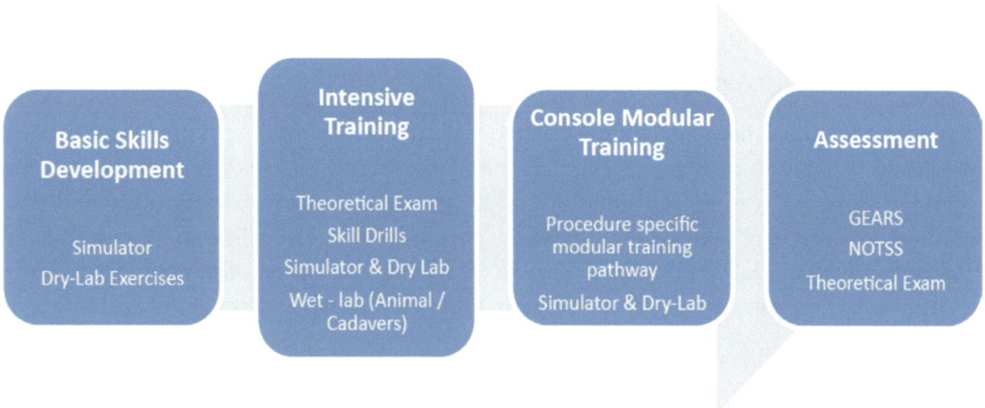

Figure 1. Proposed pathway for robotic training (reproduced with permission from BAUS robotic curriculum) [62].

Quality indicator	Proposed standard
Operative time	<200 min
Warm ischaemia time	<25 min
Estimated blood loss	<150 mL
Complication rate	<15%

Table 3. Proposed standards for outcomes on completion of robotic training.

At completion of the programme, mentors have a duty of care to the public to ensure trainees are competent. Accreditation of robotic programmes is not uniform, and formal assessment of the trainee on completion of many fellowships is not performed. Through the centralisation of programmes such as ERUS Robotic Curriculum, trainees can be assessed against a benchmark for safety and surgical quality. At a minimum, trainees should document the completed steps of procedures and meet minimum caseload requirements that correspond to the estimated learning curve for that procedure [64]. Outcome measures are a useful surrogate marker of surgical quality, and for RAPN, these are shown in **Table 3** [64].

6. Future directions

Robotic surgery is set to become even more widespread as new competitors enter the market and the demand for training will subsequently increase [65]. Surgical simulation will no doubt play a critical role meeting this demand, and an increase in the commercial availability of new platforms is anticipated. The ultimate simulation platform would be high-fidelity, low cost, readily available and translate to improved performance in the operating theatre. The validation process for new developments needs to be robust as resources are finite, and training time needs to be optimised. Even with the recent advancements in simulation, only limited evidence exists to establish the correlation between simulation performance and actual intraoperative performance [66]. This is the ultimate end-goal of the simulation process, and future research needs to focus on establishing this link.

Patient-specific simulation has already arrived with the advent of 3D printing, and progress in this field is likely to be rapid as the technology becomes more readily available and cost effective [14, 26, 58]. It is conceivable that in the near future, patient's anatomical and oncological variations will be able to be reproduced in a model with incredible accuracy and detail. Advancements in model complexity are also anticipated, and the possibility of incorporating perinephric fat and vascular perfusion will no doubt increase the utility of this technology.

Finally, artificial intelligence (AI) has had large impacts outside of medicine and is starting to be adapted into the surgical field. From autonomous surgery to virtual assistants, the possibilities are seemingly infinite. Of particular interest in training and simulation is the use of machine learning algorithms to assess and track surgical performance. These algorithms are able to rapidly analyse vast quantities of data in order to determine relationships that may not be apparent to the human eye or traditional statistical methodology [67]. Recently, Hung and colleagues [68] were able to use intraoperative data captured from a recording device (dVLogger; Intuitive Surgical, Inc.) to develop automated performance metrics (APMs) for robotic prostatectomy. Using these APMs, the authors were able to predict clinical outcomes including length of stay, procedural time and catheter duration. Such sophisticated procedural feedback could be very beneficial for training purposes and allow bespoke tailoring of training based on the identified needs of the individual.

Conflicts of interest

None declared.

Author details

Nicholas Mehan*, Nicholas Simson and Ben Challacombe

*Address all correspondence to: nicholas.mehan@gstt.nhs.uk

Guy's and St. Thomas' NHS Foundation Trust, London, United Kingdom

References

[1] Cameron JL. William Stewart Halsted. Our surgical heritage. Annals of Surgery. 1997 May; **225**(5):445-458

[2] Chikwe J, de Souza AC, Pepper JR. No time to train the surgeons. BMJ (Clinical research ed.). England. 2004;**328**:418-419

[3] European Union. European Work Time Directive. Available from: https://eur-lex.europa.eu/legal-content/EN/ALL/?uri=CELEX:32003L0088. Accessed 7th February 2019

[4] Al Bareeq R, Jayaraman S, Kiaii B, Schlachta C, Denstedt JD, Pautler SE. The role of surgical simulation and the learning curve in robot-assisted surgery. Journal of Robotic Surgery. May 2008;**2**(1):11-15

[5] Schreuder HWR, Wolswijk R, Zweemer RP, Schijven MP, Verheijen RHM. Training and learning robotic surgery, time for a more structured approach: A systematic review. BJOG: An International Journal of Obstetrics and Gynaecology. Jan 2012;**119**(2):137-149

[6] Moglia A, Ferrari V, Morelli L, Ferrari M, Mosca F, Cuschieri A. A systematic review of virtual reality simulators for robot-assisted surgery. European Urology. Jun 2016;**69**(6): 1065-1080

[7] Wass V, Van der Vleuten C, Shatzer J, Jones R. Assessment of clinical competence. Lancet. 2001;**357**(9260):945-949

[8] McDougall EM. Validation of surgical simulators. Journal of Endourology. 2007;**21**(3): 244-247

[9] Abboudi H, Khan MS, Aboumarzouk O, Guru KA, Challacombe B, Dasgupta P, et al. Current status of validation for robotic surgery simulators—A systematic review. BJU International. 2013 Feb;**111**(2):194-205

[10] Aydin A, Raison N, Khan MS, Dasgupta P, Ahmed K. Simulation-based training and assessment in urological surgery. Nature Reviews. Urology. 2016 Sep 23;**13**(9):503-519

[11] Golab A, Smektala T, Kaczmarek K, Stamirowski R, Hrab M, Slojewski M. Laparoscopic partial nephrectomy supported by training involving personalized silicone replica poured in three-dimensional printed casting mold. Journal of Laparoendoscopic & Advanced Surgical Techniques. 2017;**27**(4):420-422

[12] Fernandez A, Chen E, Moore J, Cheung C, Erdeljan P, Fuller A, et al. First prize: A phantom model as a teaching modality for laparoscopic partial nephrectomy. Journal of Endourology. 2012;**26**(1):1-5

[13] Maddox MM, Feibus A, Liu J, Wang J, Thomas R, Silberstein JL. 3D-printed soft-tissue physical models of renal malignancies for individualized surgical simulation: A feasibility study. Journal of Robotic Surgery. 2018;**12**(1):27-33

[14] Monda SM, Weese JR, Anderson BG, Vetter JM, Venkatesh R, Du K, et al. Development and validity of a silicone renal tumor model for robotic partial nephrectomy training. Urology. Apr 2018;**114**:114-120

[15] Hidalgo J, Belani J, Maxwell K, Lieber D, Talcott M, Baron P, et al. Development of exophytic tumor model for laparoscopic partial nephrectomy: Technique and initial experience. Urology. May 2005;**65**(5):872-876

[16] Hung AJ, Ng CK, Patil MB, Zehnder P, Huang E, Aron M, et al. Validation of a novel robotic-assisted partial nephrectomy surgical training model. BJU International. 2012; **110**:870-874

[17] Molinas CR, Binda MM, Mailova K, Koninckx PR. The rabbit nephrectomy model for training in laparoscopic surgery. Human Reproduction. Jan 2004;**19**(1):185-190

[18] Barret E, Guillonneau B, Cathelineau X, Validire P, Vallancien G. Laparoscopic partial nephrectomy in the pig: Comparison of three hemostasis techniques. Journal of Endourology. Apr 2001;**15**(3):307-312

[19] Ahmed K, Aydin A, Dasgupta P, Khan MS, McCabe JE. A novel cadaveric simulation program in urology. Journal of Surgical Education. Jul 1 2015;**72**(4):556-565

[20] Hung AJ, Zehnder P, Patil MB, Cai J, Ng CK, Aron M, et al. Face, content and construct validity of a novel robotic surgery simulator. The Journal of Urology. Sep 2011; **186**(3):1019-1025

[21] Brewin J, Nedas T, Challacombe B, Elhage O, Keisu J, Dasgupta P. Face, content and construct validation of the first virtual reality laparoscopic nephrectomy simulator. BJU International. Sep 2010;**106**(6):850-854

[22] Hung AJ, Shah SH, Dalag L, Shin D, Gill IS. Development and validation of a novel robotic procedure specific simulation platform: Partial nephrectomy. The Journal of Urology. Aug 2015;**194**(2):520-526

[23] Rai A, Scovell JM, Xu A, Balasubramanian A, Siller R, Kohn T, et al. Patient-specific virtual simulation—A state of the art approach to teach renal tumor localization. Urology. Oct 2018;**120**:42-48

[24] Chowriappa A, Raza SJ, Fazili A, Field E, Malito C, Samarasekera D, et al. Augmented-reality-based skills training for robot-assisted urethrovesical anastomosis: A multi-institutional randomised controlled trial. BJU International. Feb 2015;**115**(2):336-345

[25] Ahmadi H, Liu J-J. 3-D imaging and simulation for nephron sparing surgical training. Current Urology Reports. Aug 17 2016;**17**(8):58

[26] von Rundstedt F-C, Scovell JM, Agrawal S, Zaneveld J, Link RE. Utility of patient-specific silicone renal models for planning and rehearsal of complex tumour resections prior to robot-assisted laparoscopic partial nephrectomy. BJU International. Apr 2017;**119**(4):598-604

[27] Yang B, Zeng Q, Yinghao S, Wang H, Wang L, Xu C, et al. A novel training model for laparoscopic partial nephrectomy using porcine kidney. Journal of Endourology. Dec 2009;**23**(12):2029-2033

[28] Gilbody J, Prasthofer A, Ho K, Costa M. The use and effectiveness of cadaveric workshops in higher surgical training: A systematic review. Annals of the Royal College of Surgeons of England. Jul 2011;**93**(5):347-352

[29] Lendvay TS, Casale P, Sweet R, Peters C. Initial validation of a virtual-reality robotic simulator. Journal of Robotic Surgery. Sep 25 2008;**2**(3):145-149

[30] Kenney PA, Wszolek MF, Gould JJ, Libertino JA, Moinzadeh A. Face, content, and construct validity of dV-trainer, a novel virtual reality simulator for robotic surgery. Urology. 2009;**73**(6):1288-1292

[31] Schreuder HWR, Persson JEU, Wolswijk RGH, Ihse I, Schijven MP, Verheijen RHM. Validation of a novel virtual reality simulator for robotic surgery. Scientific World Journal. 2014;**2014**:1-10

[32] Alzahrani T, Haddad R, Alkhayal A, Delisle J, Drudi L, Gotlieb W, et al. Validation of the da Vinci surgical skill simulator across three surgical disciplines. Canadian Urological Association Journal. Jul 2 2013;**7**(7-8):520

[33] Kelly DC, Margules AC, Kundavaram CR, Narins H, Gomella LG, Trabulsi EJ, et al. Face, content, and construct validation of the da Vinci skills simulator. Urology. May 2012;**79**(5):1068-1072

[34] Lyons C, Goldfarb D, Jones SL, Badhiwala N, Miles B, Link R, et al. Which skills really matter? Proving face, content, and construct validity for a commercial robotic simulator. Surgical Endoscopy. Jun 7 2013;**27**(6):2020-2030

[35] Seixas-Mikelus SA, Kesavadas T, Srimathveeravalli G, Chandrasekhar R, Wilding GE, Guru KA. Face validation of a novel robotic surgical simulator. Urology. Aug 2010; **76**(2):357-360

[36] Seixas-Mikelus SA, Stegemann AP, Kesavadas T, Srimathveeravalli G, Sathyaseelan G, Chandrasekhar R, et al. Content validation of a novel robotic surgical simulator. BJU International. Apr 2011;**107**(7):1130-1135

[37] Chowriappa AJ, Shi Y, Raza SJ, Ahmed K, Stegemann A, Wilding G, et al. Development and validation of a composite scoring system for robot-assisted surgical training—The robotic skills assessment score. The Journal of Surgical Research. Dec 2013;**185**(2):561-569

[38] Whittaker G, Aydin A, Raison N, Kum F, Challacombe B, Khan MS, et al. Validation of the RobotiX mentor robotic surgery simulator. Journal of Endourology. Mar 2016; **30**(3):338-346

[39] van der Meijden OAJ, Broeders IAMJ, Schijven MP. The SEP 'robot': A valid virtual reality robotic simulator for the Da Vinci surgical system? Surgical Technology International. Apr 2010;**19**:51-58

[40] McDonough PS, Tausch TJ, Peterson AC, Brand TC. Initial validation of the ProMIS surgical simulator as an objective measure of robotic task performance. Journal of Robotic Surgery. 2011;**5**(3):195-199

[41] Kim SP, Shah ND, Weight CJ, Thompson RH, Moriarty JP, Shippee ND, et al. Contemporary trends in nephrectomy for renal cell carcinoma in the United States: Results from a population based cohort. The Journal of Urology. 2011;**186**(5):1779-1785

[42] Poon SA, Silberstein JL, Chen LY, Ehdaie B, Kim PH, Russo P. Trends in partial and radical nephrectomy: An analysis of case logs from certifying urologists. The Journal of Urology. 2013;**190**(2):464-469

[43] Capelouto CC, Kavoussi LR. Complications of laparoscopic surgery. Urology. Jul 1993;**42**(1):2-12

[44] Shalhav AL, Dabagia MD, Wagner TT, Koch MO, Lingeman JE. Training postgraduate urologists in laparoscopic surgery: The current challenge. The Journal of Urology. 2002;**167**(5):2135-2137

[45] van Velthoven RF, Piechaud PT. Training centers: An essential step to developing skills in urolaparoscopy. Current Urology Reports. 2009;**10**(2):93-96

[46] Clayman RV, Kavoussi LR, Soper NJ, Dierks SM, Meretyk S, Darcy MD, et al. Laparoscopic nephrectomy: Initial case report. The Journal of Urology. Aug 1991;**146**(2):278-282

[47] van Velthoven RF, Hoffmann P. Methods for laparoscopic training using animal models. Current Urology Reports. Mar 2006;**7**(2):114-119

[48] da Cruz JAS, Passerotti CC, Frati RMC, dos Reis ST, Okano MTR, Gouveia ÉM, et al. Surgical performance during laparoscopic radical nephrectomy is improved with training in a porcine model. Journal of Endourology. Mar 2012;**26**(3):278-282

[49] Woodrum DT, Andreatta PB, Yellamanchilli RK, Feryus L, Gauger PG, Minter RM. Construct validity of the LapSim laparoscopic surgical simulator. American Journal of Surgery. Jan 2006;**191**(1):28-32

[50] Zhang A, Hünerbein M, Dai Y, Schlag PM, Beller S. Construct validity testing of a laparoscopic surgery simulator (lap Mentor®). Surgical Endoscopy. Jun 2008;**22**(6):1440-1444

[51] Nguyen CT, Campbell SC, Novick AC. Choice of operation for clinically localized renal tumor. The Urologic Clinics of North America. Nov 2008;**35**(4):645-655

[52] Petros F, Sukumar S, Haber G-P, Dulabon L, Bhayani S, Stifelman M, et al. Multi-institutional analysis of robot-assisted partial nephrectomy for renal tumors >4 cm versus ≤4 cm in 445 consecutive patients. Journal of Endourology. Jun 4 2012;**26**(6):642-646

[53] Gill IS, Kavoussi LR, Lane BR, Blute ML, Babineau D, Colombo JR, et al. Comparison of 1800 laparoscopic and open partial nephrectomies for single renal tumors. The Journal of Urology. Jul 2007;**178**(1):41-46

[54] Thompson RH, Lane BR, Lohse CM, Leibovich BC, Fergany A, Frank I, et al. Every minute counts when the renal hilum is clamped during partial nephrectomy. European Urology. Sep 2010;**58**(3):340-345

[55] Taylor GD, Johnson DB, Hogg DC, Cadeddu JA. Development of a renal tumor mimic model for learning minimally invasive nephron sparing surgical techniques. The Journal of Urology. Jul 2004;**172**(1):382-385

[56] Deane LA, Lee HJ, Box GN, Melamud O, Yee DS, Abraham JBA, et al. Robotic versus standard laparoscopic partial/wedge nephrectomy: A comparison of intraoperative and perioperative results from a single institution. Journal of Endourology. May 2008;**22**(5):947-952

[57] Eun D, Bhandari A, Boris R, Lyall K, Bhandari M, Menon M, et al. A novel technique for creating solid renal pseudotumors and renal vein-inferior vena caval pseudothrombus in a porcine and cadaveric model. The Journal of Urology. Oct 2008;**180**(4):1510-1514

[58] Silberstein JL, Maddox MM, Dorsey P, Feibus A, Thomas R, Lee BR. Physical models of renal malignancies using standard cross-sectional imaging and 3-dimensional printers: A pilot study. Urology. Aug 2014;**84**(2):268-272

[59] Milburn JA, Khera G, Hornby ST, Malone PSC, Fitzgerald JEF. Introduction, availability and role of simulation in surgical education and training: Review of current evidence and recommendations from the Association of Surgeons in training. International Journal of Surgery. 2012;**10**(8):393-398

[60] Ahmed K, Khan R, Mottrie A, Lovegrove C, Abaza R, Ahlawat R, et al. Development of a standardised training curriculum for robotic surgery: A consensus statement from an international multidisciplinary group of experts. BJU International. 2015;**116**(1):93-101

[61] Stolzenburg J-U, Rabenalt R, Do M, Horn LC, Liatsikos EN. Modular training for residents with no prior experience with open pelvic surgery in endoscopic extraperitoneal radical prostatectomy. European Urology. Mar 2006;**49**(3):491-500

[62] British Association of Urological Surgeons. British Association of Urological Surgeons-Robotic Surgery Curriculum. Available from: https://www.baus.org.uk/_userfiles/pages/files/Publications/RoboticSurgeryCurriculum.pdf. [Accessed: 7th February 2019]

[63] Volpe A, Ahmed K, Dasgupta P, Ficarra V, Novara G, van der Poel H, et al. Pilot validation study of the European Association of Urology robotic training curriculum. European Urology. Aug 2015;**68**(2):292-299

[64] Abboudi H, Khan MS, Guru KA, Froghi S, de Win G, Van Poppel H, et al. Learning curves for urological procedures: A systematic review. BJU International. Oct 2014; **114**(4):617-629

[65] Namdarian B, Dasgupta P. What robot for tomorrow and what improvement can we expect? Current Opinion in Urology. Jan 2018:1

[66] Aghazadeh MA, Mercado MA, Pan MM, Miles BJ, Goh AC. Performance of robotic simulated skills tasks is positively associated with clinical robotic surgical performance. BJU International. 2016;**118**(3):475-481

[67] Deo RC. Machine learning in medicine. Circulation. 2015;**132**(20):1920-1930

[68] Hung AJ, Chen J, Gill IS. Automated performance metrics and machine learning algorithms to measure surgeon performance and anticipate clinical outcomes in robotic surgery. JAMA Surgery. 2018; **153**(8):770-771

Chapter 5

Augmented Reality in Kidney Cancer

Keshav Shree Mudgal and Neelanjan Das

Additional information is available at the end of the chapter

http://dx.doi.org/10.5772/intechopen.81890

Abstract

Augmented reality(AR) is the concept of a digitally created perception that enhances components of the real-world to allow better engagement with it. Within healthcare, there has been a recent expansion of AR solutions, especially in the field of surgery. Traditional renal cancer surgery has been largely replaced by minimally invasive laparoscopic (or robotic) partial nephrectomies. This has meant loss of certain intra-operative experiences such as haptic feedback and AR can aid this replacement with enhanced visual and patient-specific feedback. The kidney is a dynamic organ and current AR development has revolved around specific surgical stages such as safe arterial clamping and perfecting tumour margins. This chapter discusses the current state of AR technology in these areas with key attention to the aspects of image registration, organ tracking, tissue deformation and live imaging. The chapter then discusses limitations of AR, such as intentional blindness and depth perception and provides potential future ideas and solutions. These include inventions such as AR headsets and 3D-printed renal models (with the possibility of remote surgical intervention). AR provides a very positive outcome for the future of truly minimally invasive renal surgery. However, current AR needs validation, cost evaluation and thorough planning before being safely integrated into everyday surgical practice.

Keywords: augmented reality, AR, nephrectomies, partial nephrectomies, image registration, surface registration, organ tracking, tissue deformation, renal artery clamping, safe selective arterial clamping, precise tumour margin, live imaging, virtual reality, AR headset, 3D printing

1. What is augmented reality?

The term "augmented reality" was coined by the Boeing researcher, Thomas Caudell in 1990 to describe a projection of digital graphics onto a physical working space for use by aircraft engineers [1]. Augmented reality (AR) has come a long way since, however the fundamental idea remains the same: working in a real-world environment where the components of the environment are enhanced by a digitally-created perception. This perception can include multiple sensory inputs including visual, auditory, haptic, somatosensory and olfactory senses.

In healthcare, AR progression has involved a wide range of medical areas—from aiding clinic appointments by easy access to electronic health records and patient times, to wearable glasses that help teach life-skills to children on the autism spectrum [2]. However, it seems that the biggest expansion of AR is seen in enhancing surgical procedures. Project DR is one such development—internal organs as 3D reconstructions of the patient's anatomy are projected onto the patient's skin and this allows a constant view of the person's anatomy that moves with patient in real time. This is achieved by the amalgamation of CT/MRI imaging, motion-sensing infrared sensors and projectors all working as one unit [3]. Another example is the use of Microsoft's HoloLens glasses for trauma and plastic surgeries (Imperial College London and St Mary's Hospital). The "hologram" (made from pre-op imaging) through the lens of the glasses projects onto the patient's skin and allows a "mixed reality" which lets the surgeon track the pathways of the various blood vessels and bones to be operated upon [4]. This technology promises to let surgeons carefully plan and execute breast reconstruction surgeries in the future. Google glass is another extensively used example of AR. The 'glasses' allow an augmented field of view and surgeons have used these for all purposes from navigation tools to display ultrasound imaging, to remote videoconferencing in intraoperative communication [5].

2. Augmented reality vs. virtual reality?

Whilst augmented reality is technology that overlays on the reality that already exists around us, virtual reality (VR) is a complete replacement of the real world with a simulated one. This means that AR allows us to interact and work with the real world, whilst getting an enhanced input from an informed digital world.

VR has shown to be a great teaching tool. Moglia et al. [6] found that subjects trained on virtual simulators were better than the control group (using conventional methods). An example is the Uro Tainer, a validated simulator for teaching transurethral resection of bladder tumours [7]. VR has not only shown promise in surgery, but also other areas like simulation of shock trauma centres (where surgeons can be trained in high pressured environments) [8] and Virtual Environment for Radiotherapy Training (VERT)—a system built to reduce anxiety in breast cancer patients [9].

3. VR in kidney cancer

Within renal cancer, a VR system has been developed by Rai et al. that enhances the novice's ability to localise renal tumour margins [10]. Specific to nephrectomies, Makiyama et al. [11] have developed a VR "rehearsal" simulator for surgeons that plans for anatomical abnormalities and incorporates haptic feedback for pre-operative training. Ueno et al. have developed VR addressing another aspect of nephrectomies—reducing postoperative urine leakage by predicting open urinary tracts on preoperative 3D CT—reconstructions [12]. Whereas, VR might be a great teaching tool in simulated nephrectomies, AR is the platform for practise of medicine and surgery—on real people.

4. Augmented reality in renal cancer

In renal cancer surgery, open nephrectomies for the most part, have been replaced by minimally invasive laparoscopic surgeries. This has led to many positive outcomes, including decreased intra-op blood loss and shorter hospital stay [13]. Furthermore, partial nephrectomies have shown an overall improved survival over radical nephrectomies, [14] and this has been made possible due to crucial development in laparoscopic and robotic-assisted surgery [15]. However, there have also been some drawbacks. One of these is the loss of haptic feedback that would usually allow the surgeon to manoeuvre intra-operatively and make instinctive decisions. AR can aid the loss in this feedback sense by replacing it with an enhancement in another—the visual sense.

AR systems exist that allow surgeons to see detailed anatomical structures on the surface of the organ by projecting pre-operative CT/MRI images onto a live laparoscopic video. This allows the view of the patient-unique renal anatomy, it's neighbouring structures and its relation to the rest of the intra-abdominal anatomy [16]. Having this added information can aid the surgeon in planning and executing an accurate and precise partial or total nephrectomy. Exact areas to be incised can be planned and damage to nearby delicate structures such as

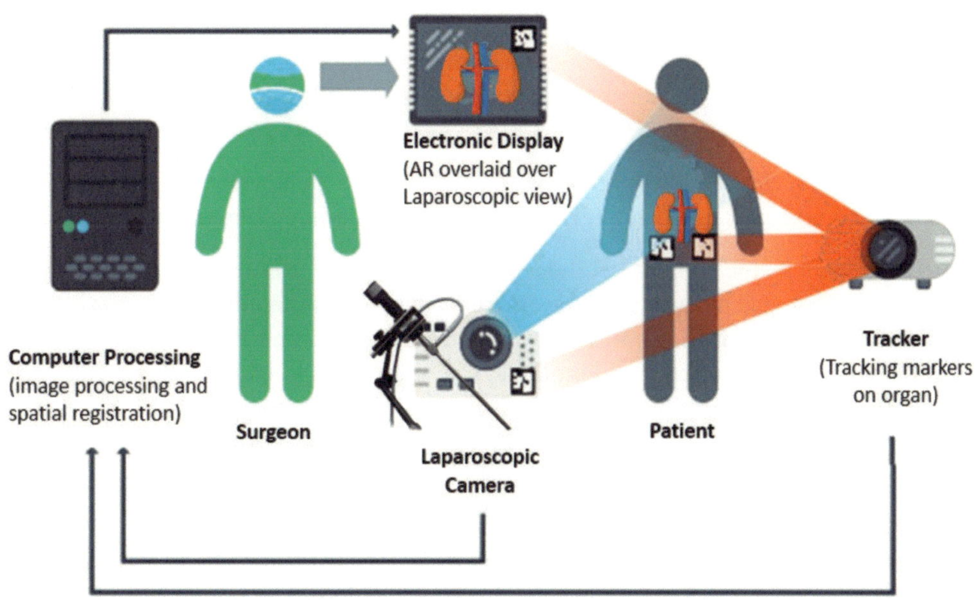

Figure 1. An illustration showing the basic components involved in AR. "the basic method is to superimpose a computer generated image on a real-world imagery captured by a camera and displaying the combination of these on a computer, tablet PC or a video projector. The main advantage of AR is that the surgeon is not forced to look away from the surgical site as opposed to common visualisation techniques." Adapted from: 'Recent Development of Augmented Reality in Surgery: A Review' [20].

renal vasculature and ureters can be reduced. AR can also reduce excision margins—to spare as many well-functioning nephrons and reduce the risk and progression of chronic renal insufficiency [17] (**Figure 1**).

For an AR system to be ideal, the full length of a surgical procedure need to be "augmented." This requires 3 essential features (as adapted by a recent review by Hughes-Hallet et al. [18]): image registration, organ tracking and adapting to intra-operative tissue deformation. In the following chapter, I will describe, in detail, these aspects of AR specific to nephrectomies.

5. Image registration

This is the process where a medical imaging is aligned with the patient's anatomy to form a visually projected overlay. This can be done through various methods, but the fundamentals rely upon multiple data points being processed to align medical imaging with the best corresponding surface-landmarks on an organ/patient's anatomy.

Image registration can be used in pre-operative planning stage and in the intra-operative stage. The planning stage involves using the combined imaging overlay (of CT scans and MRIs) onto the kidney to identify key structures of importance—hilar vasculature, the spatial attributes of the kidney and their relationship with the renal collecting system. This helps build a roadmap of what the surgery will involve and although it does not require accuracy to the millimetre (as is involved in the intra-operative phase) it allows a pretty good estimation to the planned steps in surgery.

The intra-operative stage requires higher precision image registration and more importantly, dynamic correspondence with the moving organ. This is to allow tumour resection margins that can be accurate to the millimetre.

Hughes-Hallet [18] classify image registration used by AR developers into 3 main subtypes: manual registration, surface-based registration and 3D registration (**Figure 2**).

Manual registration is the simplest method where the surgeon uses their anatomical knowledge to align a projected imaging onto the organ. Examples of this method have involved: fusing 3D reconstructions with live operative view, projecting intra-abdominal anatomy onto the skin and colour coded projection to highlight "safe zones" of resection margins. These have offered quite a hands-on approach with relatively little planning compared to other registration methods—allowing a low barrier to entry, good anatomical orientation and relatively good awareness of disease-free parenchyma. Manual registration does not allow accurate estimates of tumour margins and is mostly limited to the planning phase.

Surface based registration method involves using a tracked instrument to build a topographical map of the internal organ. This has been most extensively used in robotic partial nephrectomy—an example being the da Vinci robot. The laparoscopic instrument tip of the robot can touch a point on the live kidney and this information along with the joint positions sense of the robotic arms can calculate a position in space to build a surface anatomy of the kidney.

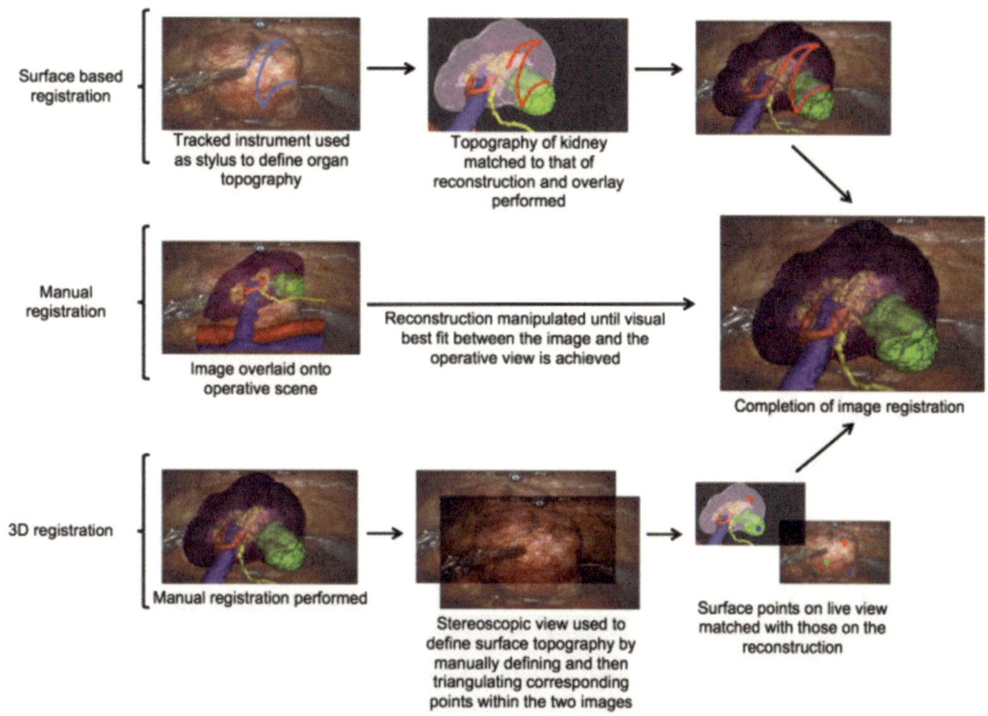

Figure 2. Different methods of image registration [18].

The surface anatomy can then be correlated with 3D reconstruction imaging of the patient and projected onto the surgeon's operating view.

This method is a form of internal tracking relying on a good tracking instrument and accurate computer algorithms to provide the correct position of the organ being operated on. Errors in the estimated spatial position of the instrument tip can create unsafe image registration that would be inaccurate for tumour margins of partial nephrectomies.

This registration method is more accurate than manual registration as it provides automation and reduces the surgical workload. However, there are still areas for improvement such as better tracking methods. External tracking, where the organ is tracked from the outside is another method. Examples include optical, magnetic and laser but there are inherent drawbacks such as optical tracking requires a direct line of sight and magnetic tracking requiring physical placement of a tracer in the organ.

A recent advancement in surface-based registration was developed by Edgcumbe et al. where a miniature laser projector called 'Pico lantern' can be dropped into the patient's abdomen. It can then be picked up by laparoscopic instruments and perform surface recognition on the abdominal organ. Using surface-based recognition, it can then project the pre-operative image on the surface of the organ. The projector is visually tracked in the laparoscopic field of view and has been tested in porcine kidneys and in detecting pulsatile motion in carotid arteries [19].

3D-CT stereoscopic image registration uses 2 cameras that focus on the same object in space and a combination of the perspectives from 2 separate viewpoints allows a spatial reference for the object. This system has been used for kidneys by isolating a point on the surface of the organ, which can then be aligned to the corresponding point on a 3D reconstruction image. Using this as the centre of rotation, the surgeon can manipulate the operative view for a better understanding of field of operation. This system has shown average target registration error of less than 1 mm and mean registration duration of 48.1 s i.e. more accurate resection margins, faster registration and reduced theatre time.

There is however, a lack of organ tracking in this system, meaning that each movement of the camera needs a new image registration. Furthermore, stereoscopic cameras are usually very expensive and require large handling computer systems, which is another limitation to adoption of this method.

6. Organ tracking

An ideal AR system would allow the organ to be tracked in real time as it is affected by respiration, tissue deformation and other complications like bleeding. The renal system is particularly vulnerable to these dynamic changes compared to other organs systems like the brain or bones where rigid image registration systems are the norm and do not require as much tracking. The registered image projected into the operative view should be locked and dynamically move with the organ and the laparoscopic camera.

There are many types of tracking studied in AR surgery. These have mainly included optical tracking where optical markers on the organ allow a measured position of the laparoscopic camera relative to the organ and move with the organ [20]. Infra-red tracking is another method which involves the use of infrared-emitting diode markers. The main issue with optical tracking is instruments obscuring the direct view of field (required for tracking) and a limited depth perception. Infra-red tracking has the issue of selecting the correct anatomical landmarks as markers—mismatches can occur due to deformations, compression and intraoperative haemorrhaging. Many studies have failed to achieve accurate registration of dynamic intra-abdominal organs with infra-red [21].

Electromagnetic tracking is another way of doing this—this has been explored by use of the wireless trackers an ex-vivo bovine partial nephrectomy model. This involved surrounding the tumour within the kidney with magnetic transponders which relayed back to the surgeon and in conjunction with optical camera tracking, a partial nephrectomy was performed [22]. There are limitations to this tracking method as magnetic fields can have interference from laparoscopic instruments and operating tables. The method also requires placement of the magnetic transponders into the target organ and it is currently hard to achieve an alignment error of less than 5 mm—a tumour margin error too great for accurate partial nephrectomies [23].

An alternative has been explored by Yip et al. where 3D stereoscopic image registration has been combined this with tracking algorithms—producing only 1.3–3.3 mm degree of error

[24]. More recently, Edgcumbe et al. have developed a tracking device called the Dynamic Augmented Reality Tracker (DART). This is a 3D-printed stainless-steel tracker that can be anchored to a fixed position on the kidney relative to the tumour. This, with the help of an ultrasound transducer, can then be used to track the location of surgical instruments relative to the tumour in real time. This system has been named ARUNS (Augmented Reality Ultrasound Navigation System) and was used in the robotic-assisted excision of a phantom kidney tumour [25].

Vávra et al., in their recent review, comment that it may be possible to track organ movement without physical markers in the future. Some of these methods explored include algorithms to predict real-time movement of organs, physics-based deformation models, natural points of reference as tracking points and the use of red-green-blue cameras to perform image registration without markers. They also comment that whilst the average marker associated registration takes 8 min, a recent marker-less system only took about 5 min [20].

7. Tissue deformation

The kidney is a dynamic organ and renal surgery involves deformation of the anatomy. Every step in the operation changes the initially projected image registration [26] and for an ideal AR system, there need to be real time feedback for tracing this. An answer to this would be the development of computer algorithms to predict changes in anatomy at crucial steps such as clamping of the renal arteries and surgical dissection at tumour margins. Algorithms can also be developed to predict the effect of ongoing influences on the organ position such as respiratory patterns and peritoneal insufflation.

There have been some tissue deformation models considering renal clamping, incision and external pressure loads to the kidney like intra-operative insufflation. Some of these have shown an improvement of 29% in the registration error when compared to a non-deformation model. However, in these models, the kidney is assumed to have a linear elastic behaviour and the models have been based on ex-vivo kidneys. Another method has been developed taking the diaphragm motion and its influence on kidney motion into consideration—this has used preoperative CT scans during inspiration and expiration and computer errors have been shown to be less than 2 mm in predicting kidney positions [27].

Although there is a scarcity of studies in this area, one study showed that mathematical models were able to predict up to 52% of the operative deformation in porcine kidneys when compared to pre and post-op CT imaging [28].

Baumhauer et al. [29] have proposed a system to answer tissue deformation by insertion of custom-designed navigation aids into the kidney and using "inside-out tracking." This is where the CT-scan can provide real-time spatial awareness by identifying the navigation aids and projecting imaging onto the laparoscopic view. Tested in a virtual environment, this system showed a visualisation error of 1.36 mm (adequately accurate). This system was replicated in the clinical setting by Teber et al. [30] where 10 patients had retroperitoneal laparoscopic partial nephrectomies. The results showed zero cases with a positive surgical margin, zero complication rate and zero conversion to open surgery. This system does however, require placement of aids (like 1.5 cm long needles) into the kidney and is dependent on at least 4 aids being present. This brings risks of damage to healthy parenchyma and aids being lost intra-op.

An answer to tissue deformation could lie closer to technology used within the commercial sector. Advanced facial recognition software used in simulating real time 'Apple animojis' [31] could be adapted to intra-operative kidneys. The software could delineate an optical real time map of the kidney which would change with the active deformation.

8. Live imaging

Live imaging is an answer to capturing tissue deformation as it allows real-time dynamic information on the kidney and removes the need to 'estimate' structural changes in the tissue. Ultrasound is one live imaging modality that has shown high sensitivity and specificity at identifying tumour margins [32, 33]. There have been several studies using live USS to aid AR. Kang et al. [34] merged live laparoscopic ultrasound images on stereoscopic video and showed accuracy of image-to-video correlation of up to 2.76 mm. Kang et al. claim this aids in depth perception and better visualisation of internal structures. Cheung et al. demonstrated that a fused video-USS model for phantom partial nephrectomy allowed for a 1.1 mm tumour resection margin (with 2D fusion) for endophytic tumours [35].

Singla et al. [36] showed in their study, that simulated healthy renal tissue excised was reduced from an average 30.6–17.5 cm^3 using intra-operative USS based AR. This technique would be especially beneficial in critical structures like endophytic renal tumours where most of the tumour lies below the organ surface—(endophytic tumours currently have complication rate of nearly 50%).

These are all however preliminary studies and are based on phantom models which does not represent the true nature of the operation in vivo. A majority of studies have involved manual registration with labour intensive methods that are unrealistic to be currently used in-vivo. Cheung et al. found that although there was 29% reduction in planning time with the USS-fused model, the tumour required longer operative times (being up to 39% slower than the conventional system) [35].

Some projects have combined all three aspects of AR named above. An example of this is PARIS (projector-based AR intracorporeal system)—a method by Edgcumbe et al. [37] where there is a combination of a tracked projector, tracked marker and laparoscopic ultrasound transducer. This has been used in 16 simulated laparoscopic partial nephrectomies, where cancerous tumours were projected onto the kidney surface and this projection moved with kidney. An ultrasound allowed live imaging of the intra-operative environment. This study showed better identification of underlying anatomy and tumour boundaries to show signification reduction in healthy tissue excised.

http://dx.doi.org/10.5772/intechopen.81890

9. Specific aspects of renal cancer surgery focused upon in AR development

There are a few aspects of renal cancer surgery (highlighted by Detmer et al. [27]), that AR development has specifically focused on. These include precise tumour resection and safe selective arterial clamping.

We have covered the issue of a precise tumour resection to preserve maximum healthy tissue throughout the chapter. However, Detmer et al. specifically mention some studies to tackle this very area. Ukimara and Gill [38] describe using different colours to signify increasing distance from the tumour and this is overlaid on the AR field of view. Another method uses contouring of the organ around the tumour margin to highlight the tumour itself. Uncertainty of the tumour margin has also been encoded by using different colours to signify certain and uncertain areas of the margin [27].

Renal artery clamping is a crucial procedural step as ischemia needs to be limited to tumour-specific parenchyma. This is done by identifying and clamping only the tumour specific arterial branches (usually tertiary or higher-order). This concept has been described as "zero-ischaemia" [39]. There have been some studies detecting renal vessels underneath the organ surface and several studies aiming to identify arterial branches for selective clamping with variable success. These have been used for pre-operative planning and some intraoperative guidance. Development has been mostly based in manual registration techniques with displays over the laparoscopic view or on a separate screen [27].

10. Current limitations

This chapter has described the different aspects of AR in renal cancer and areas that have seen progress. However, there are current limitations holding back the use of AR technology in the clinical set-up. Vavar et al. and Detmer et al. have highlighted some of these (as below):

1. Pre-operative medical imaging: currently all reconstructed images need preparing in advance by powerful processing systems. Not only is this expense, it is time consuming. With technological advancement—real-time high-resolution medical imaging and 3D reconstructions could be the norm. This would be displayed in real time intraoperatively and would markedly reduce/eliminate pre-op times.

2. Inattentional blindness: not seeing an unexpected object in the field of view. This has especially been an issue with 3D image registrations, where the surgeon does not register an object as they were not expecting it to be part of that procedural step. With the development of AR headsets, there will be more information displayed to the operating surgeon. This can be distracting and there needs to be a conscious effort towards only displaying vital information or switching between different sets of information. Further work needs to be done on reducing human factor issues and making the human-computer interface more ergonomic.

3. Depth perception: whilst current image registration involves imaging modalities such as MRI and CTs, the 2D or 3D imaging does not allow a full understanding of intraabdominal environment. Minimally invasive surgery has especially deprived the depth perception aspect of the surgical experience. Vávra et al. [20] suggest depth-sensing cameras could aid AR in the future.

4. Hardware capacities: current AR is limited by the *hardware capacities* and thus processing power of computer systems they are run on. Vizua is a company developing "cloudification" and "application roaming" where the AR applications and data can be remotely managed to get the highest computing power and access to large datasets. A platform such as this could be incorporated into AR systems and answer issues of latency in image registration and access to good quality imaging (live or pre-operative).

5. Other issues mentioned include tissue deformation studies only focusing on one source of deformation, 3D imaging requiring better image registration and the issue of simulation sickness (whilst using heavy current AR headsets).

Regardless of what aspect of AR being explored, there is little quantitative data on in-vivo procedures. Only 20 studies were found by a recent review [27] where AR had been used in clinical practice, and only 9 studies had 10 or more patients in the study. There is a crucial need for *clinical validity* to show improved patient outcomes and safety from using AR in renal interventions.

11. Future ideas/solutions

As Hughes-Hallet mention, there is a *"one-size-fits-all"* approach in most AR developments. Single imaging and imaging registration modalities have been used in isolation for many systems. Every surgical case is different however, and a combination of different modalities can provide a more accurate answer. Below are some examples of adjuncts that could aid current AR:

1. NIRF—near infrared fluorescence is a type of imaging where indocyanine green (ICG) dye is injected into the body and it can be used to illuminate intravascular renal parenchyma. This can allow the surgeon to detect blood vessels under the organ surface and detect tissue abnormalities. Although NIRF has not shown much promise in predicting malignancy in partial nephrectomies, it has shown a reduction in global renal ischaemia. NIRF has been used in robot-assisted surgery to achieve super-selective arterial clamping—avoiding main arterial clamping in 65% of patients in a recent study. Infusion of ICG dye pre and post arterial clamping ensured that there was selective ischaemia only to the tumour region and adequate renal perfusion was achieved post-clamp removal. This imaging could be used in conjunction with AR to further aid live visual feedback, organ tracking and have better post-op renal functioning [40].

2. Imperial College London's iKnife could be used in conjunction with AR [41]. This 'Intelligent knife' is a surgical scalpel that chemically tests the tissue it has contact with. It uses Rapid Evaporative Ionisation Mass Spectrometry (REIMS) for real time analysis of the aerosols created from diathermy of tissues. iKnife has been used in gynaecological

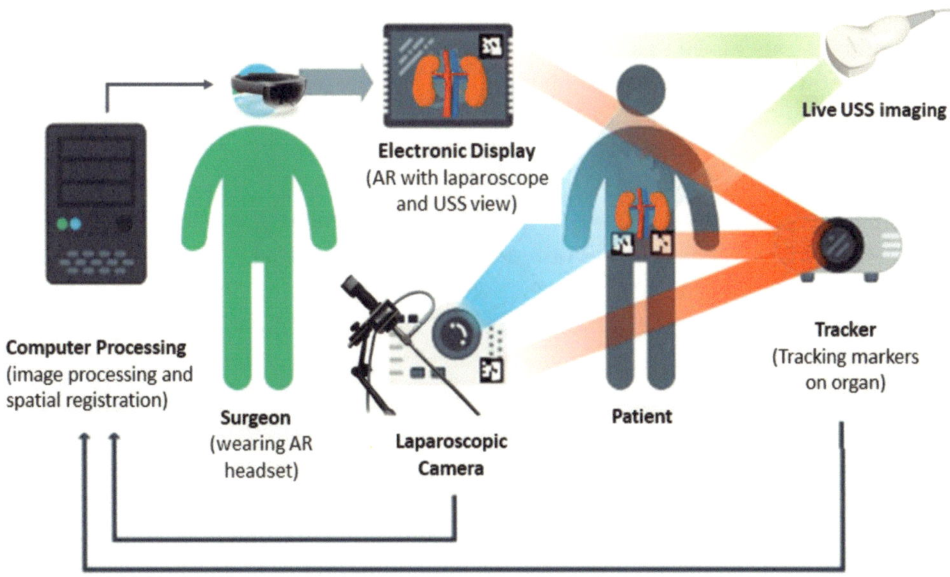

Figure 3. AR of the future. AR involving additional input from live USS imaging, organ trackers and other vital observations and patient data all being fed into the AR headset—providing a hands free platform.

tissues to distinguish between normal, borderline and malignant tissue [42] and this could be used in partial nephrectomies to give real time feedback for a precise tumour margin.

3. AR headset—this is a device that is being engineered simultaneously in many major US hospitals. Dr. Varshey and Dr. Murthi, are developing one such headset with the engineering team at the "Augmentarium" (University of Maryland). They hope to develop a system where a headset such as the Microsoft HoloLens can be worn by the surgeon and real-time USS of the patient or vital signs and patient data can be overlaid on the felid of view. This would drastically reduce the number of displays a surgeon has to usually track during an operation. Used in conjunction with dynamic image projection, the AR headset would be a good answer to cover the abovementioned 3 aspects of AR in partial nephrectomies [43].

   The AR headset hopes to eliminate any obstructions in the surgeon's view as compared to conventional methods. Furthermore, voice recognition and gesture recognition development would enable hands-free control of the device—which would allow the surgeon to interact with the AR whilst maintaining a sterile environment [20] (**Figure 3**).

4. 3D printing—model replications of the patient's kidney can be printed using pre-operative CT/MRIs and these can be used to perform simulated operations prior to placing a knife onto the patient's skin. SIMPeds 3D Print at the Boston Children's Hospital offers exactly this—rapid printing and prototyping for nearly any organ in the human body [44]. Examples of this have been used to replicate and operate on difficult paediatric brain tumours [45], facial reconstructions and orthopaedic surgeries amongst many others [46]. This has allowed surgeons to simulate a realistic assessment of the individual's organ where it can be felt, touched and cut at precise margins. 3D printed surgical planning of partial

nephrectomies has been explored by Zhang et al. [46] where face and content validity was obtained by 4 experienced laparoscopic urologists. A pilot study by Silberstein et al. [47] envisioned that 3D models could enhance the surgeon's (and patient's) understanding of the individual's renal malignancy anatomy—this would be especially beneficial in difficulties such as anatomical anomalies and precise segmental artery clamping [48].

Extrapolating further from this idea, 3D printed kidneys could also allow remote surgical procedures. An idea in conjunction with this was put forward by Dr. Murthi at a recent VR and AR applications gathering at Newseum, Washington, D.C [8]. She foresaw VR and AR working together to support patient care. An initial AR on the patient including imaging and medical data would allow the clinician to assess the patient's condition (in this case, anatomy) and a remote VR system could allow the clinician to see what the initial AR has shown and consequently advise and provide insight. An augmented nephrectomy system could benefit surgeons where instead of advising, they could operate remotely on replicated 3D models (representing in-vivo kidneys). Initial AR collected locally from the patient could be remotely projected as VR onto a 3D model and a surgeon could perform a partial nephrectomy which could be translated to the real kidney with the help of local robotic da Vinci machines. This model would allow constant feedback between the AR and VR systems and remote operations could be an answer to lack of surgical resources in healthcare deprived areas around the world.

12. Conclusion

Being the 7th most common cancer in the UK [49], renal cancer surgery can really benefit from this emerging symbiotic relationship between surgeon and AR. Since the first uses of AR for partial nephrectomy, there have been reported improvements in the familiarisation of the patient's anatomy and practicality of AR [38]. However, as Bernhardt et al. discuss in a laparoscopic AR review, there is much advancement to be made in image registration, live tracking and depth perception. Detmer et al. in their review (of AR and VR technology in renal cancers) also highlight the need for resolution of human factors and the need for large scale clinical studies that are currently sparse. In conclusion, recent AR development has worked towards systems aiming to be on par with conventional navigational techniques. Whilst some technology is achieving this in isolation, there still lie barriers of validation, cost evaluation and practical application in the way. In summary, there is much to be achieved before AR systems are precise and safe enough to be integrated into regular clinical practise.

Author details

Keshav Shree Mudgal[1*] and Neelanjan Das[2]

*Address all correspondence to: keshav.mudgal@nhs.net

1 King's College Hospital Foundation Trust, London, United Kingdom

2 East Kent Hospitals Foundation Trust, Canterbury, Kent, United Kingdom

References

[1] Interaction Design Foundation. Augmented Reality—The Past, The Present and The Future [Accessed 01/10/2018]

[2] Mesko B. The Top 9 Augmented Reality Companies in Healthcare. Available from: http://scholar.aci.info/view/156566a01ed00110002/15e38d4c7c500013f25998b

[3] Augmented reality system lets doctors see under patients' skin without the scalpel. Medical Devices & Surgical Technology Week. 2018. pp. 164

[4] Augmented reality helps surgeons to 'see through' tissue and reconnect blood vessels. Medical Devices & Surgical Technology Week. 2018. pp. 213

[5] Wei NJ, Dougherty B, Myers A, Badawy SM. Using Google glass in surgical settings: Systematic review. JMIR mHealth and uHealth. 2018;**6**(3):e54. DOI: 10.2196/mhealth.9409. Available from: https://www.ncbi.nlm.nih.gov/pubmed/29510969

[6] Moglia A, Ferrari V, Morelli L, Ferrari M, Mosca F, Cuschieri A. A systematic review of virtual reality simulators for robot-assisted surgery. 2016. Available from: http://discovery.dundee.ac.uk/portal/en/theses/a-systematic-review-of-virtual-reality-simulators-for-robot-assisted-surgery(00243bee-f90b-486d-95cd-e0fcb51d8d15).html

[7] Schulz GB, Grimm T, Buchner A, Jokisch F, Casuscelli J, Kretschmer A, et al. Validation of a high-end virtual reality simulator for training transurethral resection of bladder tumors. Journal of Surgical Education. 2018. DOI: 10.1016/j.jsurg.2018.08.001. Available from: https://www.sciencedirect.com/science/article/pii/S1931720418304021

[8] Likowski A. Augmenting Reality in the Operating Room. Available from: https://www.umaryland.edu/news/archived-news/march-2017/newspressreleaseshottopics/augmenting-reality-in-the-operating-room.php [Accessed September 12, 2018]

[9] Jimenez Y, Cumming S, Wang W, Stuart K, Thwaites D, Lewis S. Patient education using virtual reality increases knowledge and positive experience for breast cancer patients undergoing radiation therapy. Supportive Care in Cancer. 2018;**26**(8):2879-2888. Available from. DOI: 10.1007/s00520-018-4114-4. Available from: https://www.ncbi.nlm.nih.gov/pubmed/29536200

[10] Rai A, Scovell JM, Xu A, Balasubramanian A, Siller R, Kohn T, et al. Patient-specific virtual simulation—A state of the art approach to teach renal tumor localization. Urology. 2018;**120**:42-48. Available from: doi: 10.1016/j.urology.2018.04.043 Available from: https://www.sciencedirect.com/science/article/pii/S0090429518305405

[11] Makiyama K, Nagasaka M, Inuiya T, Takanami K, Ogata M, Kubota Y. Development of a patient-specific simulator for laparoscopic renal surgery. International Journal of Urology. 2012;**19**(9):829-835. DOI: 10.1111/j.1442-2042.2012.03053.x

[12] Ueno D, Makiyama K, Yamanaka H, Ijiri T, Yokota H, Kubota Y. Prediction of open urinary tract in laparoscopic partial nephrectomy by virtual resection plane visualization.

BMC Urology. 2014;**14**(1):47. DOI: 10.1186/1471-2490-14-47. Available from: https://www.ncbi.nlm.nih.gov/pubmed/24927795

[13] Gill IS, Kavoussi LR, Lane BR, Blute ML, Babineau D, Colombo JR, et al. Comparison of 1,800 laparoscopic and open partial nephrectomies for single renal tumors. The Journal of Urology. 2007;**178**(1):41-46. DOI: 10.1016/j.juro.2007.03.038. Available from: https://www.clinicalkey.es/playcontent/1-s2.0-S0022534707005502

[14] Tan H, Norton EC, Ye Z, Hafez KS, Gore JL and Miller DC. Long-term Survival Following Partial vs Radical Nephrectomy Among Older Patients With Early-Stage Kidney Cancer. JAMA. 2012;**307**(15):1629-1635. Available from: doi: 10.1001/jama.2012.475 Available from: http://dx.doi.org/10.1001/jama.2012.475

[15] Ellison JS, Montgomery JS, Wolf JS, Hafez KS, Miller DC, Weizer AZ. A matched comparison of perioperative outcomes of a single laparoscopic surgeon versus a multisurgeon robot-assisted cohort for partial nephrectomy. The Journal of Urology. 2012;**188**(1):45-50. DOI: 10.1016/j.juro.2012.02.2570. Available from: https://www.clinicalkey.es/playcontent/1-s2.0-S0022534712029692

[16] Chauvet P, Collins T, Debize C, Novais-Gameiro L, Pereira B, Bartoli A, et al. Augmented reality in a tumor resection model. Surgical Endoscopy. 2018;**32**(3):1192-1201. DOI: 10.1007/s00464-017-5791-7. Available from: https://www.ncbi.nlm.nih.gov/pubmed/28812157

[17] Gill IS, Aron M, Gervais DA, Jewett MAS. Small renal mass. The New England Journal of Medicine. 2010;**362**(7):624-634. DOI: 10.1056/NEJMcp0910041. Available from: http://content.nejm.org/cgi/content/extract/362/7/624

[18] Hughes-Hallett A, Mayer EK, Marcus HJ, Cundy TP, Pratt PJ, Darzi AW, et al. Augmented reality partial nephrectomy: Examining the current status and future perspectives. Urology. 2014;**83**(2):266-273. DOI: 10.1016/j.urology.2013.08.049. Available from: https://www.clinicalkey.es/playcontent/1-s2.0-S0090429513011333

[19] Edgcumbe P, Pratt P, Yang G, Nguan C, Rohling R. Pico lantern: Surface reconstruction and augmented reality in laparoscopic surgery using a pick-up laser projector. Medical Image Analysis. 2015;**25**(1):95-102. DOI: 10.1016/j.media.2015.04.008. Available from: https://www.sciencedirect.com/science/article/pii/S1361841515000584

[20] Vávra P, Roman J, Zonča P, Ihnát P, Němec M, Kumar J, et al. Recent development of augmented reality in surgery: A review. Journal of Healthcare Engineering. 2017;**2017**: 4574172-4574179. DOI: 10.1155/2017/4574172. Available from: https://www.ncbi.nlm.nih.gov/pubmed/29065604

[21] Okamoto T, Onda S, Yanaga K, Suzuki N, Hattori A. Clinical application of navigation surgery using augmented reality in the abdominal field. Surgery Today. 2015;**45**(4):397-406. DOI: 10.1007/s00595-014-0946-9. Available from: https://www.ncbi.nlm.nih.gov/pubmed/24898629

[22] Nakamoto M, Ukimura O, Gill I, Mahadevan A, Miki T, Hashizume M, et al. Realtime organ tracking for endoscopic augmented reality visualization using miniature wireless magnetic tracker. In: Medical Imaging and Augmented Reality. Berlin, Heidelberg: Springer Berlin Heidelberg; 2008. pp. 359-366

[23] Sutherland SE, Resnick MI, Maclennan GT, Goldman HB. Does the size of the surgical margin in partial nephrectomy for renal cell cancer really matter? The Journal of Urology. 2002;**167**(1):61-64. DOI: 10.1016/S0022-5347(05)65383-9. Available from: https://www.sciencedirect.com/science/article/pii/S0022534705653839

[24] Yip MC, Lowe DG, Salcudean SE, Rohling RN, Nguan CY. Tissue tracking and registration for image-guided surgery. IEEE Transactions on Medical Imaging. 2012;**31**(11): 2169-2182. DOI: 10.1109/TMI.2012.2212718. Available from: https://ieeexplore.ieee.org/document/6264103

[25] Edgcumbe P, Singla R, Pratt P, Schneider C, Nguan C, Rohling R. Augmented Reality Imaging for Robot-Assisted Partial Nephrectomy Surgery. Vol. 9805. Switzerland: Springer International Publishing; 2016. pp. 139-150. Available from: https://link.springer.com/content/pdf/10.1007%2F978-3-319-43775-0_13.pdf

[26] Schneider C, Nguan C, Longpre M, Rohling R, Salcudean S. Motion of the kidney between preoperative and intraoperative positioning. IEEE Transactions on Biomedical Engineering. 2013;**60**(6):1619-1627. DOI: 10.1109/TBME.2013.2239644. Available from: https://ieeexplore.ieee.org/document/6410004

[27] Detmer FJ, Hettig J, Schindele D, Schostak M, Hansen C. Virtual and augmented reality systems for renal interventions: A systematic review. IEEE Reviews in Biomedical Engineering. 2017;**10**:78-94. DOI: 10.1109/RBME.2017.2749527. Available from: https://ieeexplore.ieee.org/document/8026164

[28] Altamar HO, Ong RE, Glisson CL, Viprakasit DP, Miga MI, Herrell SD, et al. Kidney deformation and Intraprocedural registration: A study of elements of image-guided kidney surgery. Journal of Endourology. 2011;**25**(3):511-517. DOI: 10.1089/end.2010.0249. Available from: http://www.liebertonline.com/doi/abs/10.1089/end.2010.0249

[29] Baumhauer M, Simpfendörfer T, Müller-Stich B, Teber D, Gutt C, Rassweiler J, et al. Soft tissue navigation for laparoscopic partial nephrectomy. International Journal of Computer Assisted Radiology and Surgery. 2008;**3**(3):307-314. DOI: 10.1007/s11548-008-0216-7

[30] Teber D, Guven S, Simpfendörfer T, Baumhauer M, Güven EO, Yencilek F, et al. Augmented reality: A new tool to improve surgical accuracy during laparoscopic partial nephrectomy? Preliminary In vitro and In vivo results. European Urology. 2009;**56**(2):332-338. DOI: 10.1016/j.eururo.2009.05.017. Available from: https://www.clinicalkey.es/playcontent/1-s2.0-S0302283809005211

[31] Apple's Animoji Will Teach You To Love Face Tracking, For Better or Worse. Available from: http://scholar.aci.info/view/1476b1d538930fb01bd/15e7d4ac4f8000153c16f41

[32] Doerfler A, Cerantola Y, Meuwly J-Y, Lhermitte B, Bensadoun H, Jichlinski P. Ex vivo ultrasound control of resection margins during partial nephrectomy. The Journal of Urology. 2011;**186**(6):2188-2193. DOI: 10.1016/j.juro.2011.07.100. Available from: https://www.clinicalkey.es/playcontent/1-s2.0-S0022534711045307

[33] Choyke PL, Pavlovich CP, Daryanani KD, Hewitt SM, Linehan WM, Walther MM. Intraoperative ultrasound during renal parenchymal sparing surgery for hereditary renal cancers: A 10-year experience. The Journal of Urology. 2001;**165**(2):397-400. DOI: 10.1097/00005392-200102000-00010. Available from: https://www.sciencedirect.com/science/article/pii/S0022534705667079

[34] Kang X, Azizian M, Wilson E, Wu K, Martin A, Kane T, et al. Stereoscopic augmented reality for laparoscopic surgery. Surgical Endoscopy. 2014;**28**(7):2227-2235. DOI: 10.1007/s00464-014-3433-x. Available from: https://www.ncbi.nlm.nih.gov/pubmed/24488352

[35] Cheung CL, Wedlake C, Moore J, Pautler SE, Peters TM. Fused video and ultrasound images for minimally invasive partial nephrectomy: A phantom study. Medical Image Computing and Computer-assisted Intervention: MICCAI ... International Conference on Medical Image Computing and Computer-Assisted Intervention. 2010;**13**(Pt 3):408. Available from: https://www.ncbi.nlm.nih.gov/pubmed/20879426

[36] Singla R, Edgcumbe P, Pratt P, Nguan C, Rohling R. Intra-operative ultrasound-based augmented reality guidance for laparoscopic surgery. Healthcare Technology Letters. 2017;**4**(5):204-209. DOI: 10.1049/htl.2017.0063. Available from: https://www.ncbi.nlm.nih.gov/pubmed/29184666

[37] Edgcumbe P, Singla R, Pratt P, Schneider C, Nguan C, Rohling R. Follow the light: Projector-based augmented reality intracorporeal system for laparoscopic surgery. Journal of Medical Imaging. 2018;**5**(2):021216. DOI: 10.1117/1.JMI.5.2.021216. Available from: http://www.dx.doi.org/10.1117/1.JMI.5.2.021216

[38] Ukimura O, Gill IS. Imaging-assisted endoscopic surgery: Cleveland clinic experience. Journal of Endourology. 2008;**22**(4):803-810. DOI: 10.1089/end.2007.9823. Available from: https://www.ncbi.nlm.nih.gov/pubmed/18366316

[39] Ukimura O, Nakamoto M, Gill IS. Three-dimensional reconstruction of renovascular-tumor anatomy to facilitate zero-ischemia partial nephrectomy. European Urology. 2011;**61**(1):211-217. DOI: 10.1016/j.eururo.2011.07.068. Available from: https://www.clinicalkey.es/playcontent/1-s2.0-S030228381100978X

[40] Krane LS, Hemal AK. Is indocyanine green dye useful in robotic surgery? Nature Reviews Urology. 2014;**11**(1):12-14. DOI: 10.1038/nrurol.2013.303

[41] Imperial College London. Imperial's iKnife inspires future doctors. ENP Newswire. 2017

[42] Phelps DL, Balog J, Gildea LF, Bodai Z, Savage A, El-Bahrawy MA, et al. The surgical intelligent knife distinguishes normal, borderline and malignant gynaecological tissues using rapid evaporative ionisation mass spectrometry (REIMS). The British Journal of

Cancer. 2018;**118**(10):1349-1358. DOI: 10.1038/s41416-018-0048-3. Available from: https://www.ncbi.nlm.nih.gov/pubmed/29670294

[43] Murthi S, Varshney A. How augmented reality will make surgery safer. Available from: https://hbr.org/2018/03/how-augmented-reality-will-make-surgery-safer [Accessed 03/10/2018]

[44] Boston Children's Hospital, Simulator Program. SIMPeds 3D Print [Accessed 12/08/2018]

[45] Verge Staff, Boston Children's Hospital, Simulator Program. A 3D Printed Brain Saved this Toddler's Life. Available from: http://simpeds.org/news/a-3d-printed-brain-saved-this-toddlers-life/ [Accessed September 12, 2018]

[46] Zhang Y, Ge H-w, Li N-c, Yu C-f, Guo H-f, Jin S-h, et al. Evaluation of three-dimensional printing for laparoscopic partial nephrectomy of renal tumors: A preliminary report. World Journal of Urology. 2016;**34**(4):533-537. DOI: 10.1007/s00345-015-1530-7. Available from: https://www.ncbi.nlm.nih.gov/pubmed/25841361

[47] Silberstein JL, Maddox MM, Dorsey P, Feibus A, Thomas R, Lee BR. Physical models of renal malignancies using standard cross-sectional imaging and 3-dimensional printers: A pilot study. Urology. 2014;**84**(2):268-273. DOI: 10.1016/j.urology.2014.03.042. Available from: https://www.clinicalkey.es/playcontent/1-s2.0-S0090429514004555

[48] Chen Y, Li H, Wu D, Bi K, Liu C. Surgical planning and manual image fusion based on 3D model facilitate laparoscopic partial nephrectomy for intrarenal tumors. World Journal of Urology. 2014;**32**(6):1493-1499. DOI: 10.1007/s00345-013-1222-0. Available from: https://www.ncbi.nlm.nih.gov/pubmed/24337151

[49] Series MB1 Number 47 Cancer Statistics Registrations. Registrations of cancer diagnosed in 2016, England. Key Non Parliamentary Papers 2018

Chapter 6

Renal Tumor Biopsies: A Shift towards Improving Outcomes in the Management of Small Renal Masses

Menazir Sha and Faiz Mumtaz

Additional information is available at the end of the chapter

http://dx.doi.org/10.5772/intechopen.85781

Abstract

This chapter reviews the current literature in view of varying clinical practices surrounding the diagnostic role of renal tumor biopsies of small renal masses. Surgical management of small renal masses without pretreatment biopsy is a routine strategy in many urological centres around the world. This is in spite of improvements in techniques, accuracies and biomarkers to diagnose the neoplasm. Apart from its effectiveness, renal tumor biopsies avoid the risks of surgically treating benign renal masses and may also prove cost-effective to healthcare systems. Interdisciplinary communication between urologists, interventional radiologists and pathologists will facilitate the process of making this biopsy-driven management the standard of care.

Keywords: active surveillance, biopsy, diagnostic accuracy, intratumour heterogeneity, kidney neoplasms, renal cell carcinoma, renal tumor biopsy, partial nephrectomies, renal mass biopsy, small renal mass

1. Introduction

The surgical disposition towards partial nephrectomies and ablative techniques in the management of small renal masses (**SRMs**) urges the use of biopsies to overcome preoperative misclassifications.

SRMs are defined to be T1a tumors ≤4 cm in greatest dimension, limited to the kidneys. With improved medical imaging, the incidence of patients with SRMs has been rising. These patients tend to be asymptomatic and show a good prognosis. The current European Association of Urology (**EAU**) guidelines promote nephron-sparing techniques, especially partial nephrectomies (**PN**) in the management of T1a tumors. Other approaches such as radiofrequency ablation (**RFA**), cryotherapy and active surveillance (**AS**) are also considered.

However, it has been shown that a large proportion of SRMs treated are benign incidentalomas. Twenty percent of surgically removed SRMs have proven to be benign [1, 2] (angiomyolipoma, oncocytoma, metanephric adenoma, etc.), with the figure rising to 29% for tumors <2.5 cm [3]. Thus, it is necessary for current practices to be reevaluated to avoid unnecessary overtreatment.

Surgical management based on CT imaging, without pretreatment biopsy, is considered appropriate in most centres. Such an approach not only leads to the patient undertaking unnecessary surgical risks but also places a significant burden on the healthcare system. Premanagement renal tumour biopsies (**RTBs**) have the potential to not only offer holistic approach to their management but can equally be cost-effective.

Opponents to RTBs believe that concordance rates of the final pathology with radiological imaging, false-negative rates and potential seeding make this an unreliable procedure. However, the safety and outcomes of RTBs have improved significantly over the last decade. Improved imaging techniques allow for a specific localized tissue to be biopsied. Samples taken from percutaneous needle biopsies also now utilize biomarkers that can lend further insights to the heterogeneous nature of renal neoplasms.

It is important to recognize that avoiding unnecessary surgical treatments is more cost-effective and negates associated risks. In this chapter, we will discuss the improvements of RTBs and the merits of incorporating them to deliver better outcome measures.

2. Protocol of SRM management

It is estimated that 60% of all diagnosed renal cell carcinomas (**RCCs**) are SRMs that are discovered as incidentalomas on ultrasound and/or abdominal CT scans [4]. The current protocol in many urological renal centres, following the discovery of a SRM, is to offer the patient treatment options without a biopsy. Generally, unless contraindicated, these options include PN, RFA, or AS. This approach to treating a SRM is done without a clear histological diagnosis.

There should be a paradigm shift on how SRMs are approached. In some centres, RTBs are now performed upon the discovery of an incidentaloma. Here, patients are referred to an interventional radiologist who will then perform a RTB before their consultation with their urologist. Following the biopsy results from the pathologist, the urologist will meet the patient and offer better informed treatment options.

3. Contemporary indications and contraindications for biopsy

The EAU guidelines recommend RTBs to be performed for AS on selected patients with SRMs, prior to ablative treatments and patients suffering from renal metastatic disease before embarking on systemic treatment.

The American Urological Association (**AUA**) guidelines stipulate that biopsies should be considered when a renal mass is suspected to be metastatic, hematological, inflammatory or infectious. RTBs are also expected to be performed before ablative procedures.

Historically, absolute contraindications to RTBs include uncontrolled severe hypertension, inability to cooperate with biopsy, solitary kidney and uncontrollable bleeding diathesis [5]. Relative contraindications may include a lack of a safe pathway to the lesion and pregnancy where imaging guidance involves ionizing radiation.

4. Prevalence of biopsies

Recent studies have shown that RTBs are still not widely adopted among urologists in clinical practice. A survey in 2010 by Barwari et al. [6] showed that 73% of urologists never take biopsies and only 9% take biopsies in more than 25% of cases. Another survey in 2016 by Richard et al. [7], investigating the prevalence of biopsies for SRMs, showed that only 12% perform RTBs in >75% of cases, while 53% never perform or perform RTBs in <25% of cases.

In both surveys the main reasons urologists cited for not performing biopsies were the lack of influence in clinical management, the risk of false negatives and safety. There is also a radiology-related concern of a lack of expertise with RTBs [7]. These concerns will have to be tackled.

4.1. Prevalence of RTBs in active surveillance

In current literature, many patients undergoing AS have not had a biopsy [8–10]. AS is usually indicated for elderly patients with significant comorbidities or those refusing surgery. Though considered a safe option for patients with SRMs, the risk of developing metastatic disease during surveillance is not ruled out. A systematic review performed by Prins et al. [9] showed that though 1.12% (0–3.2%) of the pooled AS population (968 patients) incurred delayed intervention, only a small proportion of the said population had undergone a RTB. If a biopsy had been performed, it could have led to an earlier appropriate intervention [11]. A systematic review performed by Smaldone et al. [10] looked at the incidence of metastases in AS strategies. In this review of 880 patients, 18 patients (2.05%) progressed to metastatic disease. Unfortunately, only three of these patients had undergone a RTB.

RTBs can also pave the way for a more refined AS strategy and are strongly recommended [8, 10, 12, 13]. If the SRM proves to be histologically benign, a less stringent follow-up protocol can be adopted, or the patient may even be discharged. Higher metastatic potential masses that are better suited for surgical intervention can also be identified. Thus, RTBs can stratify patients into a low-risk or high-risk surveillance strategy.

4.2. Prevalence of RTBs in radiofrequency ablation

In some centres performing RFA, RTBs are either done at the time of the procedure or not performed at all [14–16]. These patients continue to be treated with a presumptive diagnosis of renal cancer based on CT/US imaging. This increases the rate of RFA performed for benign or indeterminate pathology [15]. Performing RTBs prior to ablative techniques can also be used to stratify patients—where those with unfavorable histology can be triaged to surgery instead.

5. Addressing barriers

In order to facilitate the shift in managing SRMs (be it in AS, RFA or systemic treatment), it is important for us to address these barriers in adopting RTBs. We will now assess the reliability and improvements of RTBs.

5.1. Improved techniques for biopsy

RTBs are performed percutaneously under local anesthesia. It can be with needle core biopsy or fine needle aspiration (FNA) with US or CT guidance.

Core needle biopsies yield a higher diagnostic rate and a more accurate histological examination over FNA. This was exemplified by a systematic review performed by Marconi et al. [17] (57 studies recruiting 5228 patients)—showing superior sensitivities and specificities over diagnostic FNAs. A coaxial technique allows multiple biopsies to be taken through a coaxial canula, avoiding potential tumor seeding. Comparing needle sizes used, 18-gauge needles are preferred over 14- and 20-gauge needles—showing safer and more accurate histological results [18, 19].

With regard to imaging modalities, US and CT possess their own merits. CT has the advantage of a better resolution that is ideal to locate lesions that are in proximity to critical structures. US has the advantage of lower radiation and lower cost. More importantly it allows real-time needle placement that is suited for nonfocal renal lesions [20].

In spite of acknowledging preferred techniques of RTBs, there are other technical factors that affect their success: amount of adipose tissue in the patient, echogenicity and location of lesion. The challenge of performing a successful biopsy can thus vary from lesion to lesion. Effective communication between the interventional radiologist and urologist is necessary to ensure that a RTB would be reliable in managing a specific SRM.

5.2. Improvements in accuracy

Recent literature lends support to the diagnostic accuracies of RTBs, challenging the notions some urologists believe. The meta-analysis performed by Marconi et al. [17] showed that initial RTBs yielded a diagnosis in >90% of cases. Core biopsies showed a high sensitivity and specificity of 99.1 and 99.7%, respectively. In cases where both a RTB and surgical pathology were available, good concordance ($k = 0.683$) for tumor histotype and fair concordance ($k = 0.34$) for tumor grade were shown.

A systematic review by Patel et al. [21] (including 20 studies with 2979 patients) showed a high diagnostic accuracy of RTB with a sensitivity of 97.5% and a specificity of 96.2%. There was also a high histological concordance observed. Patel's study highlighted the concern of a reasonable non-diagnostic rate (14.1%).

However, repeat biopsy led to diagnosis in 80% of previously undiagnostic biopsies. It is reported that following a non-diagnostic biopsy, a repeat biopsy has a high rate of rendering a diagnosis—ranging from 67 to 85% [22]. Therefore, in the case of a non-diagnostic biopsy, there is merit in performing a repeat biopsy.

With overall improved diagnostic accuracies of RTBs, urologists should be more reassured about their successes.

5.3. Managing complications

Reported concerns regarding the safety of RTBs stem from the risks of bleeding, pneumothorax and tumor seeding [7]. Rising literature appraising the choice of gauge needles, imaging modality and preference for core biopsies over FNA have improved the safety of RTBs.

In Patel's et al. study [21], complication rates observed were quite low. The rate of haematomas was 4.9%, while the occurrence of any clinically significant pain was 1.2%. Pneumothorax was only detected in 0.6% of cases, and no study reported any cases of tumor seeding. In Marconi's et al. study [17], the median complication rate was 8.1% with only three Clavien grade ≥2 complications to be reported.

Tumor seeding along the needle tract is anecdotal and very rare. As per the EAU reported guidelines, to avoid any such complication, coaxial sheaths should be used. This allows multiple passes through the renal mass with only one through surrounding tissue.

5.4. Discerning tumour heterogeneity

Despite the high concordance rates in identifying tumor subtypes (as mentioned above), the heterogeneous nature of RCC in itself is an identified barrier in adopting RTB. It is essential for clinicians to identify the challenges in discerning between specific tumor subtypes in order to have a comprehensive grasp on the reliability of a RTB.

The four main subtypes of RCC include clear cell RCC (**ccRCC**), papillary RCC (**pRCC**), chromophobe RCC (**chRCC**) and collecting duct carcinoma (**CDC**). There are over 10 such subtypes with many inherited syndromes [23]. Each subtype is associated with its own prognostic factors from clinically indolent (pRCC type 1, chRCC) to highly metastatic (pRCC type 2 or ccRCC). Thus, it is valuable for a subtype to be distinguished from benign lesions and also to be reliably identified for a more tailored management.

Another systematic review by Patel et al. [24] investigated the success of identifying oncocytomas. Of the 48 lesions that were diagnostic of oncocytoma on RTB, 64.6% was in concordance with analysis following surgical treatment. Meta-analysis determined the PPV of oncocytoma on RTB to be 67% with a notable proportion to be identified as chRCC. Histologically, they are hard to distinguish as both have an eosinophilic cytoplasm. Clinical diagnostic dilemmas between chRCC and oncocytomas still remain. Clinicians should factor this in tailoring an altered AS for oncocytomas.

6. Investigating biomarkers

Recent studies have explored the merits of molecular biomarkers to improve diagnostic classification of RTBs. A recent systematic evaluation by Gulati et al. [25] assessed cancer-specific survival (**CSS**) in 350 ccRCC patients with 28 published genetic biomarkers. Seventeen of these genetic and transcriptomic prognostic ccRCC markers were validated as predictors of CSS. A comprehensive review article by Farber et al. [26] shows the many other areas where biomarkers are being developed: PET imaging, MRI, serum biomarkers, urine biomarkers, liquid biopsy and immunohistochemistry. Of particular interest is the staining method for CK7 that is expressed in both chRCC and oncocytoma. In the former it is strongly and diffusely positive, while in the latter, only focal positivity or no staining is observed [18, 26, 27]. With further prospective clinical studies, a combinatorial approach can be adopted to discern the heterogeneous nature of renal lesions.

7. Cost-effectiveness

It is critical to stress on the cost-effectiveness of integrating RTBs in the management of SRMs. A cost-effectiveness study by Pandharipande et al. [28] showed that a strategy of pretreatment biopsies of SRMs leads to a minimally greater difference of quality-adjusted life expectancy (4 days) than empiric surgery. This is at a lower lifetime cost of ($3466). Avoiding unnecessary surgery in cases of resecting indolent SRMs is in the interests of both the patient and the healthcare system. With similar outcomes and lower cost, the use of biopsy to triage patients facilitates this.

8. Conclusion

RTBs have the strong potential to avoid unnecessary surgeries, preventing treatment-related morbidities in patients and saving healthcare costs. RTBs have high diagnostic accuracies, high concordance rates and low complication rates. Therefore, RTBs should be integrated in the pretreatment management of SRMs when their results can alter the treatment options for the patient. Further studies in improving diagnostic biomarkers are worthwhile in supplementing the classification of RCC subtypes.

This shift in management away from empiric surgical treatment requires support from interventional radiologists, histopathologists and urologists. An interventional radiologist would be suited in identifying the preferred imaging modality for a specific RTB and explaining the difficulty to obtain an adequate amount for a reliable diagnosis. A histopathologist can raise concerns on potential misclassifications of specific tumor subtypes.

Integrated clinical communication between these disciplines can optimize the effective use of a RTB in crafting a well-suited treatment plan for the patient.

Author details

Menazir Sha and Faiz Mumtaz*

*Address all correspondence to: faiz.mumtaz@nhs.net

Specialist Kidney Centre, Royal Free Hospital, London, United Kingdom

References

[1] Frank I et al. Solid renal tumors: An analysis of pathological features related to tumor size. The Journal of Urology. 2003;**170**(6 Pt 1):2217-2220

[2] Johnson DC et al. Preoperatively misclassified, surgically removed benign renal masses: a systematic review of surgical series and United States population level burden estimate. The Journal of Urology. 2015;**193**(1):30-35

[3] Fernando A, Fowler S, O'Brien T, (BAUS) BAoUS. Nephron-sparing surgery across a nation—Outcomes from the British Association of Urological Surgeons 2012 national partial nephrectomy audit. BJU International. 2016;**117**(6):874-882

[4] Hollingsworth JM, Miller DC, Daignault S, Hollenbeck BK. Rising incidence of small renal masses: A need to reassess treatment effect. Journal of the National Cancer Institute. 2006;**98**(18):1331-1334

[5] Bandari J, Fuller TW, Turner Ii RM, D'Agostino LA. Renal biopsy for medical renal disease: Indications and contraindications. The Canadian Journal of Urology. 2016;**23**(1): 8121-8126

[6] Barwari K, de la Rosette JJ, Laguna MP. The penetration of renal mass biopsy in daily practice: A survey among urologists. Journal of Endourology. 2012;**26**(6):737-747

[7] Richard PO et al. Identifying the use and barriers to the adoption of renal tumour biopsy in the management of small renal masses. Canadian Urological Association Journal. 2018;**12**(8):260-266

[8] Joice GA, Pierorazio PM, Allaf ME. Update on active surveillance for clinical T1 renal tumors. Current Opinion in Urology. 2016;**26**(5):405-409

[9] Prins FM et al. Renal cell carcinoma: Alternative nephron-sparing treatment options for small renal masses, a systematic review. Journal of Endourology. 2017;**31**(10):963-975

[10] Smaldone MC et al. Small renal masses progressing to metastases under active surveillance: A systematic review and pooled analysis. Cancer. 2012;**118**(4):997-1006

[11] Finelli A et al. Management of small renal masses: American society of clinical oncology clinical practice guideline. Journal of Clinical Oncology. 2017;**35**(6):668-680

[12] Liaw CW, Winoker JS, Mehrazin R. Imaging protocols for active surveillance in renal cell carcinoma. Current Urology Reports. 2018;**19**(10):81

[13] Campbell SC et al. Guideline for management of the clinical T1 renal mass. The Journal of Urology. 2009;**182**(4):1271-1279

[14] Iguchi T et al. Simultaneous biopsy and radiofrequency ablation of T1a renal cell carcinoma. Diagnostic and Interventional Imaging. 2016;**97**(11):1159-1164

[15] Wells SA et al. Renal mass biopsy and thermal ablation: should biopsy be performed before or during the ablation procedure? Abdominal Radiology (New York). 2017;**42**(6): 1773-1780

[16] Tuncali K et al. Evaluation of patients referred for percutaneous ablation of renal tumors: Importance of a preprocedural diagnosis. AJR. American Journal of Roentgenology. 2004;**183**(3):575-582

[17] Marconi L et al. Systematic review and meta-analysis of diagnostic accuracy of percutaneous renal tumour biopsy. European Urology. 2016;**69**(4):660-673

[18] Breda A et al. Comparison of accuracy of 14-, 18- and 20-G needles in ex-vivo renal mass biopsy: A prospective, blinded study. BJU International. 2010;**105**(7):940-945

[19] Maturen KE et al. Renal mass core biopsy: Accuracy and impact on clinical management. AJR. American Journal of Roentgenology. 2007;**188**(2):563-570

[20] Uppot RN, Harisinghani MG, Gervais DA. Imaging-guided percutaneous renal biopsy: Rationale and approach. AJR. American Journal of Roentgenology. 2010;**194**(6):1443-1449

[21] Patel HD et al. Diagnostic accuracy and risks of biopsy in the diagnosis of a renal mass suspicious for localized renal cell carcinoma: Systematic review of the literature. The Journal of Urology. 2016;**195**(5):1340-1347

[22] Capretz T, Patel RM, Okhunov Z. Percutaneous renal biopsy: Approach, diagnostic accuracy and risks. Current Opinion in Urology. 2018;**28**(4):369-374

[23] Shuch B et al. Understanding pathologic variants of renal cell carcinoma: Distilling therapeutic opportunities from biologic complexity. European Urology. 2015;**67**(1):85-97

[24] Patel HD et al. Surgical histopathology for suspected oncocytoma on renal mass biopsy: A systematic review and meta-analysis. BJU International. 2017;**119**(5):661-666

[25] Gulati S et al. Systematic evaluation of the prognostic impact and intratumour heterogeneity of clear cell renal cell carcinoma biomarkers. European Urology. 2014;**66**(5):936-948

[26] Farber NJ et al. Renal cell carcinoma: The search for a reliable biomarker. Translational Cancer Research. 2017;**6**(3):620-632

[27] Ng KL et al. Differentiation of oncocytoma from chromophobe renal cell carcinoma (RCC): Can novel molecular biomarkers help solve an old problem? Journal of Clinical Pathology. 2014;**67**(2):97-104

[28] Pandharipande PV et al. Renal mass biopsy to guide treatment decisions for small incidental renal tumors: A cost-effectiveness analysis. Radiology. 2010;**256**(3):836-846

Chapter 7

Harmonic Contrast-Enhanced Ultrasound (CEUS) of Kidney Tumors

Lidia Ciobanu, Attila Tamas Szora,
Alexandru Florin Badea, Mihai Suciu and
Radu Badea

Additional information is available at the end of the chapter

http://dx.doi.org/10.5772/intechopen.77376

Abstract

Nowadays, kidney tumor diagnosis benefits from large and highly accurate imagistic methods. A new imagistic method is contrast-enhanced ultrasound (CEUS) that accurately depicts the circulatory pattern of tumors. In kidney pathology, any mass or even capsular deformation depicted by B mode ultrasound represents an indication for CEUS. The kidney is completely and uniformly vascularized. In cystic tumors, there is a lack of contrast loading. In "impure" cystic masses (Bosnian 3 and 4), CEUS reveals vascularized septa and walls. In malignant tumors, accelerated and heterogeneous loading of contrast agent is observed in arterial phase followed by early, inhomogeneous washout of the contrast agent compared to normal renal parenchyma. In the abscesses, the appearance is the early loading of the walls associated with moderate hyperemia of the normal circulatory bed. This chapter details the CEUS in kidney tumor pathology, emphasizing the accurate information for the circulatory pattern of renal masses. It requires correlations with clinical data and information provided by other imaging explorations to make a final diagnosis.

Keywords: contrast-enhanced ultrasonography, Doppler ultrasonography, kidney tumors, kidney cysts, kidney abscesses

1. Introduction

Ultrasonography (US) is a diagnostic method based on the transmission and reception of ultrasounds in biological media, being frequently used in the "native" version without added procedures. It is the most widely available imaging method. In recent years, "conventional" ultrasound was optimized by numerous procedures, including those using "contrast agents." It consists of intravenous administration of specific substances in order to improve the diagnostic information. The technique is called "contrast-enhanced ultrasound" (CEUS). It allows simultaneously visualization of the flows from the large vessels and from the microcirculation [1]. CEUS is independent of the characteristics of blood column movement (velocity and angle of incidence of the ultrasound beam), being more sensitive than the Doppler technique. It permits the study of capillary circulation and detection of blood extravasations.

The CEUS method was first used for hepatic tumor pathology, but also for abdominal emergencies (detection of infarct or parenchymal dilacerations). The indication of CEUS has evolved and expanded rapidly in recent years, with the development of new contrast agents as well as the identification of new directions called "clinical applications" [2]. In urology, CEUS may have clinical implications with diagnostic values added to the detection and characterization of focal and diffuse renal, prostatic, testicular, and bladder lesions.

2. Principles

Ultrasound contrast agents are gas-filled microbubbles and are used clinically as blood pool tracers to significantly enhance the acoustic backscatter from blood. Definity (Lantheus Medical Imaging, North Billerica, MA, USA) and SonoVue (Bracco S.P.A., Milan, Italy) are two clinically licensed ultrasound contrast agents. MicroMarker (targeted and untargeted) (Bracco, Geneva, Switzerland; VisualSonics, Toronto, ON, Canada) is marketed as a preclinical UCA for contrast enhancement and molecular imaging in small animals. The microbubbles are made up of a lipid coating and a gaseous content (sulfur hexafluoride). The substance has a much lower solubility than air, which gives it good blood balance [3]. The diameter of the microbubbles is similar to that of the red blood cells (7 microns), which allow the passage of the contrast agent through the pulmonary and peripheral capillary circulation without any impediment. One of the main physic principles relies on the compressibility of the gases exposed to the pressure of an ultrasound beam. Microbubbles generate (through the mechanism called "non-linear vibration") harmonic echoes (higher frequency multiples) that are recorded by the transducer. This behavior is significantly different from that of tissues. Ultrasound devices use ultrasound emissions to cancel the tissue signals and to accentuate the microbubble signals.

After intravenously administration of the contrast agent, an increased intensity signal coming from the vessels is depicted on the ultrasound screen. This enhanced signal can be evaluated in the gray scale, in the color-coded modes or in the hybrid mode (the combination of the two). The CEUS technique has a dynamic character, being possible a continuous tracking of the contrast agent through a region of interest (ROI). In the case of the kidney, the contrast agent is initially visualized in the renal artery, progressing to the sinus, the renal cortical, and after a delay of several seconds to the renal medulla. The first 30–40 s (sec) postinjection is appropriate for the arterial phase and then 30–40 s for the venous phase [4] (**Figure 1**).

The CEUS examination might be focused on a region of interest (ROI). The operator might analyze this ROI in real time, during the examination or through a dedicated soft that traces the time-intensity curves. The parameters obtained describe the vascular and temporal behavior, depending on the different postadministration phases (<30–40 sec = arterial time; >30–40 sec = venous time). The time-intensity curve (TIC) represents a quantitative analysis of the variability of the mean intensity within the selected sample over a period of time (**Figure 2**). They can be postprocessed on any video clip saved during CEUS [5].

Other qualitative useful information is represented by: the intensity of fill-in with contrast agent, the sense of fill-in, the fill-in pattern, the degree of wash-out of the contrast agent, the sense of wash-out, and the pattern of wash-out [6]. The evaluation of the lesions of interest is carried out as compared to the normal parenchyma.

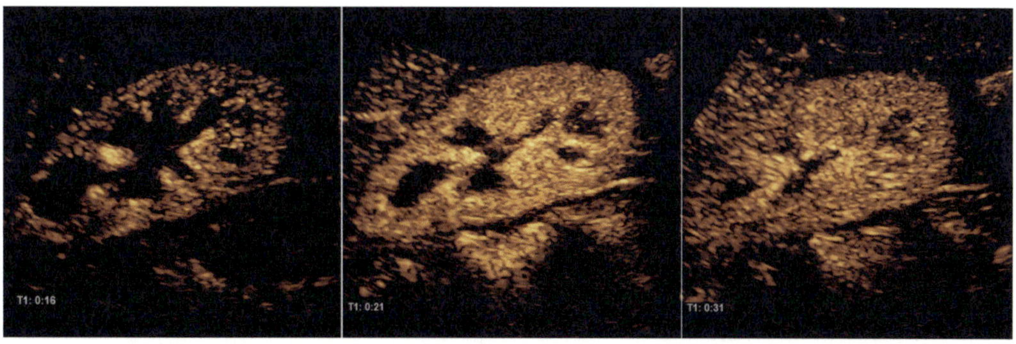

Figure 1. CEUS evaluation of the kidney. In very short time, there is a replenishment with microbubbles of cortex (periphery), cortex (columns), and the medulla.

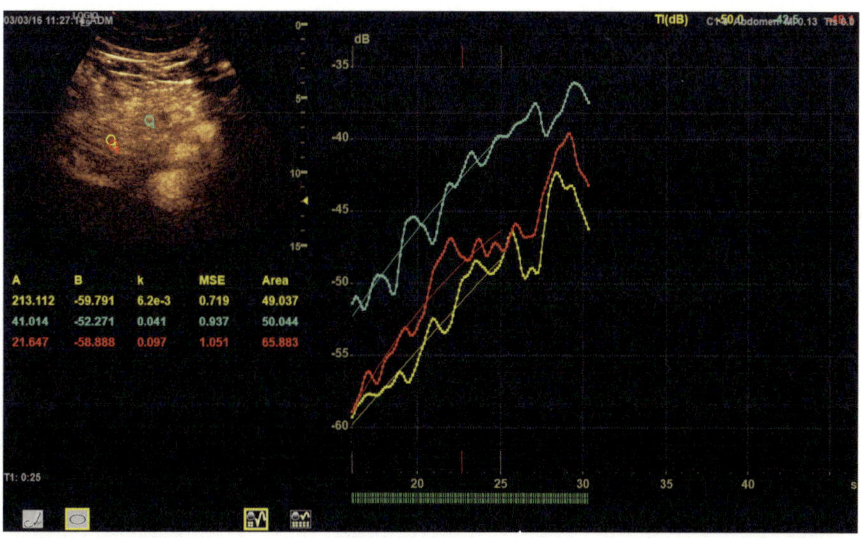

Figure 2. Representation of time-intensity transit curves. A sample area mounted in a specific area considered "target." Special software is representing the characteristics of perfusion.

3. Equipment

For CEUS technique, the ultrasound device must be capable of functioning in harmonic mode and benefit from the acoustic power adjustment. The transducers, similar to those currently used for B and Doppler mode examinations, differ in the ability to operate in contrast mode. The harmonic mode allows a real and effective discrimination of the echoes from the blood column to those from the tissues. The acoustic power regulation is set to a value of 0.09–0.11, which leads to the generation of harmonic echoes at the microbubble level, minimizing the harmonic echoes at the tissue level and the artifacts.

4. The examination technique

Prior to the examination, a peripheral vein (preferably the antecubital vein) is catheterized with a 20–22 Gauge needle. The examination methodology goes through the following steps: gray scale (for ROI detection), Doppler technique (for circulatory specificity assessment), and contrast media assessment (for ROI characterization).

The patient's position is adapted for examination of the organ of interest. For retroperitoneal organs, it is recommended that the patient adopts a shallow breath to facilitate the maintenance of the area of interest in the ultrasound examination plan.

After activating the contrast mode, the following settings of the ultrasound equipment must be done: the "Focus" position below the region of interest, the mechanical index at 0.09–0.11, and reduce "Gain" function.

The injection of the contrast agent (at an average dose of 2.4 ml) is followed by 10 ml of saline solution is bolus. At the time of injection, the ultrasound timer and record videos are started. The region of interest is dynamically tracked for up to 5 min postinjection. Theoretically, a second injection can be made immediately, although this is rarely necessary in clinical practice [7].

The quality of the CEUS image is limited, as in the case of the B mode ultrasound, by the localization of the region of interest, the presence of the intestinal gas or bone margins, and the patient weight [7].

For kidney CEUS examination, the literature proposed various contrast phase terminologies. One is similar to the terminology used by multiphase contrast-enhanced computer tomography (CE-CT) and magnetic resonance imaging (MRI) [8]. This terminology uses three phases: corticomedullary (enhancing cortex with medullary pyramids not yet perfused, approximately 15–30 s after contrast agent injection), nephrographic (homogenously enhancing renal parenchyma, approximately 30–70 s postinjection), and delayed (>70 s postinjection) [8]. Other groups used the following terminology: arterial phase <30 s postinjection and delayed phase 30–90 s postinjection [9]. Other authors proposed other terminologies: cortical (8–35 s after injection), corticomedullary (36–120 s), and delayed (>120 s) [10].

5. Precautions

The sulfur hexafluoride, the gaze part of the contrast agent is inert, nontoxic, with biocompatible membranes and easily eliminated by breathing. The metabolism of the membranes covering the microbubbles is done in the liver. These features make CEUS exploration independent of renal or thyroid functions, being an alternative to computer tomography in cases of renal failure or patients with history of thyrotoxicosis.

Very rare side effects are possible due to the interaction of ultrasound with microbubbles. These interactions may be mechanical or chemical. Mechanical features include bubble expansion and capillary rupture. Transient hyperthermia during bubbles recovering after expansion can generate free radicals. The precipitating factor for these reactions is the use of a mechanical index of about 0.4 [11]. Anaphylactic reactions were reported in 0.002% of examinations [12, 13].

6. Contraindications

CEUS contraindications are: severe coronary artery disease and pulmonary hypertension, unstable ischemic heart disease, age <18 years, and pregnancy [14]. No renal side effects have been reported so far after using CEUS.

7. CEUS in renal pseudo-tumors

Renal pseudotumors refer to persistent fetal lobulation, dromedary hump, and hypertrophied column of Bertin. These mass-like lesions are frequently detected on conventional ultrasound. The characteristic features are: location between overlapping portions of two renal sinus systems, clear demarcation from the renal sinus, size <3 cm, similar echogenicity to renal parenchyma, and lesions being bordered by a junctional parenchyma line; the Doppler mode demonstrates the regular, branch-like blood flow in the lesion [15].

There are, however, a number of situations in which their diagnosis is difficult—they may be miss-interpreted as kidney tumors through 2D gray scale techniques. This confounding is found in the following circumstances: modified echogenicity compared to the parenchymal environment, infiltrative tumor formations (metastases and lymphomas) [16], abnormal vascular tracts [17], and obese or noncooperative patients (**Figure 3**).

As CEUS is able to depict the microcirculation, this procedure could make the differential diagnosis between a pseudotumor and a solid mass. The vascular pattern of the "pseudotumors" is similar to adjacent parenchyma [18] (**Figures 4** and **5**). The accuracy of CEUS is similar to contrast-enhanced computer tomography (CE-CT) or magnetic resonance imaging (MRI) for the depiction of a normal vascular pattern in a pseudotumor mass [18].

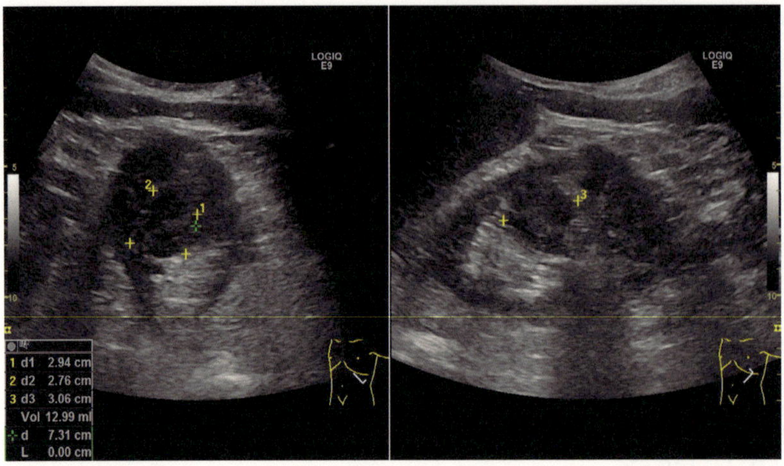

Figure 3. (a and b) Pseudotumor of the left kidney. In the middle part of the kidney, there is an area of parenchyma with hypoechoic and heterogeneous pattern suggesting a tumor. The aspect is uncertain and needs additional data especially from the vascular point of view.

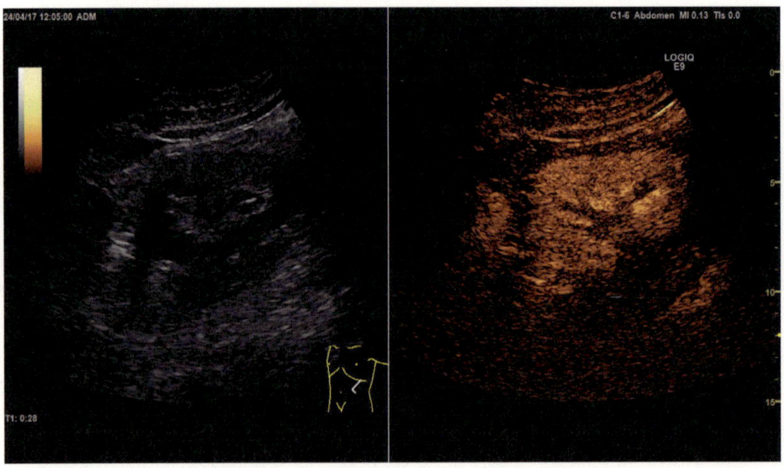

Figure 4. (a and b) Pseudotumor of the left kidney (same case as previous). Evaluation with microbubbles demonstrates no tumor in the middle of the kidney. This is a proof of how useful can be CEUS in suspicion of tumors of the kidney.

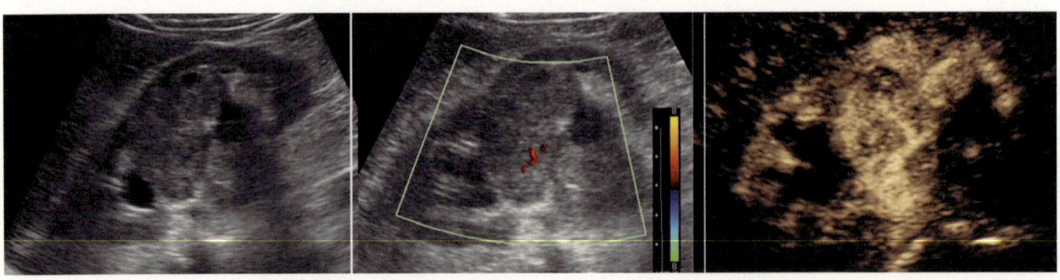

Figure 5. (a–c) Pseudotumor of the left kidney. In gray scale ultrasonography (a), there is a suspicion of a tumor in the middle of the organ. In Doppler color mode (b), there is a small vessel in the suspected tumor, insufficient for an accurate diagnosis. In CEUS focused on the middle of the kidney, there is no specific pattern for neoplasia.

8. CEUS for solid renal lesions

For solid renal masses, revealed by mode B ultrasonography, the differentiation between benign and malignant lesions is very important. The most frequent malignant lesion is renal cell carcinoma (RCC). Angiomyolipoma (AML) and oncocytoma are renal benign lesions [19]. The vascular pattern is a major criterion of differentiation and might be done with CEUS. A different vascular behavior of the renal mass compared with the adjacent parenchyma is specific for a tumor lesion and might be suggestive for malignancy [20]. CEUS has a higher accuracy than Doppler technique for renal cancer detection (100% compared to 71%) [21].

Tumor thrombus in the renal vein is a parenchymal structure with similar vascularization as the origin tumor. CEUS identifies the arterial vessels inside this parenchymal structure developed in the renal vein for the identification of the tumor's nature due to the presence of arterial time within the thrombus of the vascular signal (**Figure 6**). However, an emphasis on this character depicted in the renal vein regions of interest requires an experienced operator [11].

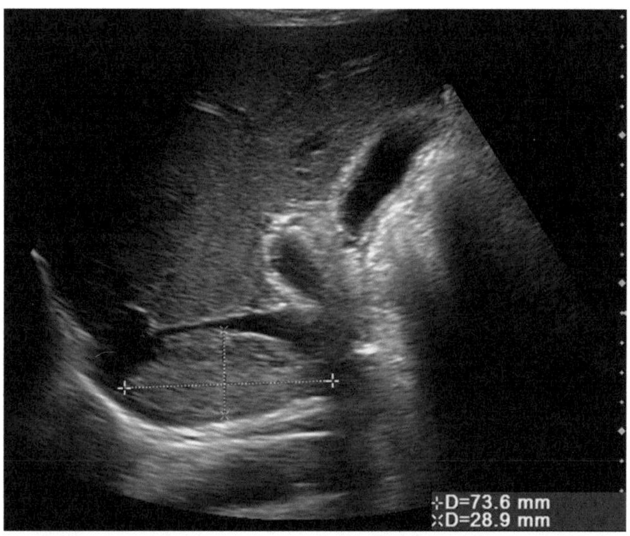

Figure 6. Malignant thrombus in inferior vena cava. Sagital evaluation of the retroperitoneal space with representation of inferior vena cava and a large parenchymal structure in the vessel. The aspect is typical for a thrombus. In the presence of a kidney tumor, the aspect suggests a vascular invasion.

9. Renal cell carcinoma (RCC)

The clear cell renal cell carcinoma (ccRCC) is the most frequent common variant of renal cancer. Histologically is characterized by numerous thin-walled blood vessels with rich blood flow. The frequent morphological features correspond to intratumoral necrosis, hemorrhage, and calcifications [22]. In ultrasound B mode, the small tumors are often hyperechoic, corresponding to the thin-walled blood vessels with rich blood flow and can mimic angiomyolipoma (**Figure 7**) [8]. Larger tumors are hypoechoic and exophytic, with central anechoic necrosis (**Figure 8**) [8].

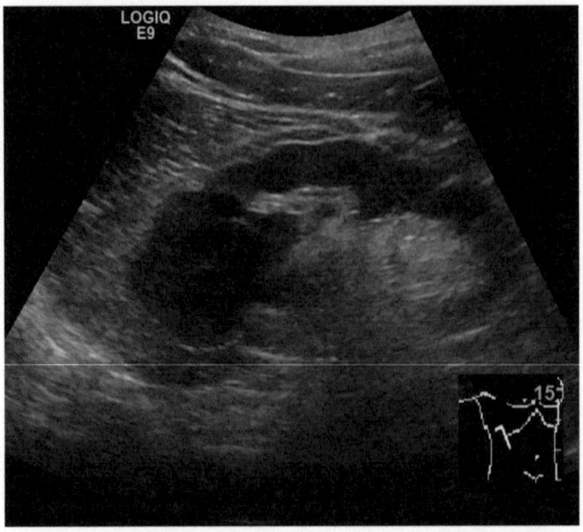

Figure 7. Renal cell carcinoma. Gray scale ultrasonography of the right kidney. At the upper pole, there is a hypoechoic tumor, relatively well defined.

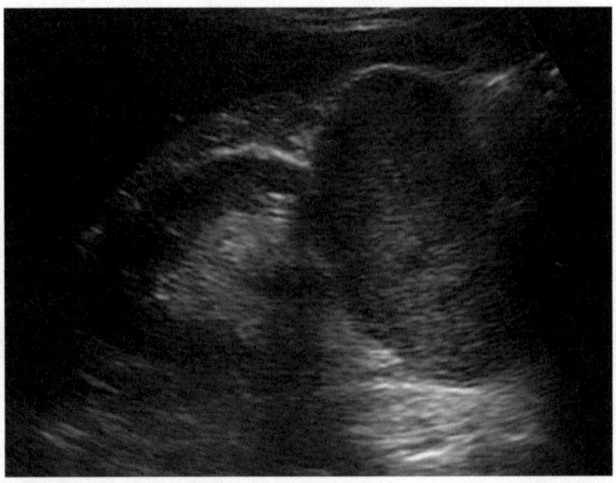

Figure 8. Renal cell carcinoma. Gray scale ultrasonography of the right kidney. At the lower pole, there is a round, well defined parenchymal tumor. The aspect is typical for a renal cell carcinoma.

The accuracy of CEUS to predict malignancy was intensively studied, but the results were not similar among authors. These confounding results are due in part to different terminology regarding the arterial and delayed phases, in part due to different contrast agents, and in part due to different features corresponding to natural development of the tumor (different CEUS characteristics depending on size) [8]. Reviewing the literature, ccRCC shows on CEUS the following vascular pattern: early hyperenhancement compared no normal adjacent parenchyma, wash-out on delayed phase, and perilesional enhancement, rim-like, corresponding to a pseudocapsule. There is also a heterogeneous enhancement, which increases with the lesion size [8].

A meta-analysis studied 11 comparable studies (including 567 malignant lesions and 313 benign lesions) and found a sensitivity of 88% and a specificity of 80% for CEUS to differentiate between malignant and benign renal tumors [23].

The papillary renal cell carcinoma are described in B mode ultrasound as unilocular and hypoechoic. The CEUS features of this type of RCC are: hypoenhance to renal parenchyma throughout examination and homogeneous [8].

10. Angiomyolipoma

Typically, AMLs contain macroscopic fat and in B mode ultrasound, there are homogeneously echogenic. There are lipid-poor AMLs that correspond to isoechoic feature on B mode ultrasound. The CEUS reveals for AMLs the following vascular pattern: homogeneous, hypoenhanced compared to adjacent renal parenchyma (**Figure 9**). The contrast agent persists in delayed phases. This characteristic is very important in differential algorithm for RCC [8].

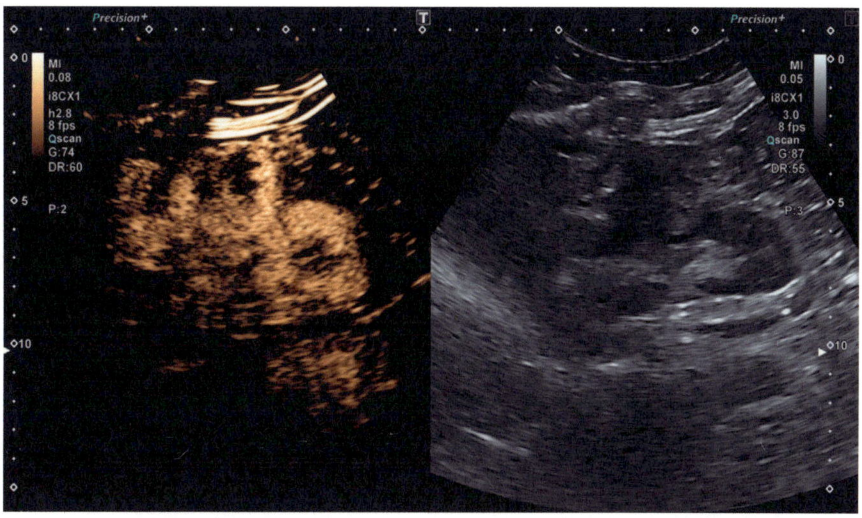

Figure 9. (a and b) Angiomyolipoma. CEUS (left) and gray scale ultrasonography (right). There is a tumor, round, well defined, and hypoechoic, with peripheral vascularity. The aspect suggests the presence of a neoplasia, but is not entirely typical for angiomyolipoma.

11. Oncocytoma

Oncocytoma are considered benign lesions. In B mode ultrasound, a hypoechoic central scar might be present, and color Doppler might show central radiating vessels (**Figure 10**) [8]. The differential diagnosis with chromophobe RCC of low malignant potential might be difficult. The vascular pattern depicted on CEUS was described differently in published case reports. It was documented a spoke wheel configuration of vessels on CEUS in an oncocytoma [20]. But other authors depicted an enhancement from periphery to center [8, 23]. The majority of the reports found hyperenhancement early compared with normal renal parenchyma and persistent (greater delayed) compared to ccRCC [8, 23].

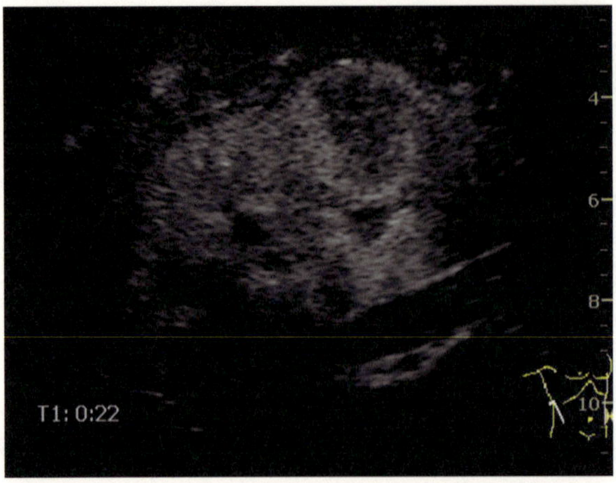

Figure 10. Oncocytoma. Round, parenchymal mass with enhancement of the peripheral vascular bed in the arterial time (Section 22).

12. Metastases and lymphoma

Imaging features suggestive for metastasis or lymphoma are: size <3 cm, lack of spherical shape, "infiltrative" growth, multiplicity, and bilaterality. There are no capsules or calcifications [8].

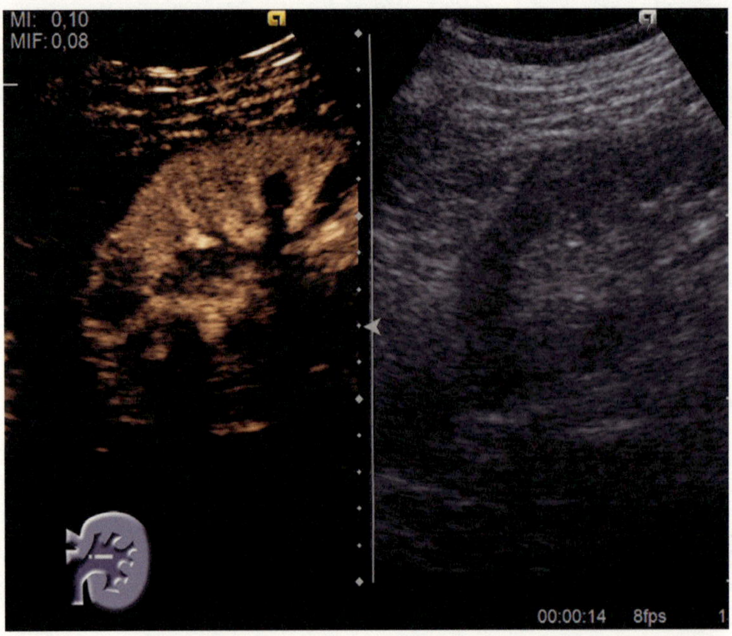

Figure 11. Renal lymphoma. CEUS evaluation (left) with an area of hypoenhancement at the upper pole; gray scale evaluation (right) with no signs of tumor. Vascular evaluation seems to be superior for the diagnostic than the morphometric pattern.

Few case reports depicted CEUS vascular pattern of renal metastasis, which are hypovascular on all phases [8]. Renal lymphoma was also described as hypovascular throughout renal perfusion after contrast agent administration on ultrasound (**Figure 11**) [8].

13. Cystic renal lesions

At imaging studies, approximately 10% of kidney cancers have a complex cystic appearance. Nonmalignant renal tumors may also have a complex appearance. This is most commonly due to the hemorrhage, infection, inflammation or ischemia. Differentiation between complex cysts requiring surgical treatment or monitoring is essential. The identification of vascularity in the solid area or septa of cystic lesions by CEUS simplifies the diagnosis of lesions with high malignancy potential [24].

The Bosniak classification differentiates five categories of renal cysts named I, II, IIf, III, and IV based on the imaging criteria (ultrasound and CT), being used for further clinical management of the patient [8, 25].

First Bosniak category, called I, depicts thin walls of the cyst, without septa and sharp margins. There are no solid components or calcifications. No enhancement is depicted on CEUS. There is no malignancy potential (**Figure 12**) [8, 25].

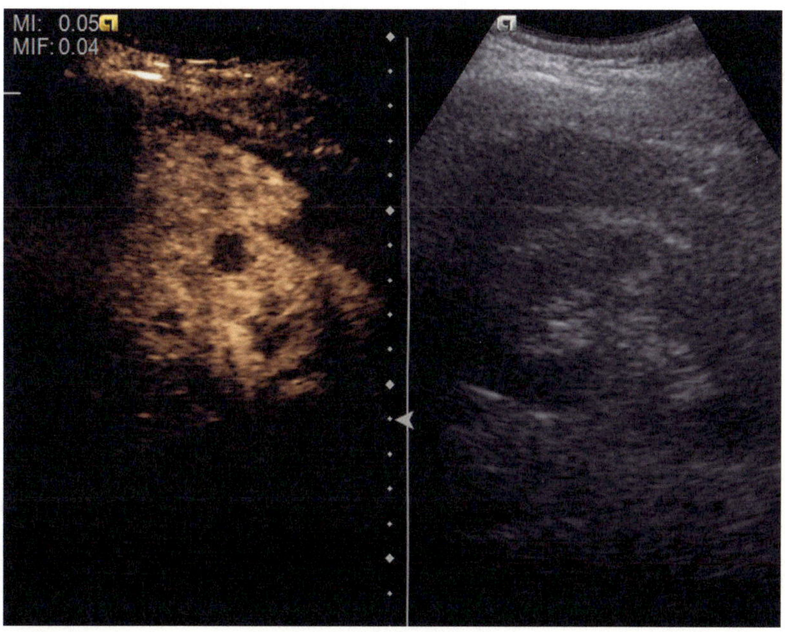

Figure 12. (a and b) Renal cyst. CEUS evaluation (a); an gray scale evaluation (b). In CEUS (asterisc), the lack of vascular signal suggests an avascular lesion compatible with the diagnosis of cyst.

Renal cysts from second category, II, are characterized by septa thinner than 1 mm, which might have fine calcifications. No contrast enhancement or very discrete enhancement is observed. The malignant potential is 0% [8, 25].

In the third category, called IIF, the cysts have multiple septa, minimally thickened walls, thin or thick calcifications. On CEUS, a discrete enhancement of the walls and septa is depicted. The malignant potential is 5%, and these lesions need regular monitoring for 6 months [8, 25].

Renal cysts from the fourth category, called III, present homogeneous of irregular thickening of the walls and/or septa and irregular calcifications. The CEUS examination reveals multiple contrast enhancing septa. The malignant potential is 50% [8, 25].

In the last category, called IV, the cysts present solid components together with homogeneous of irregular thickening of the walls and/or septa and irregular calcifications. The CEUS examination depicts multiple contrast enhancing septa and irregular contrast enhancing soft tissue components. These lesions are considered malignant [8, 25].

The accuracy of CEUS in differentiating renal cystic lesions as benign or malignant is similar to CE-CT [11]. The sensitivity of CEUS for depicting the vascular signal at the level of the cystic components (septa, walls, and nodules) is superior to CE-CT [26]. However, CEUS does not have the same sensitivity as CT in detecting calcifications, a confounding factor for the measurement of wall thickness and septum [27].

14. CEUS for monitoring renal interventions

CEUS is a very accurate method to depict blood extravasation after kidney surgery.

In the last years, CEUS became a useful tool for monitoring during and after radiofrequency ablations (RFA) and cryoablation (CA). The CEUS score system for monitoring after these interventions was proposed by Wink et al. [28] in which 0 = no enhancement, 1 = rim enhancement, 2 = diffuse enhancement, 3 = localized enhancement, and 4 = no defect in enhancement. The accuracy of CEUS compared to CE-CT or MRI was lower at 3 months post-treatment, but similar to these procedures at 12 month after [29].

15. Future expectations and developments in the field of kidney CEUS

A better quantification of blood flow could be achieved using contrast enhanced three-dimensional (3D) harmonic ultrasound imaging (HI) and subharmonic ultrasound imaging (SHI) [30]. In this preliminary study, 3D contrast-enhanced nonlinear ultrasound was able to quantify perfusion in vivo, in canine kidneys. Three-dimensional SHI resulted in better overall agreement with the reference standard than 3D HI did and was superior to previously reported 2D SHI results. Three-dimensional SHI outperformed the other methods for estimating blood perfusion because of the improved visualization of the complete perfused vascular networks [30]. This 3D technique based on CEUS proved an accurate examination for detecting renal transplant perfusion defects [31].

Another future application is related to robotic-assisted partial nephrectomy, which has gained prominence recently, as this approach has a shorter learning curve and a shorter warm ischemia time as compared to laparoscopic partial nephrectomy [32]. CEUS is capable of dynamic evaluation and quantification of microvasculature blood (capillary perfusion) in real time, without affecting renal function. When used in conjunction with a robotic ultrasound probe, CEUS can facilitate better visualization of renal vasculature and tumor and ultimately improving acumen and precision. CEUS is a valuable and a cost-effective tool for the identification of renal blood flow in robotic-assisted partial nephrectomy, especially with complex, challenging tumors [32].

16. Conclusions

The CEUS examination is an important progress for ultrasonography. The procedure depicts dynamic angio-perfusion. It is valuable in strengthening the diagnosis of renal cancer by evidencing neo-angiogenesis. It is useful in detecting tumor and nontumor circulatory abnormalities.

Acknowledgement

This work was supported by a grant of the Romanian Ministry of Research and Innovation, CCDI-UEFISCDI, project number PN-III-P1-1.2-PCCDI-2017-0056/3, within PNCDI III.

Author details

Lidia Ciobanu*, Attila Tamas Szora, Alexandru Florin Badea, Mihai Suciu and Radu Badea

*Address all correspondence to: ciobanulidia@yahoo.com

University of Medicine and Pharmacy "Iuliu Hatieganu", Cluj-Napoca, Romania

References

[1] Badea R, Ciobanu L. Contrast enhanced and Doppler ultrasonography in the characterization of the microcirculation. Expectancies and performances. Medical Ultrasonography. 2012;**14**(4):307-317

[2] Cosgrove D, Eckersley R. Contrast-enhanced ultrasound: Basic physics and technology overview. In: Lencioni R, editor. Enhancing the Role of Ultrasound with Contrast Agents. Milan: Springer; 2006. pp. 3-14

[3] Kono Y, Mattrey RF. Ultrasound of the liver. Radiologic Clinics of North America. 2005; **43**(5):815-826

[4] Nilsson A. Contrast-enhanced ultrasound of the kidneys. European Radiology. 2004; **14**(Suppl 8):104-109

[5] Cosgrove D, Lassau N. Imaging of perfusion using ultrasound. European Journal of Nuclear Medicine and Molecular Imaging. 2010;**37**(Suppl 1):S65-S85

[6] Tranquart F, Mercier L, Frinking P, Gaud E, Arditi M. Perfusion quantification in contrast-enhanced ultrasound (CEUS)—Ready for research projects and routine clinical use. Ultraschall in der Medizin. 2012;**33**(Suppl 1):S31-S38

[7] Setola SV, Catalano O, Sandomenico F, Siani A. Contrast-enhanced sonography of the kidney. Abdominal Imaging. 2007;**32**(1):21-28

[8] Gulati M, King KG, Gill IS, Pham V, Grant E, Duddalwar VA. CEUS of cystic and solid renal lesions. Abdominal Imaging. 2015;**40**(6):1982-1996

[9] Fan L, Lianfang D, Jinfang X, Yijin S, Ying W. Diagnostic efficacy of contrast-enhanced ultrasonography in solid renal parenchymal lesions with maximum diameters of 5 cm. Journal of Ultrasound in Medicine. 2008;**27**(6):875-885

[10] Xu ZF, Xu HX, Xie XY, Liu GJ, Zheng YL, Liang JY, Lu MD. Renal cell carcinoma: Real-time contrast-enhanced ultrasound findings. Abdominal Imaging. 2010;**35**(6):750-756

[11] Piscaglia F, Nolsøe C, Dietrich CF, et al. The EFSUMB guidelines and recommendations on the clinical practice of contrast enhanced ultrasound (CEUS): Update 2011 on non-hepatic applications. Ultraschall in der Medizin. 2012;**33**(1):33-59

[12] Piscaglia F, Bolondi L. Italian society for ultrasound in medicine and biology (SIUMB) study group on ultrasound contrast agents. The safety of Sonovue in abdominal applications: Retrospective analysis of 23188 investigations. Ultrasound in Medicine & Biology. 2006;**32**(9):1369-1375

[13] Ter Haar G. Safety and bio-effects of ultrasound contrast agents. Medical & Biological Engineering & Computing. 2009;**47**(8):893-900

[14] Main ML, Goldman JH, Grayburn PA. Ultrasound contrast agents: Balancing safety versus efficacy. Expert Opinion on Drug Safety. 2009;**8**(1):49-56

[15] Leekam RN, Matzinger MA, Brunelle M, Grey RR, Grosman H. The sonography of renal columnar hypertrophy. Journal of Clinical Ultrasound. 1983;**11**(9):491-494

[16] Ascenti G, Zimbaro G, Mazziotti S, Gaeta M, Lamberto S, Scribano E. Contrast-enhanced power Doppler US in the diagnosis of renal pseudotumors. European Radiology. 2001;**11**(12):2496-2499

[17] Robbin ML, Lockhart ME, Barr RG. Renal imaging with ultrasound contrast: Current status. Radiologic Clinics of North America. 2003;**41**(5):963-978

[18] Mazziotti S, Zimbaro F, Pandolfo A, Racchiusa S, Settineri N, Ascenti G. Usefulness of contrast-enhanced ultrasonography in the diagnosis of renal pseudotumors. Abdominal Imaging. 2010;**35**(2):241-245

[19] Ignee A, Straub B, Schuessler G, Dietrich CF. Contrast enhanced-ultrasound of renal masses. World Journal of Radiology. 2010;**2**(1):15-31

[20] Tamai H, Takiguchi Y, Oka M, et al. Contrast-enhanced ultrasonography in the diagnosis of solid renal tumors. Journal of Ultrasound in Medicine. 2005;**24**(12):1635-1640

[21] Dong XQ, Shen Y, Xu LW, Xu CM, Bi W, Wang XM. Contrast-enhanced ultrasound for detection and diagnosis of renal clear cell carcinoma. Chinese Medical Journal. 2009;**122**(10):1179-1183

[22] Reese JH. Renal cell carcinoma. Current Opinion in Oncology. 1992;**4**(3):427-434

[23] Wang C, Yu C, Yang F, Yang G. Diagnostic accuracy of contrast-enhanced ultrasound for renal cell carcinoma: A meta-analysis. Tumor Biology. 2014;**35**(7):6343-6350

[24] Aoki S, Hattori R, Yamamoto T, Funahashi Y, Matsukawa Y, Gotoh M, Yamada Y, Honda N. Contrast-enhanced ultrasound using a time-intensity curve for the diagnosis of renal cell carcinoma. BJU International. 2011;**108**(3):349-354

[25] Rubenthaler J, Bogner F, Reiser M, Clevert DA. Contrast-enhanced ultrasound (CEUS) of the kidney by using the Bosniak classification. Ultraschall in der Medizin. 2016;**37**:234-252

[26] Park BK, Kim B, Kim SH, Ko K, Lee HM, Choi HY. Assessment of cystic renal masses based on Bosniak classification: Comparison of CT and contrast-enhanced US. European Journal of Radiology. 2007;**61**(2):310-314

[27] Israel GM, Hindman N, Bosniak MA. Evaluation of cystic renal masses: Comparison of CT and MR imaging by using the Bosniak classification system. Radiology. 2004; **231**(2):365-371

[28] Wink MH, Laguna MP, Lagerveld BW, de la Rosette JJ, Wijkstra H. Contrast-enhanced ultrasonography in the follow-up of cryoablation of renal tumours: A feasibility study. BJU International. 2007;**99**(6):1371-1375

[29] Barwari K, Wijkstra H, van Delden OM, de la Rosette JJ, Laguna MP. Contrast-enhanced ultrasound for the evaluation of the cryolesion after laparoscopic renal cryoablation: An initial report. Journal of Endourology. 2013;**27**(4):402-407

[30] Sridharan A, Eisenbrey JR, Liu JB, Machado P, Halldorsdottir VG, Dave JK, Zhao H, He Y, Park S, Dianis S, Wallace K, Thomenius KE, Forsberg F. Perfusion estimation using contrast-enhanced 3-dimensional subharmonic ultrasound imaging: An in vivo study. Investigative Radiology. 2013;**48**(9):654-660. DOI: 10.1097/RLI.0b013e3182925160

[31] Stenberg B, Chandler C, Wyrley-Birch H, Elliott ST. Post-operative 3-dimensional contrast-enhanced ultrasound (CEUS) versus Tc99m-DTPA in the detection of post-surgical perfusion defects in kidney transplants—Preliminary findings. Ultraschall in der Medizin. 2014;**35**(3):273-278. DOI: 10.1055/s-0033-1355964

[32] Alenezi AN, Karim O. Role of intra-operative contrast-enhanced ultrasound (CEUS) in robotic-assisted nephron-sparing surgery. Journal of Robotic Surgery. 2015;**9**(1):1-10. DOI: 10.1007/s11701-015-0496-1

Section 3

Medical Management of Kidney Cancer

Chapter 8

Target Therapy for Kidney Cancer

Yang Wang and Lingxiang Liu

Additional information is available at the end of the chapter

http://dx.doi.org/10.5772/intechopen.73386

Abstract

Renal cell carcinoma (RCC) is considered a chemotherapy-resistant tumor; the landscape of metastatic RCC (mRCC) is rapidly changing due to the development of target therapy. By now, 10 novel agents have dramatically improved the prognosis of mRCC. The purpose of this chapter is to provide an updated overview of the clinical data, which support the use of these agents. We conducted a systematic review using PubMed and ClinicalTrials.gov about target therapy in RCC according to the existing guidelines, made analysis of the clinic trials, and discussed their mechanism, impact on quality of life (QoL), and patient selection algorithms. A total of 11 completed phase III trials were included in our research data. Agreement was correlated with the availability of data in seven trials, contributing to the category 1 option of first-line therapy for patients with mRCC. Three completed phase III trials contributed for the subsequent therapy as the evidence. Target therapy shows promise in clinical practice. Guidelines and algorithms should be revised and adapted to the new target drugs. However, more research is needed in parallel to discover biomarkers that enable the prediction of a treatment response and therefore lead to better patient selection.

Keywords: renal cell cancer, target therapy, tyrosine kinase inhibitor, immune checkpoint inhibitors, clinical trial

1. Introduction

About 25–30% of renal cell carcinoma patients are in locally advanced or metastatic stage when diagnosed, an additional third patients with localized tumor will recur after rational surgery. Before 2005, treatment option for advanced renal cell carcinoma (RCC) was limited to cytokines and clinical trial. With both IFN and IL-2, the response rate was only 5–27% [1, 2], while associated with substantial side effect. The last decade witnessed the important advance in the development of renal cell carcinoma (RCC) molecular biology, which leads to the improvement in the survival of patients with advanced RCC, Nowadays, half of the patients with advance RCC are likely to survive more than 2 years. Currently, 10 targeted agents are approved for first-line or later-line use in the treatment of patients with RCC including one monoclonal antibody targeting vascular endothelial growth factor (VEGF; bevacizumab), six multi-targeted tyrosine kinase inhibitors (TKIs; sunitinib, sorafenib, axitinib, pazopanib, cabozantinib, and lenvatinib), two target the mammalian target of rapamycin (mTOR) pathway (everolimus and temsirolimus), and one target the immune checkpoint programmed death-1 (PD-1) pathway (nivolumab) (**Figure 1**). The guidelines of kidney cancer recommend first-line pazopanib, sunitinib, bevacizumab (plus interferon-2b [IFN-2b]) as category 1 recommended for patients with clear cell histology and good or intermediate Memorial Sloan Kettering Cancer Center (MSKCC) prognosis (NCCN category 1 preferred, European Society for Medical Oncology (ESMO) level I evidence of activity and grade A recommendation). Temsirolimus is only recommended as first-line treatment for poor-prognosis patients, and in the latest version of NCCN 2018, cabozantinib was added to the first-line therapy for poor- and intermediate-risk patients based on modified MSKCC criteria [3]. For patients who experience disease progression during (or who are intolerant to) treatment with a first-line target treatment, subsequent therapy with the highest level of evidence include cabozantinib, nivolumab, axitinib, or lenvatinib plus everolimus. Although several targeted agents were recommended, the optimal sequence has not been determined. The goal of therapy for patients with mRCC is to prolong survival while maintaining good quality of life, which should be taken into consideration when choosing second-line and third-line agents. Choosing a sequence of targeted agents with nonoverlapping safety profiles might improve quality of life by improving tolerability. Looking forward, identification of the optimal sequence of targeted agents might be achieved through identification of biomarkers and individualization of treatment for patients with mRCC.

Prognostic scoring systems used in some clinical trials is from the Memorial Sloan Kettering Cancer Center (MSKCC), which was derived from evaluating prognostic factors in patients with mRCC in clinical trials [4]. The validated MSKCC model includes the following five independent predictors of short survival: time from diagnosis to treatment less than 1 year; Karnofsky performance status less than 80%; lactate dehydrogenase level more than 1.5 times ULN; low serum hemoglobin level, and corrected serum calcium level more than 10 mg/dL). Patients with 0, 1–2, or 3 risk factors are stratified into categories as low risk with good

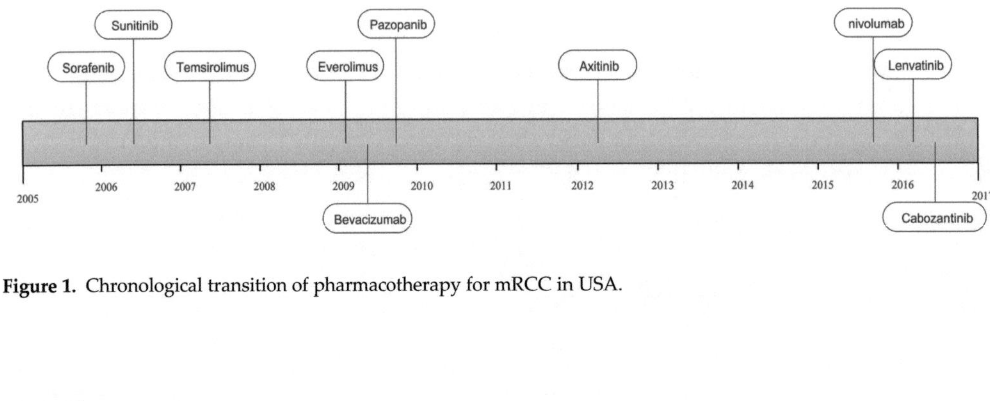

Figure 1. Chronological transition of pharmacotherapy for mRCC in USA.

prognosis, intermediate risk, or poor risk, respectively. The MSKCC model has been validated by an independent group at the Cleveland Clinic, and has been valuable in identifying the most effective treatment strategy [5].

2. Approved drugs

2.1. Targeting VEGF/VEGFR

Angiogenesis is a key target in the treatment of advanced RCC. Therapeutic strategies include the inhibition of the receptor of the vascular endothelial growth factor (VEGFR) by tyrosine kinase inhibitors and the blockage of the ligand (VEGF) by monoclonal antibodies.

2.1.1. Sorafenib

Sorafenib is a small molecule multi-tyrosine kinase inhibitor that targets RAF, MEK, ERK, VEGFR1–3, PDGFR-β, c-KIT, RET, CRAF, and BRAF, which are involved in tumor cell proliferation and angiogenesis [6].

A randomized phase II trial investigated the efficacy and safety of sorafenib vs. IFN-2α in previously untreated patients with clear cell RCC. One hundred and eighty nine patients were randomized to receive oral sorafenib (400 mg twice daily) or subcutaneous IFN-2α. When the disease progressed, the dose of sorafenib escalated to 600 mg twice daily for sorafenib patients and IFN-2α patients had to crossover to sorafenib (400 mg twice daily). The primary endpoint was PFS.

Ninety seven patients in the sorafenib arm received treatment and had a median of 5.7 months PFS vs. 5.6 months for IFN-2α. More sorafenib-treated patients had tumor regression (68.2 vs. 39.0%). Overall, sorafenib-treated patients show fewer symptoms and better quality of life [7].

The clinical efficacy of sorafenib has also been shown in the phase III randomized TARGET trial [8, 9]. Nine hundred and five cytokine-refractory mRCC patients with favorable or intermediate MSKCC risk were randomly assigned to receive sorafenib vs. placebo. The median PFS was longer in the experimental arm at the time of the interim analysis (5.5 vs. 2.8 months; hazard ratio (HR) 0.44; $p < 0.01$) and a median overall survival (OS) of 17.8 months, which was statistically identical with that of the placebo group, 15.2 months. The most common grade 3 or 4 adverse events (AEs) sorafenib was associated with were as follows: hand-foot-syndrome (86%), fatigue (5%), dyspnea (4%), and hypertension (4%).

Sorafenib was approved by the U.S. Food and Drug Administration (FDA) and the European Medicines Agency (EMA) in December 2005 and July 2006, respectively. It was listed as a category 2A option as first-line treatment for patients with relapse or unresectable stage IV predominantly clear cell renal carcinoma.

In second line, efficacy of sorafenib was studied in patients who progressed to a previous tyrosine kinase inhibitor (TKI). The international phase III trial INTORSECT [10] randomized

512 mRCC patients with progressive disease after sunitinib in two groups: temsirolimus 25 mg once weekly (n = 259) or sorafenib 400 mg twice a day (n = 253). The median PFS did not differ statistically (4.2 vs. 3.9 months) but the secondary endpoint, the OS, favored sorafenib (12.3 vs. 16.6 months).

Sorafenib has also been evaluated in the adjuvant therapy in ASSURE trial [11], however, no clinical benefit both in the PFS and OS was showed compared to placebo. There are still several clinical trials that are ongoing in order to verify the role of sorafenib in the adjuvant setting of RCC, the SORCE trial compares sorafenib to placebo for 1 or 3 years after surgery (NCT00492258) and The RESORT trial is assessing the clinical value of sorafenib for 1 year after radical resection of the metastases (NCT01444807) [12].

2.1.2. Sunitinib

Sunitinib is an oral multikinase inhibitor that targets VEGFR 1–3, c-Kit, PDGFR, FMS-like tyrosine kinase-3 (Flt3), and neurotrophic factor receptor (RET). A large multinational phase III trial compared sunitinib vs. IFN in 750 untreated patients with mRCC. Patients selected for the trial had no prior treatment, and around 90% of the patients in the trial had either favorable or intermediate MSKCC risk features. They were randomized 1:1 to receive oral sunitinib or subcutaneous IFN. This trial showed a statistically significant benefit for experimental arm in both objective response rate (ORR) (39 vs. 6%; $p < 0.001$) and median PFS (11 vs. 5 months; HR 0.54; $p < 0.001$). However, no difference in median OS was seen, maybe it is due to the crossover occurring in more than 50% of placebo-assigned patients. The most common grade 3–4 adverse events (AEs) reported were neutropenia (12%), thrombocytopenia (8%), hypertension (8%), hyperamylasemia (5%), hand foot syndrome (5%), and diarrhea (5%) [13]. Updated results of the trial demonstrate a strong trend toward median OS in the sunitinib group than in the IFN-α group (26.4 vs. 21.8 months, $p = 0.051$) [14].

Based on these studies, this drug received full approval in February 2007 from both the FDA and the EMA due to the study findings in untreated patients with advanced RCC. And the NCCN Kidney Cancer Panel has also listed sunitinib as a preferred category 1 option for first-line treatment for patients with relapsed or medically unresectable predominantly clear cell stage IV renal carcinoma.

Sunitinib also has demonstrated substantial anti-tumor activity in the subsequent-line therapy of metastatic RCC after progression on cytokine therapy [15, 16]. Studies investigating the sequential use of sunitinib and sorafenib are mostly retrospective, along with limited prospective data, showing their differences in target specificities and slightly different toxicity spectra that sometimes permit tolerance of one agent over another [17–19]. Sunitinib is considered a category 2A subsequent therapy option and was registered by the FDA in January 2006 for patients with mRCC refractory to cytokine therapy.

2.1.3. Pazopanib

Pazopanib is an oral second-generation multitarget receptor tyrosine kinase inhibitor that targets VEGFR1–3, PDGFR, and c-Kit [20].

The safety and efficacy of pazopanib was evaluated in a double blind, phase III, international study. Four hundred and thirty five patients with locally advance and/or mRCC were enrolled with no prior treatment or with one prior cytokine-based treatment. All the patients were randomized 2:1 to pazopanib 800 mg daily or placebo. Pazopanib was significantly associated with a longer median PFS compared with the placebo arm (9.2 vs. 4.2 months; $p < 0.0001$) [21]. And in the treatment-naive subgroup of 233 patients, pazopanib arm also showed survival advantage with median PFS of 11.1 months vs. 2.8 months on placebo. The ORR was 30% with pazopanib and 3% with placebo. The most common grade 3/4 AEs related to pazopanib was hypertension and diarrhea. The most common grade 3/4 chemistry abnormalities were ALT elevation and AST elevation.

Another phase III noninferiority study (COMPARZ) compared randomly pazopanib to sunitinib as first-line therapy for advanced RCC [22], the PFS being the primary endpoint. One thousand one hundred and ten patients with mRCC were randomized to receive pazopanib or sunitinib. The predefined criterion for noninferiority was reached with a median PFS of 8.4 and 9.5 months for pazopanib arm and sunitinib arm respectively (HR 1.05; 95% CI 0.90–1.22), and ORRs were 31% for pazopanib, and 25% for sunitinib. This trial showed a different safety profile between both drugs: diarrhea and hepatotoxicity being more frequent with pazopanib, while fatigue, hand-foot syndrome, and alteration in taste were most seen with sunitinib.

Based on the above evidence, Pazopanib was approved as first-line therapy by the FDA for the treatment of advanced/metastatic RCC in 2009. And the NCCN Kidney Cancer Panel has listed pazopanib as a preferred category 1 option for first-line treatment of patients with relapsed or medically unresectable predominantly clear cell stage IV renal carcinoma.

2.1.4. *Axitinib*

Axitinib is a second-generation multitarget TKI that inhibits the receptors VEGFR1–3 and with low inhibitory activities against PDGFR-α, $-\beta$ and c-Kit.

Some preclinical and clinical data suggested that axitinib might have an increased efficacy when compared with first-line VEGFR inhibitors. Two phase II trials evaluated axitinib in patients with cytokine refractory mRCC after sorafenib, the ORR reached 44 and 22.6%, respectively. The phase III AXIS trial compared axitinib and sorafenib in the second-line therapy of mRCC, 723 patients in 22 countries were enrolled in the trial. Patients who had progressed after an initial systemic therapy including sunitinib (54%), cytokines (35%), and bevacizumab-IFN or temsirolimus (11%) were randomized to 1:1 to axitinib 5 mg twice daily and sorafenib 400 mg twice daily as a second-line option. Dose of axitinib was predefined to escalate to 10 mg twice daily according to the toxicity profile of each patient. PFS was the primary endpoint, patients in the axitinib group showed significantly longer PFS than in the sorafenib group (6.7 vs. 4.7 months; HR 0.67; $p < 0.001$). The type of prior treatment did not impact those study findings. The ORR differed significantly in both arms (19.4 vs. 9.4%; $p < 0.001$). The most common adverse events were diarrhea (55%), hypertension (40%), and fatigue (39%) in the axitinib arm. However, the updated result showed no difference in the terms of OS between the two groups (20.1 vs. 19.2 months, $p = 0.3744$) [23].

To determine its effectiveness in the first-line setting, a randomized, phase III study was carried out. Around 288 patients were randomized 2:1 to receive axitinib and sorafenib, and the result indicated that axitinib was associated with improvements in both median PFS: 6.5 vs. 10.1 months (HR 0.767; p = 0.0377) and ORR 14.6 versus 32.3% (p = 0.0006), respectively, while these results were inferior to those of sunitinib or pazopanib [24].

Based on these results, the NCCN panel listed axitinib as a first-line treatment option (category 2A) and second-line treatment option (category 1).

Axitinib is also being evaluated in the adjuvant setting in the ATLAS trial (NCT01599754), a prospective, randomized, double blind placebo-controlled phase III trial, axitinib was given orally at 5 mg twice daily for 3 years vs. placebo. The study has completed recruitment and the results are awaited.

2.1.5. Lenvatinib

Lenvatinib is an oral active multikinase inhibitor that shows inhibitory activity against VEGFR1–3, FGFR 1–4, PDGFR-β, RET, and KIT.

A phase Ib clinical trial evidenced that the combination of daily lenvatinib 18 mg and everolimus at 5 mg was a potential therapeutic option for mRCC patients who had disease progression after antiangiogenics therapy: the OR was 30% and the median PFS reached 330 days (95%CI 157-446) [25].

A multicenter phase II trial that randomized 153 patients with metastatic, unresectable, or locally advanced mRCC whose disease progressed after a first-line treatment of anti-angiogenic agents. Patients were randomized to lenvatinib plus everolimus or single agent of lenvatinib or everolimus. Patients treated with the combination therapy experienced better PFS than patients treated by everolimus alone (14.6 vs. 5.5 months; HR, 0.40; 95% CI 0.24–0.68), and also with superiority in OS (25.5 vs. 15.4 months; HR, 0.67; 95% CI 0.42–1.08). Grade 3–4 AEs occur in fewer patients with everolimus alone compared with lenvatinib alone and combination therapy (everolimus 50%, lenvatinib 79%, combination 71%) [26].

In March 2016, the FDA approved the combination of lenvatinib with everolimus for the treatment of patients with advanced RCC following one prior antiangiogenic therapy, and it was listed as a category 1 recommendation for subsequent therapy by the NCCN Cancer Panel. In July 2016, the EMA registered the combination under accelerated assessment program.

2.1.6. Cabozantinib

Cabozantinib is an oral small molecule TKI of MET, VEGFR2, RET, and AXL with promising antitumor activity evidenced in preclinical studies. The clinical effectiveness of cabozantinib focused in patients who had already progressed to previous treatment. METEOR is a randomized open-label phase III clinical trial, which compared cabozantinib vs. everolimus in the patients with advanced RCC that had disease progression after prior antiangiogenics. All the patients were allocated into two arms: cabozantinib at a dose of 60 mg daily and everolimus at 10 mg daily. Median PFS and ORR were superior in the experimental arm: 7.4 vs. 3.8 months (HR 0.58; 95% CI 0.45–0.75), and ORR 21 vs. 5%, respectively. A planned interim analysis showed that OS was improved in the cabozantinib arm (HR 0.67; 95% CI 0.51–0.89; P = 0.005). Grade 3–4 AEs were reported in 74% of cabozantinib arm and 65% of the everolimus arm.

In April and July 2016, the FDA and the EMA approved cabozantinib for the treatment of patients with an advanced RCC refractory to antiangiogenics, respectively.

The most recent CABOSUN phase II multicenter trial evaluated cabozantinib in a population of patients with intermediate or poor prognosis mRCC. Patients are randomized 1:1 to cabozantinib of 60 mg daily or sunitinib 50 mg daily. The primary endpoint was PFS. Cabozantinib associated with a better median PFS than sunitinib in the first line setting (8.2 vs. 5.6 months; HR, 0.66; 95% CI, 0.46–0.95; one-sided p = 0.012). ORR was 46% for cabozantinib vs. 18% for sunitinib. Grade 3–4 AEs of all causality were 67% for cabozantinib and 68% for sunitinib that comprised fatigue, hypertension, diarrhea palmar-plantar erythrodysesthesia, and hematological toxicity. Sixty-seven percentage of the patient allocated to cabozantinib caused grade 3 or 4 AEs, which included hypertension (28%), diarrhea (10%), and fatigue (6%) [3].

Based on the data of CABOSUN trial, cabozantinib has been listed in the first-line setting for poor- and intermediate- risk of mRCC patients in the updated version 2018 NCCN guideline.

2.1.7. *Bevacizumab along with interferon*

Bevacizumab is an endovenous recombinant human monoclonal antibody that binds and neutralizes VEGF-A, which are biologically active. It was also the first antiangiogenic treatment to show clinical efficacy in advanced RCC.

In a randomized double-blind phase II trial, 116 patients with mRCC with measurable metastatic disease were randomized into three arms: placebo, low-dose (3 mg/kg), or high-dose of bevacizumab (10 mg/kg) every 2 weeks. The results demonstrated a significant prolongation of PFS in the high-dose bevacizumab comparing to the placebo group (HR 2.55; P < 0.001) [27]. A multicenter phase III trial (AVOREN) compared bevacizumab in combination with IFN-α to IFN-α in the first line of treatment. Six hundred and forty nine patients were enrolled. The median PFS was significantly longer in the arm with combination arm than in the arm with the monotherapy (10.2 vs. 5.4 months), and ORR (30.6 vs. 12.4%) was significantly different. A trend toward improved OS was observed although not statistical significantly (23.3 vs. 21.3 months). These results could be due to the crossover to the bevacizumab plus IFN-α group before progression. The main side effects related to the combination included asthenia (11%), fatigue (13%), proteinuria (8%), and hypertension (6%) [28].

The CALGB90206, which is a prospective, randomized, phase III trial clinical carried out in United States showed the similar results with the AVOREN trial, with 732 treat-naïve patients randomized 1:1 to monotherapy of IFN-α or bevacizumab plus IFN-α. The combination group produced better PFS (8.5 vs. 5.2 months) and ORR (25.5 vs. 13.1%). Also, no significant differences exist in OS between the two groups [29].

Bevacizumab plus IFN was registered in November 2007 and in August 2009 by the EMA and the FDA, respectively, for untreated patients with mRCC of good or intermediate risk (Memorial Sloan Kettering Cancer Center (MSKCC) classification.

2.2. Targeting the mammalian target of rapamycin (mTOR) pathway

TORC1 and TORC2 are two multiprotein complexes, which include a serine threonine kinase called mTOR, and they can regulate micronutrients, cell growth, apoptosis, and angiogenesis. mTOR inhibitor can inhibit small-molecule kinase, which lies downstream in the phosphatidylinositol 3-kinase (PI3K)-AKT pathway.

2.2.1. Temsirolimus

Temsirolimus is an intravenous mTOR inhibitor, which inhibits the TORC1 complex by binding FKBP12 protein. Temsirolimus showed promising effectiveness in patients with mRCC in the early phase clinical trials [30, 31].

A phase III, multicenter open-label, clinical trial in untreated mRCC patients were carried out with three of six unfavorable prognosis factors. Six hundred and twenty six patients were randomized equally to three arms of treatment: IFN, temsirolimus, or IFN plus temsirolimus. The primary endpoint was OS. Patents were stratified with prior nephrectomy and geographic region. Patients who received temsirolimus alone experienced the best clinical outcome, showed a significant improvement in OS for 10.9 months ($p = 0.008$ vs. IFN 7.3 months) while the toxicity profile was acceptable. The combination group failed to improve the OS and PFS and also with increased adverse reactions [32]. About 20% of the patients included in this trial with nonclear cell RCC also benefited from temsirolimus.

Based on these data, in 2007, this drug was approved by both the FDA and the EMA as a category 1 recommendation for first-line treatment of poor-risk patients with relapsed or medically unresectable predominantly clear cell stage IV renal carcinoma.

2.2.2. Everolimus

Everolimus is an orally administered inhibitor of mTOR, and it showed promising antitumor activity in patients with advanced RCC previously treated with cytokines [33]. Based on the results, a phase III, randomized, double-blind trial was designed (RECORD1) to evaluate the efficacy and toxicity of everolimus vs. placebo for the treatment of mRCC patients whose disease had progressed on the treatment of VEGFR inhibitors (sorafenib or sunitinib) [34]. The primary endpoint was PFS, and the secondary endpoints included OS and safety. The results of the second interim analysis indicated that the everolimus arm was associated with better PFS than the placebo arm (4.9 vs. 1.9 months; HR 0.33; $p < 0.001$). However, no significant differences exist in median OS between both arms (14.8 vs. 14.4 months; HR 0.87; $p = 0.162$). The most commonly AEs observed in the everolimus treatment arm were stomatitis (40%), rash (25%), and fatigue (20%), which were mostly mild or moderate in severity. Pneumonitis was caused in 8% of the patients with everolimus treated, eight of them reaching a grade 3 of severity.

A recent randomize phase III trial compares nivolumab with everolimus in patients with advanced mRCC who were previously treated, indicated that the OS was longer occurred with nivolumab than with everolimus (25.0 vs. 19.6 months, $p = 0.002$) [35]. In METEOR trial, which is also a phase III trial, randomized 658 patients to receive cabozantinib or everolimus; the result showed longer PFS with cabozantinib compared to everolimus (7.4 vs. 3.8 months; HR:0.58; $p < 0.001$) [36].

Based on the above data, in 2009, everolimus was approved by both the FDA and the EMA as a category 2A subsequent therapy option for the treatment of mRCC after antiangiogenics.

2.3. Immunotherapy

T cells play an important role in anti-tumor activity through stimulatory and inhibitory system. Due to high mutation and other factors, immune system has been made to be self-tolerant by cancer cells, the most active immunotherapy recently be studied include: anti-PD1, anti-PDL1, and anti-CTLA-4. Immunotherapy with monoclonal antibodies against the programmed cell death 1 (PD-1) protein has become an important and effective therapy of advanced melanoma and nonsmall cell lung cancer and also is now being tested in a large number of malignancies. It has been tested in RCC with success results.

2.3.1. Nivolumab

Nivolumab is a fully human IgG4 antibody against PD-1. A phase I clinical trial was designed to determine the safety and tolerability of nivolumab with treatment-refractory solid tumor, one RCC patient previously treated experienced an overall PR that lasted more than 16 months after only three infusions of nivolumab [37]. These findings prompted the clinical development of this compound in the treatment of mRCC.

A randomized open-label phase III study CheckMate 025 compared nivolumab with everolimus in patients with previously treated mRCC. Eight hundred and twenty one patients were randomly assigned 1:1 to receive nivolumab or everolimus. The primary end point was OS. Patients in the experimental arm experienced better median OS of 25 vs. 19 months (HR 0.73; $p = 0.002$) and greater ORR (25 vs. 5%; $p<0.001$). Grade 3–4 toxicities occurred in 19 and 37% for patients receiving nivolumab and everolimus, respectively [35].

Based on the results of the CheckMate 025, nivolumab was approved by the FDA and the EMA as a category 1, preferred subsequent therapy option in November 2015 and February 2016, respectively for the treatment of RCC after progression to TKI therapy.

The clinical development of nivolumab in RCC is currently very intense, and multiple studies are testing the value of strategies in several ways. Phase I CheckMate 016 clinical trial evaluated the efficacy and safety of the combination of nivolumab with the anti-CTLA4 ipilimumab [38]. CheckMate 214 (NCT02231749) evaluates the role of ipilimumab in combination with nivolumab in patients who do not response after monotherapy of nivolumab, and results are highly awaited.

2.4. Target therapy for nonclear cell RCC

The only available category 1 preferred recommendation for systemic treatment of nonclear cell RCC (nccRCC) is temsirolimus, and it was commended in patients with poor-risk features [32]. Although other targeted agents against the VEGF and mTOR pathways are frequently used in the treatment of nccRCC, optimal first-line agent is much less defined and the outcomes are inferior to that in patients with ccRCC [39, 40]. Immune checkpoint inhibitors appear promising effect in early clinical trials and we look forward to a good result in the updating clinical trial.

3. Upcoming therapies in RCC

3.1. Last generation for targeting VEGF/VEGFR

3.1.1. Dovitinib

Dovitinib (TKI-258) is an oral tyrosine-kinase inhibitor that inhibits VEGF and FGF receptors. In a multicenter phase III study, patients who previously received VEGF-targeted therapy or mTOR inhibitor were randomized to dovitinib or sorafenib. The results indicated that the mPFS was 3.7 months in dovitinib group vs. 3.6 months in sorafenib group, showing improvement in mPFS, however, with no significant difference [41]. A phase II clinical trial has been designed to find out the usefulness of dovitinib in the initial treatment for patients with advanced kidney cancer, and the study will additionally look for changes in the genetic makeup of tumor cells.

3.1.2. Trebananib

Angiopoietin-2 (Ang2) exhibits broad expression in the remodeling vasculature of tumors but not in the normal tissues. Trebananib (AMG-386) can bind to angiopoietin 1 and 2 and block their union with the Tie2 receptor tyrosine kinase, showing its antiangiogenic effect. In preclinical and clinical phase I studies, AMG-386 showed a good safety profile in inhibiting tumor growth [42]. A randomized phase II trial showed that AMG-386 plus sorafenib reach a RR of 38% in RCC patients previously treated [43].

3.2. Immunotherapy

3.2.1. Pembrolizumab

Pembrolizumab (MK-3475) is a highly selective IgG4-humanized monoclonal antibody, which prevents the binding of PD-1 with PD-L1 and PD-L2. A phase I study evaluated the safety, tolerated does, and antitumor effect of pembrolizumab in patients with advanced solid tumors. It showed durable antitumor activity in multiple solid tumors including RCC [44]. There are two clinical trials NCT02212730 and NCT02853344, both of which are currently recruiting, are going to test the effect of pembrolizumab in the neoadjuvant treatment for localized RCC and in untreated mRCC, respectively as monotherapy.

3.2.2. *Avelumab*

Avelumab (MSB0010718C) is a human IgG1 monoclonal antibody against PD-L1. Avelumab binds to PD-L1 inhibiting its binding to PD-1 and therefore inhibiting its activation of T cells and restoring anticancer immune function. In an open-label, single-center, phase 1a trial, safety and activity of this compound was tested in multiple solid tumors including RCC and prompted the further research for this drug [45]. An open, randomized phase II trial SUAVE, which is recruiting is going to compare avelumab followed by sunitinib with the opposite sequence. The effect of avelumab in the combination therapy is also being evaluated. A phase III, multinational, randomized trial is going to compare avelumab with axitinib vs. sunitinib in advance renal cell cancer which is currently recruiting (NCT02684006).

3.2.3. *Atezolizumab*

Atezolizumab (MPDL-3280A) is a PD-L1-specific monoclonal antibody, which inhibits the binding of PD-L1 to PD-1. Based on the promising date in the phase I clinical trial [46], a further phase II clinical trial IMmotion 150 enrolled untreated mRCC patients, and randomized them into three arms, atezolizumab alone, atezolizumab with bevacizumab, and sunitinib alone. Preliminary result showed no significant difference in PFS between the two arms with immunotherapy, PD-1+ patients showed a trend of survival benefit, although with no significant difference. The IMmotion 151 phase III trial is ongoing to assess the combination of atezolizumab with sunitinib in mRCC.

3.2.4. *Ipilimumab*

Ipilimumab is an antibody against CTLA-4 and it shows powerful antitumor activity and clinical experience in the treatment of patients with metastatic melanoma. Therefore, a phase II trial was conducted in patients with mRCC, observing a 10% partial RR, 33% of the patients experienced a grade III or IV immune-mediated toxicity [47]. The efficacy of ipilimumab combine with other drugs is also being evaluated in some trials, like the phase III, randomized study CheckMate 214, comparing the combination of nivolumab and ipilimumab with sunitinib monotherapy in previously untreated local advanced RCC or mRCC. Ipilimumab is also being investigated in association with other drugs for the treatment of advanced RCC, like CheckMate 214 study or Keynote-29 study.

Due to the remarkable development of the advanced in the molecular mechanism and cytogenetic of tumor in the last decade, targeted agents directed against VEGF, VEGFR, and mTOR have been important therapy in mRCC. Immune checkpoint inhibitors also appear promising power, and a lot of novel targets including small molecule TKIs and immunotherapies are entering clinical trials, which will update the treatment paradigms in the future time. It is hoped that with better understanding of the molecular diversity of RCC, more effective and personalized therapeutic strategies can be developed against mRCC to make the patients obtain the maximum benefit.

Author details

Yang Wang[1] and Lingxiang Liu[2]*

*Address all correspondence to: llxlau@163.com

1 Department of Oncology, The Second Affiliated Hospital of Nanjing Medical University, Nanjing, China

2 Department of Oncology, The First Affiliated Hospital of Nanjing Medical University, Nanjing, China

References

[1] Fyfe G, Fisher RI, Rosenberg SA, Sznol M, Parkinson DR, Louie AC. Mint: Results of treatment of 255 patients with metastatic renal cell carcinoma who received high-dose recombinant interleukin-2 therapy. Journal of Clinical Oncology : Official Journal of the American Society of Clinical Oncology. 1995;**13**:688-696. DOI: 10.1200/jco.1995.13.3.688

[2] McDermott DF, Regan MM, Clark JI, Flaherty LE, Weiss GR, Logan TF, Kirkwood JM, Gordon MS, Sosman JA, Ernstoff MS, Tretter CP, Urba WJ, Smith JW, Margolin KA, Mier JW, Gollob JA, Dutcher JP, Atkins MB. Mint: Randomized phase iii trial of high-dose interleukin-2 versus subcutaneous interleukin-2 and interferon in patients with metastatic renal cell carcinoma. Journal of Clinical Oncology : Official Journal of the American Society of Clinical Oncology. 2005;**23**:133-141. DOI: 10.1200/jco.2005.03.206

[3] Choueiri TK, Halabi S, Sanford BL, Hahn O, Michaelson MD, Walsh MK, Feldman DR, Olencki T, Picus J, Small EJ, Dakhil S, George DJ, Morris MJ. Mint: Cabozantinib versus sunitinib as initial targeted therapy for patients with metastatic renal cell carcinoma of poor or intermediate risk: The alliance a031203 cabosun trial. Journal of Clinical Oncology : Official Journal of the American Society of Clinical Oncology. 2017;**35**:591-597. DOI: 10.1200/jco.2016.70.7398

[4] Motzer RJ, Bacik J, Murphy BA, Russo P, Mazumdar M. Mint: Interferon-alfa as a comparative treatment for clinical trials of new therapies against advanced renal cell carcinoma. Journal of Clinical Oncology : Official Journal of the American Society of Clinical Oncology. 2002;**20**:289-296. DOI: 10.1200/JCO.2002.20.1.289

[5] Mekhail TM, Abou-Jawde RM, Boumerhi G, Malhi S, Wood L, Elson P, Bukowski R. Mint: Validation and extension of the memorial sloan-kettering prognostic factors model for survival in patients with previously untreated metastatic renal cell carcinoma. Journal of Clinical Oncology : Official Journal of the American Society of Clinical Oncology. 2005; **23**:832-841. DOI: 10.1200/JCO.2005.05.179

[6] Mendel DB, Laird AD, Xin X, Louie SG, Christensen JG, Li G, Schreck RE, Abrams TJ, Ngai TJ, Lee LB, Murray LJ, Carver J, Chan E, Moss KG, Haznedar JO, Sukbuntherng J, Blake RA, Sun L, Tang C, Miller T, Shirazian S, McMahon G, Cherrington JM. Mint: In

vivo antitumor activity of su11248, a novel tyrosine kinase inhibitor targeting vascular endothelial growth factor and platelet-derived growth factor receptors: Determination of a pharmacokinetic/pharmacodynamic relationship. Clinical Cancer Research : An Official Journal of the American Association for Cancer Research. 2003;**9**:327-337

[7] Escudier B, Szczylik C, Hutson TE, Demkow T, Staehler M, Rolland F, Negrier S, Laferriere N, Scheuring UJ, Cella D, Shah S, Bukowski RM. Mint: Randomized phase ii trial of first-line treatment with sorafenib versus interferon alfa-2a in patients with metastatic renal cell carcinoma. Journal of Clinical Oncology : Official Journal of the American Society of Clinical Oncology. 2009;**27**:1280-1289. DOI: 10.1200/jco.2008.19.3342

[8] Escudier B, Eisen T, Stadler WM, Szczylik C, Oudard S, Staehler M, Negrier S, Chevreau C, Desai AA, Rolland F, Demkow T, Hutson TE, Gore M, Anderson S, Hofilena G, Shan M, Pena C, Lathia C, Bukowski RM. Mint: Sorafenib for treatment of renal cell carcinoma: Final efficacy and safety results of the phase iii treatment approaches in renal cancer global evaluation trial. Journal of Clinical Oncology : Official Journal of the American Society of Clinical Oncology. 2009;**27**:3312-3318. DOI: 10.1200/JCO.2008.19.5511

[9] Escudier B, Eisen T, Stadler WM, Szczylik C, Oudard S, Siebels M, Negrier S, Chevreau C, Solska E, Desai AA, Rolland F, Demkow T, Hutson TE, Gore M, Freeman S, Schwartz B, Shan M, Simantov R, Bukowski RM. Mint: Sorafenib in advanced clear-cell renal-cell carcinoma. New England Journal of Medicine. 2007;**356**:125-134. DOI: 10.1056/NEJMoa060655

[10] Hutson TE, Escudier B, Esteban E, Bjarnason GA, Lim HY, Pittman KB, Senico P, Niethammer A, DR L, Hariharan S, Motzer RJ. Mint: Randomized phase iii trial of temsirolimus versus sorafenib as second-line therapy after sunitinib in patients with metastatic renal cell carcinoma. Journal of Clinical Oncology : Official Journal of the American Society of Clinical Oncology. 2014;**32**:760-767. DOI: 10.1200/JCO.2013.50.3961

[11] Haas NBMJ, Uzzo RG, Atkins MB, Wilding G, Pins M, et al. Mint: Initial results from assure (e2805): Adjuvant sorafenib or sunitinib for unfavorable renal carcinoma, an ecog-acrin-led, nctn phase iii trial. Journal of Clinical Oncology. 2015;**33** (suppl 7; abstr 403)

[12] Procopio G, Grassi P, Cognetti F, Milella M, Mosca A, Chiuri VE, et al. A randomized, opne label, multicenter phase 2 study to evaluate the efficacy of sorafenib in patients (pts) with advanced renal cell carcinoma (rcc) after radical resection of metastases: Resort trial. Journal of Clinical Oncology. 2016;**34** (suppl; abstr tps4582)

[13] Motzer RJ, Hutson TE, Tomczak P, Michaelson MD, Bukowski RM, Rixe O, Oudard S, Negrier S, Szczylik C, Kim ST, Chen I, Bycott PW, Baum CM, Figlin RA. Mint: Sunitinib versus interferon alfa in metastatic renal-cell carcinoma. The New England Journal of Medicine. 2007;**356**:115-124. DOI: 10.1056/NEJMoa065044

[14] Motzer RJ, Hutson TE, Tomczak P, Michaelson MD, Bukowski RM, Oudard S, Negrier S, Szczylik C, Pili R, Bjarnason GA, Garcia-del-Muro X, Sosman JA, Solska E, Wilding G, Thompson JA, Kim ST, Chen I, Huang X, Figlin RA. Mint: Overall survival and updated results for sunitinib compared with interferon alfa in patients with metastatic renal cell carcinoma. Journal of Clinical Oncology : Official Journal of the American Society of Clinical Oncology. 2009;**27**:3584-3590. DOI: 10.1200/JCO.2008.20.1293

[15] Motzer RJ, Michaelson MD, Redman BG, Hudes GR, Wilding G, Figlin RA, Ginsberg MS, Kim ST, Baum CM, DePrimo SE, Li JZ, Bello CL, Theuer CP, George DJ, Rini BI. Mint: Activity of su11248, a multitargeted inhibitor of vascular endothelial growth factor receptor and platelet-derived growth factor receptor, in patients with metastatic renal cell carcinoma. Journal of Clinical Oncology : Official Journal of the American Society of Clinical Oncology. 2006;**24**:16-24. DOI: 10.1200/JCO.2005.02.2574

[16] Motzer RJ, Rini BI, Bukowski RM, Curti BD, George DJ, Hudes GR, Redman BG, Margolin KA, Merchan JR, Wilding G, Ginsberg MS, Bacik J, Kim ST, Baum CM, Michaelson MD. Mint: Sunitinib in patients with metastatic renal cell carcinoma. JAMA : The Journal of the American Medical Association. 2006;**295**:2516-2524. DOI: 10.1001/jama.295.21.2516

[17] Dudek AZ, Zolnierek J, Dham A, Lindgren BR, Szczylik C. Mint: Sequential therapy with sorafenib and sunitinib in renal cell carcinoma. Cancer. 2009;**115**:61-67. DOI: 10.1002/cncr.24009

[18] Eichelberg C, Heuer R, Chun FK, Hinrichs K, Zacharias M, Huland H, Heinzer H. Mint: Sequential use of the tyrosine kinase inhibitors sorafenib and sunitinib in metastatic renal cell carcinoma: A retrospective outcome analysis. European Urology. 2008;**54**:1373-1378. DOI: 10.1016/j.eururo.2008.07.051

[19] Shepard DR, Rini BI, Garcia JA, et al. A multicenter prospective rial of sorafenib in patients (pts) with metastatic clear cell renal cell carcinoma (mccrcc) refractory to prior sunitinib or bevacizumab[abstract]. Journal of Clinical Oncology. 2008;**26**:Abstract 5123

[20] Hamberg P, Verweij J, Sleijfer S. Mint: (pre-)clinical pharmacology and activity of pazopanib, a novel multikinase angiogenesis inhibitor. The Oncologist. 2010;**15**:539-547. DOI: 10.1634/theoncologist.2009-0274

[21] Sternberg CN, Davis ID, Mardiak J, Szczylik C, Lee E, Wagstaff J, Barrios CH, Salman P, Gladkov OA, Kavina A, Zarba JJ, Chen M, McCann L, Pandite L, Roychowdhury DF, Hawkins RE. Mint: Pazopanib in locally advanced or metastatic renal cell carcinoma: Results of a randomized phase iii trial. Journal of Clinical Oncology : Official Journal of the American Society of Clinical Oncology. 2010;**28**:1061-1068. DOI: 10.1200/jco.2009.23.9764

[22] Motzer RJ, Hutson TE, Cella D, Reeves J, Hawkins R, Guo J, Nathan P, Staehler M, de Souza P, Merchan JR, Boleti E, Fife K, Jin J, Jones R, Uemura H, De Giorgi U, Harmenberg U, Wang J, Sternberg CN, Deen K, McCann L, Hackshaw MD, Crescenzo R, Pandite LN, Choueiri TK. Mint: Pazopanib versus sunitinib in metastatic renal-cell carcinoma. The New England Journal of Medicine 2013;**369**:722-731. DOI: 10.1056/NEJMoa1303989

[23] Motzer RJ, Escudier B, Tomczak P, Hutson TE, Michaelson MD, Negrier S, Oudard S, Gore ME, Tarazi J, Hariharan S, Chen C, Rosbrook B, Kim S, Rini BI. Mint: Axitinib versus sorafenib as second-line treatment for advanced renal cell carcinoma: Overall survival analysis and updated results from a randomised phase 3 trial. The Lancet Oncology. 2013;**14**:552-562. DOI: 10.1016/s1470-2045(13)70093-7

[24] Hutson TE, Lesovoy V, Al-Shukri S, Stus VP, Lipatov ON, Bair AH, Rosbrook B, Chen C, Kim S, Vogelzang NJ. Mint: Axitinib versus sorafenib as first-line therapy in patients with metastatic renal-cell carcinoma: A randomised open-label phase 3 trial. The Lancet Oncology. 2013;**14**:1287-1294. DOI: 10.1016/s1470-2045(13)70465-0

[25] Molina AM, Hutson TE, Larkin J, Gold AM, Wood K, Carter D, Motzer R, Michaelson MD. Mint: A phase 1b clinical trial of the multi-targeted tyrosine kinase inhibitor lenvatinib (e7080) in combination with everolimus for treatment of metastatic renal cell carcinoma (rcc). Cancer Chemotherapy and Pharmacology. 2014;**73**:181-189. DOI: 10.1007/s00280-013-2339-y

[26] Motzer RJ, Hutson TE, Glen H, Michaelson MD, Molina A, Eisen T, Jassem J, Zolnierek J, Maroto JP, Mellado B, Melichar B, Tomasek J, Kremer A, Kim HJ, Wood K, Dutcus C, Larkin J. Mint: Lenvatinib, everolimus, and the combination in patients with metastatic renal cell carcinoma: A randomised, phase 2, open-label, multicentre trial. The Lancet Oncology. 2015;**16**:1473-1482. DOI: 10.1016/s1470-2045(15)00290-9

[27] Yang JC, Haworth L, Sherry RM, Hwu P, Schwartzentruber DJ, Topalian SL, Steinberg SM, Chen HX, Rosenberg SA. Mint: A randomized trial of bevacizumab, an anti-vascular endothelial growth factor antibody, for metastatic renal cancer. The New England Journal of Medicine. 2003;**349**:427-434. DOI: 10.1056/NEJMoa021491

[28] Escudier B, Bellmunt J, Negrier S, Bajetta E, Melichar B, Bracarda S, Ravaud A, Golding S, Jethwa S, Sneller V. Mint: Phase iii trial of bevacizumab plus interferon alfa-2a in patients with metastatic renal cell carcinoma (avoren): Final analysis of overall survival. Journal of Clinical Oncology : Official Journal of the American Society of Clinical Oncology. 2010;**28**:2144-2150. DOI: 10.1200/jco.2009.26.7849

[29] Rini BI, Halabi S, Rosenberg JE, Stadler WM, Vaena DA, Archer L, Atkins JN, Picus J, Czaykowski P, Dutcher J, Small EJ. Mint: Phase iii trial of bevacizumab plus interferon alfa versus interferon alfa monotherapy in patients with metastatic renal cell carcinoma: Final results of calgb 90206. Journal of Clinical Oncology : Official Journal of the American Society of Clinical Oncology. 2010;**28**:2137-2143. DOI: 10.1200/jco.2009.26.5561

[30] Atkins MB, Hidalgo M, Stadler WM, Logan TF, Dutcher JP, Hudes GR, Park Y, Liou SH, Marshall B, Boni JP, Dukart G, Sherman ML. Mint: Randomized phase ii study of multiple dose levels of cci-779, a novel mammalian target of rapamycin kinase inhibitor, in patients with advanced refractory renal cell carcinoma. Journal of Clinical Oncology : Official Journal of the American Society of Clinical Oncology. 2004;**22**:909-918. DOI: 10.1200/jco.2004.08.185

[31] Raymond E, Alexandre J, Faivre S, Vera K, Materman E, Boni J, Leister C, Korth-Bradley J, Hanauske A, Armand JP. Mint: Safety and pharmacokinetics of escalated doses of weekly intravenous infusion of cci-779, a novel mtor inhibitor, in patients with cancer. Journal of Clinical Oncology : Official Journal of the American Society of Clinical Oncology. 2004;**22**:2336-2347. DOI: 10.1200/jco.2004.08.116

[32] Hudes G, Carducci M, Tomczak P, Dutcher J, Figlin R, Kapoor A, Staroslawska E, Sosman J, McDermott D, Bodrogi I, Kovacevic Z, Lesovoy V, Schmidt-Wolf IG, Barbarash O, Gokmen E, O'Toole T, Lustgarten S, Moore L, Motzer RJ. Mint: Temsirolimus, interferon alfa, or both for advanced renal-cell carcinoma. The New England Journal of Medicine. 2007;**356**:2271-2281. DOI: 10.1056/NEJMoa066838

[33] O'Donnell A, Faivre S, Burris HA 3rd, Rea D, Papadimitrakopoulou V, Shand N, Lane HA, Hazell K, Zoellner U, Kovarik JM, Brock C, Jones S, Raymond E, Judson I. Mint: Phase i pharmacokinetic and pharmacodynamic study of the oral mammalian target of rapamycin inhibitor everolimus in patients with advanced solid tumors. Journal of Clinical Oncology : Official Journal of the American Society of Clinical Oncology. 2008;**26**:1588-1595. DOI: 10.1200/JCO.2007.14.0988

[34] Motzer RJ, Escudier B, Oudard S, Hutson TE, Porta C, Bracarda S, Grunwald V, Thompson JA, Figlin RA, Hollaender N, Urbanowitz G, Berg WJ, Kay A, Lebwohl D, Ravaud A, Group R-S. Mint: Efficacy of everolimus in advanced renal cell carcinoma: A double-blind, randomised, placebo-controlled phase iii trial. Lancet. 2008;**372**:449-456. DOI: 10.1016/S0140-6736(08)61039-9

[35] Motzer RJ, Escudier B, McDermott DF, George S, Hammers HJ, Srinivas S, Tykodi SS, Sosman JA, Procopio G, Plimack ER, Castellano D, Choueiri TK, Gurney H, Donskov F, Bono P, Wagstaff J, Gauler TC, Ueda T, Tomita Y, Schutz FA, Kollmannsberger C, Larkin J, Ravaud A, Simon JS, Xu LA, Waxman IM, Sharma P. Mint: Nivolumab versus everolimus in advanced renal-cell carcinoma. The New England Journal of Medicine. 2015;**373**:1803-1813. DOI: 10.1056/NEJMoa1510665

[36] Choueiri TK, Escudier B, Powles T, Mainwaring PN, Rini BI, Donskov F, Hammers H, Hutson TE, Lee JL, Peltola K, Roth BJ, Bjarnason GA, Geczi L, Keam B, Maroto P, Heng DY, Schmidinger M, Kantoff PW, Borgman-Hagey A, Hessel C, Scheffold C, Schwab GM, Tannir NM, Motzer RJ, Investigators M. Mint: Cabozantinib versus everolimus in advanced renal-cell carcinoma. The New England Journal of Medicine. 2015;**373**:1814-1823. DOI: 10.1056/NEJMoa1510016

[37] Brahmer JR, Drake CG, Wollner I, Powderly JD, Picus J, Sharfman WH, Stankevich E, Pons A, Salay TM, McMiller TL, Gilson MM, Wang C, Selby M, Taube JM, Anders R, Chen L, Korman AJ, Pardoll DM, Lowy I, Topalian SL. Mint: Phase i study of single-agent anti-programmed death-1 (mdx-1106) in refractory solid tumors: Safety, clinical activity, pharmacodynamics, and immunologic correlates. Journal of Clinical Oncology : Official Journal of the American Society of Clinical Oncology. 2010;**28**:3167-3175. DOI: 10.1200/JCO.2009.26.7609

[38] Hammers HJ, Plimack ER, Infante JR, Rini BI, McDermott DF, Lewis LD, Voss MH, Sharma P, Pal SK, Razak ARA, Kollmannsberger C, Heng DYC, Spratlin J, McHenry MB, Amin A. Mint: Safety and efficacy of nivolumab in combination with ipilimumab in metastatic renal cell carcinoma: The checkmate 016 study. Journal of Clinical Oncology : Official Journal of the American Society of Clinical Oncology. 2017:JCO2016721985. DOI: 10.1200/JCO.2016.72.1985

[39] Singer EA, Bratslavsky G, Linehan WM, Srinivasan R. Mint: Targeted therapies for non-clear renal cell carcinoma. Targeted Oncology. 2010;**5**:119-129. DOI: 10.1007/s11523-010-0148-3

[40] Kroeger N, Xie W, Lee JL, Bjarnason GA, Knox JJ, Mackenzie MJ, Wood L, Srinivas S, Vaishamayan UN, Rha SY, Pal SK, Yuasa T, Donskov F, Agarwal N, Kollmannsberger CK, Tan MH, North SA, Rini BI, Choueiri TK, Heng DY. Mint: Metastatic non-clear cell renal cell carcinoma treated with targeted therapy agents: Characterization of survival outcome and application of the international mrcc database consortium criteria. Cancer. 2013;**119**:2999-3006. DOI: 10.1002/cncr.28151

[41] Motzer RJ, Porta C, Vogelzang NJ, Sternberg CN, Szczylik C, Zolnierek J, Kollmannsberger C, Rha SY, Bjarnason GA, Melichar B, De Giorgi U, Grunwald V, Davis ID, Lee JL, Esteban E, Urbanowitz G, Cai C, Squires M, Marker M, Shi MM, Escudier B. Mint: Dovitinib versus sorafenib for third-line targeted treatment of patients with metastatic renal cell carcinoma: An open-label, randomised phase 3 trial. The Lancet Oncology. 2014;**15**:286-296. DOI: 10.1016/S1470-2045(14)70030-0

[42] Oliner J, Min H, Leal J, Yu D, Rao S, You E, Tang X, Kim H, Meyer S, Han SJ, Hawkins N, Rosenfeld R, Davy E, Graham K, Jacobsen F, Stevenson S, Ho J, Chen Q, Hartmann T, Michaels M, Kelley M, Li L, Sitney K, Martin F, Sun JR, Zhang N, Lu J, Estrada J, Kumar R, Coxon A, Kaufman S, Pretorius J, Scully S, Cattley R, Payton M, Coats S, Nguyen L, Desilva B, Ndifor A, Hayward I, Radinsky R, Boone T, Kendall R. Mint: Suppression of angiogenesis and tumor growth by selective inhibition of angiopoietin-2. Cancer Cell. 2004;**6**:507-516. DOI: 10.1016/j.ccr.2004.09.030

[43] Rini B, Szczylik C, Tannir NM, Koralewski P, Tomczak P, Deptala A, Dirix LY, Fishman M, Ramlau R, Ravaud A, Rogowski W, Kracht K, Sun YN, Bass MB, Puhlmann M, Escudier B. Mint: Amg 386 in combination with sorafenib in patients with metastatic clear cell carcinoma of the kidney: A randomized, double-blind, placebo-controlled, phase 2 study. Cancer. 2012;**118**:6152-6161. DOI: 10.1002/cncr.27632

[44] Patnaik A, Kang SP, Rasco D, Papadopoulos KP, Elassaiss-Schaap J, Beeram M, Drengler R, Chen C, Smith L, Espino G, Gergich K, Delgado L, Daud A, Lindia JA, Li XN, Pierce RH, Yearley JH, Wu D, Laterza O, Lehnert M, Iannone R, Tolcher AW. Mint: Phase i study of pembrolizumab (mk-3475; anti-pd-1 monoclonal antibody) in patients with advanced solid tumors. Clinical Cancer Research : An Official Journal of the American Association for Cancer Research. 2015;**21**:4286-4293. DOI: 10.1158/1078-0432.CCR-14-2607

[45] Heery CR, O'Sullivan-Coyne G, Madan RA, Cordes L, Rajan A, Rauckhorst M, Lamping E, Oyelakin I, Marte JL, Lepone LM, Donahue RN, Grenga I, Cuillerot JM, Neuteboom B, Heydebreck AV, Chin K, Schlom J, Gulley JL. Mint: Avelumab for metastatic or locally advanced previously treated solid tumours (javelin solid tumor): A phase 1a, multicohort, dose-escalation trial. The Lancet Oncology. 2017;**18**:587-598. DOI: 10.1016/S1470-2045(17)30239-5

[46] Brahmer JR, Tykodi SS, Chow LQ, Hwu WJ, Topalian SL, Hwu P, Drake CG, Camacho LH, Kauh J, Odunsi K, Pitot HC, Hamid O, Bhatia S, Martins R, Eaton K, Chen S, Salay TM, Alaparthy S, Grosso JF, Korman AJ, Parker SM, Agrawal S, Goldberg SM, Pardoll DM, Gupta A, Wigginton JM. Mint: Safety and activity of anti-pd-l1 antibody in patients with advanced cancer. The New England Journal of Medicine. 2012;**366**:2455-2465. DOI: 10.1056/NEJMoa1200694

[47] Yang JC, Hughes M, Kammula U, Royal R, Sherry RM, Topalian SL, Suri KB, Levy C, Allen T, Mavroukakis S, Lowy I, White DE, Rosenberg SA. Mint: Ipilimumab (anti-ctla4 antibody) causes regression of metastatic renal cell cancer associated with enteritis and hypophysitis. Journal of Immunotherapy. 2007;**30**:825-830. DOI: 10.1097/CJI.0b013e318156e47e

Chapter 9

Medical Management of Renal Cell Cancer

Jennifer Turner, Adrian Simoes, Albert Edwards and
Rakesh Raman

Additional information is available at the end of the chapter

http://dx.doi.org/10.5772/intechopen.85931

Abstract

In 2018, there were an estimated 400,000 new cases of renal cell carcinoma (RCC) worldwide—with 64,000 cases in the United States and 12,600 in the United Kingdom (UK). The medical management of RCC is an integral part of treatment as between one-quarter and one-third of patients will present with metastatic disease. There has been a rapid evolution of targeted and novel treatments for RCC over the last two decades. This chapter explores the biology of renal cell carcinoma and current treatment strategies.

Keywords: renal cell carcinoma, metastatic renal cell carcinoma, tyrosine kinase inhibitor, targeted treatment, risk stratification

1. Introduction

Renal cell carcinoma (RCC) is the fourteenth most common cancer internationally [1]. There were estimated to be around 400,000 new cases worldwide in 2018, with 64,000 cases in the United States of America and 12,600 in the United Kingdom (UK) [1–3]. The increasing incidence of RCC worldwide over the past three decades has been attributed to increasing obesity, increasing height, and increasing tobacco smoking [4, 5]. RCC is also noted to be twice as prevalent in men than women [4]. Overall, 25–30% of patients have locally advanced RCC or metastatic disease at presentation [6], although in the UK, the proportion is 40% [3]. Systemic therapy and, in selected cases, surgical intervention has an important role in the management of metastatic RCC. The landscape of available systemic treatment options has developed rapidly over the past 10 years with a wide variety of systemic strategies now being employed. This chapter will review current therapies in the metastatic setting, consider the evidence for adjuvant systemic treatment, as well as look at some of the promising new therapies that are likely to emerge in the coming years.

2. Histological subtypes

Renal cell carcinoma is divided into several histological subtypes, of which the most common is clear cell renal cell carcinoma (ccRCC), accounting for approximately three-quarters of all kidney cancers [7]. Clear cell RCC originates from the epithelium of the proximal convoluted tubules. Most are sporadic, but there is a strong familial connection with those with a first-degree relative more likely to be effected and around 5% are associated with hereditary conditions such as Von Hippel–Lindau disease, tuberous sclerosis, and adult polycystic disease. The next most prevalent histological subtypes are papillary (10%) and chromophobe (5%) [7]. These three histological subtypes make up 90% of renal cell carcinomas and are also most common in patients over the age of 50 years. Other rarer subtypes, such as medullary and Xp11 translocation, are typically seen in younger people. A better understanding of the genetic drivers for renal cell carcinoma has led to the development of targeted systemic agents and revolutionised the metastatic treatment landscape.

3. Staging and risk stratification in renal cell carcinoma

Staging for RCC is based on the TNM 8 classification and staging groups [8]. The staging takes into account the size and loco-regional extent of the tumour in addition to lymph node and distant metastatic spread [9]. **Table 1** illustrates this is in further detail.

In metastatic renal cell carcinoma, the decision to treat and, more importantly the choice of initial treatment, is based on risk stratification of the patients into three groups. The choice of initial systemic therapy in metastatic RCC may be informed by risk stratification using the International Metastatic Renal Cell Carcinoma Database Consortium (IMDC) prognostic model [10–12].

The six adverse risk factors in the IMDC model are as follows [11]:

- time from original diagnosis to initiation of targeted therapy <1 year;
- Karnofsky performance score < 80;
- haemoglobin < lower limit of normal;
- neutrophil > upper limit of normal;
- platelet > upper limit of normal; and
- serum calcium > upper limit of normal.

Patients with none of these risk factors are considered to be in the favourable-risk group, those with one or two are considered to be in the intermediate-risk group, and those with three or more risk factors are considered to be in the poor-risk group. These groups correlate with median overall survival: 43.2 months in the favourable-risk group, 22.5 months in the

TX	Primary tumour cannot be assessed
T0	No evidence of primary tumour
T1	Tumour ≤7 cm in greatest dimension, limited to the kidneys
T1a	Tumour ≤4 cm in greatest dimension, limited to the kidneys
T1b	Tumour >4 and ≤7 cm in greatest dimension, limited to the kidneys
T2	Tumour >7 cm in greatest dimension, limited to the kidneys
T2a	Tumour >7 and ≤10 cm in greatest dimension, limited to the kidneys
T2b	Tumour >10 cm in greatest dimension, limited to the kidneys
T3	Tumour extends into major veins or perinephric tissues, but not into the ipsilateral adrenal gland and not beyond Gerota's fascia
T3a	Tumour extends into the renal veins or its segmental branches, or invades the pelvicalyceal system, or invades perirenal and/or renal sinus fat but not beyond Gerota's fascia
T3b	Tumour extends into the vena cava below the diaphragm
T3c	Tumour extends into the vena cava above the diaphragm or invades the wall of the vena cava
T4	Tumour invades beyond Gerota's fascia (including contiguous extension into the ipsilateral adrenal gland)
NX	Regional lymph nodes cannot be assessed
N0	No regional lymph nodes metastasis
N1	Metastasis in regional lymph node(s)
M0	No distant metastasis
M1	Distant metastasis

Prognostic groups

T stage	N stage	M stage	Stage group
T1	N0	M0	I
T1	N1	M0	III
T2	N0	M0	II
T2	N1	M0	III
T3	Nx, N0	M0	III
T3	N1	M0	III
T4	Any N	M0	IV
Any T	Any N	M1	IV

Table 1. TNM staging of renal cell carcinoma [8].

intermediate-risk group, and 7.8 months in the poor-risk group [11]. Oncologists use this, or similar risk stratification, to decide upon the most appropriate treatment from the systemic options available. The advantage of the IMDC-model-based risk stratification is that it has been validated in both clear cell and non-clear cell histopathological groups and after first line and subsequent lines of treatment [11–14].

4. Metastatic systemic treatment options

4.1. Overview

The treatment objective in metastatic cancer is different to the primary setting. Treatment is palliative and the benefits, in terms of progression-free and overall survival, must be carefully balanced against the quality of life of the patient and potential side effects that any treatment may cause. The evolution of therapies has led to an increase in the median overall survival in metastatic RCC to beyond 2 years, and is likely to increase further as more treatments are developed [15–17].

4.2. Tyrosine kinase inhibitors

Tyrosine kinase inhibitors (TKIs) are a mainstay of targeted treatment in renal cell carcinoma. The drugs are designed to inhibit tyrosine kinases and enzymes, which themselves activate pathways of growth within the tumour cell. There are many different targets for TKIs, and in renal cell carcinoma, agents are targeted at vascular endothelial growth factor (VEGF), platelet-derived growth factor (PDGF), and the mammalian target of rapamycin (mTOR). Over half of patients have abnormalities in the von Hippel Lindau (VHL) gene, which leads to an increased expression of hypoxia inducible factors (HIF) [18]. In turn, accumulation of HIF switches on hypoxia-inducible genes such as VEGF and PDGF, and further downstream, mTOR. Expression of VEGF and mTOR drives tumour growth and angiogenesis [18].

The most commonly used TKIs employing VEGF are sorafenib, sunitinib, pazopanib, axitinib, and cabozantinib, and employing mTOR everolimus and temsirolimus. The action of these agents at a cellular level is illustrated in **Image 1**. Multiple clinical trials have shown the efficacy of these agents in RCC and are summarised in **Table 2**. The most commonly observed side effects for TKI therapy are rash, diarrhoea, hypertension, fatigue, and palmar-plantar erythrodysesthesia syndrome (hand-foot syndrome) [19–26].

Bevacizumab has also been used in renal cell cancer. Bevacizumab is a monoclonal antibody, which blockades the VEGF ligand, binding with VEGF-A. Initial trials of bevacizumab versus interferon alpha (IFN-**α**) showed a progression-free survival (PFS) benefit, but no OS benefit as crossover was allowed on progression [27]. When used in combination, IFN-**α** bevacizumab showed a higher response rate and PFS, but again OS was not demonstrated, and there was also significant toxicity [27]. Although it remains a first-line treatment option, in practice, due to the high toxicity of the treatment and efficacy of other first-line treatment options, it is rarely used. Trials also explored the combination of bevacizumab and mTOR inhibitors; however, no clinical benefit was determined and toxicity proved to be a limiting factor [28–31].

4.3. Immunotherapy

One of the most exciting areas of development in systemic therapy has been immunotherapy. The purpose of immunotherapy is to unmask the cancer to the body's own immune system. Historically, IFN-**α** has been used in RCC with a modest effect, and overall response rates

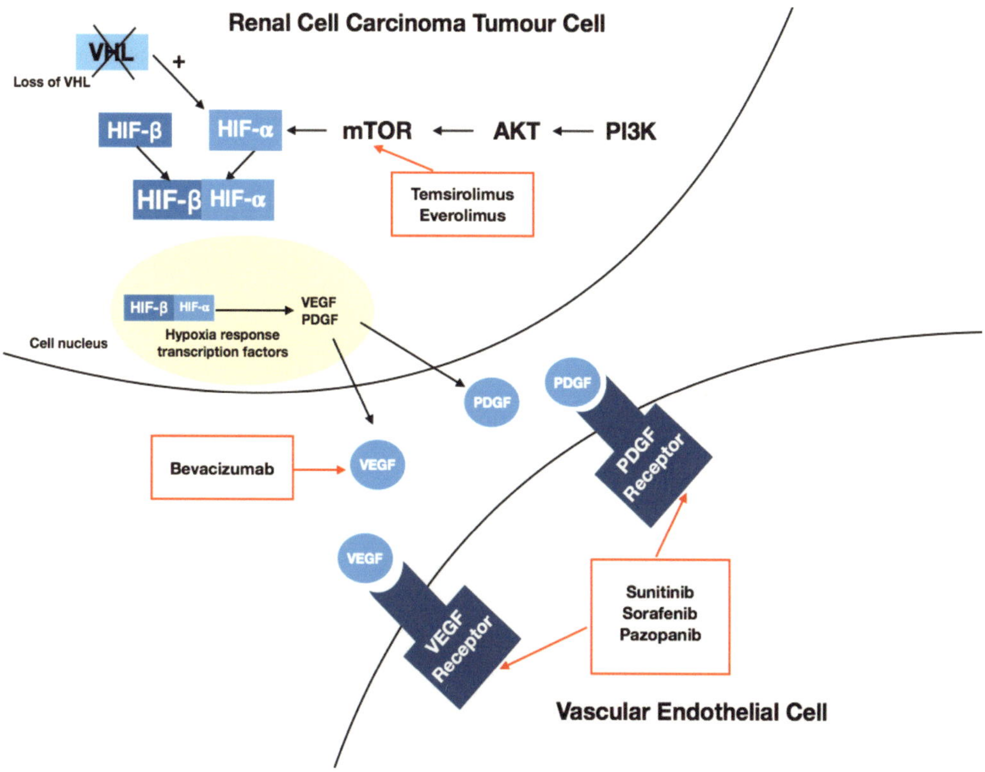

Image 1. A graphic showing how loss of the von Hippel Lindau (VHL) protein results in up regulation of hypoxia induced factors (HIF) and in turn vascular endothelial growth factor (VEGF) and platelet derived growth factor (PDGF) and the actions of targeted therapies.

(ORR) were around 10–15% [17]. More recently, studies have investigated Nivolumab, a fully human IgG4 anti-programmed cell death-1 antibody (anti-PD-1) that selectively blocks the interaction between PD-1 and its ligands PD-L1 and PD-L2 and RCC [17, 32]. In the CheckMate 025 study, patients were randomised to receive either nivolumab or everolimus, OS was 25 vs. 19 months in favour of nivolumab, and less grade 3 or 4 toxicity was seen in the nivolumab arm [33]. This trial led to the FDA approval of nivolumab for RCC in 2015 with European approval quickly following.

After the success of single agent immunotherapy, attention turned to the investigation of combination immunotherapy in metastatic RCC. Here, nivolumab was used in combination with a second agent ipilimumab, a monoclonal antibody, which targets cytotoxic T lymphocyte-associated antigen 4 (CTLA-4). CheckMate 214 trial randomised nivolumab and ipilimumab against sunitinib. Median OS was not reached in the combination immunotherapy arm compared to the immunotherapy used for 26 months with sunitinib, and PFS was 11.6 vs. 8.4 months in favour of combination immunotherapy [16].

The mechanism of action of the various immunotherapy agents can be complex. In short, they upregulate the body's own immune response against the 'foreign' tumour cells. For those

Trial	Drug	Number of patients (n)	Line of treatment	Disease-free survival (DFS) (months)	Overall survival (OS) (months)
Motzer et al.: sunitinib versus interferon alpha in metastatic renal cell carcinoma [19]	Sunitinib versus interferon alpha	750	First line	Sunitinib 11 interferon alpha 5 HR 0.42 $p < 0.001$	Sunitinib 28.7 Interferon alpha 23.7 HR 0.8209 $p = 0.051$
Sternberg et al.: pazopanib in locally advanced or metastatic renal cell carcinoma: results of a randomised phase III trial [20]	Pazopanib versus placebo	435	Treatment naive or cytokine pretreated	Pazopanib 9.2 placebo 4.2 HR 0.46 $P < 0.001$	Not available
Motzer et al.: pazopanib versus sunitinib in metastatic renal cell carcinoma [21]	Sunitinib versus pazopanib	1110	First line	Sunitinib 9.5 Pazopanib 8.8 HR 1.05	Sunitinib 29.3 Pazopanib 28.4
Hudes et al.: temsirolimus, interferon alpha, or both for advanced renal cell carcinoma [22]	Interferon alpha versus temsirolimus versus temsirolimus plus interferon alpha	626 (poor prognosis)	First line	Interferon alpha 3.1 temsirolimus 5.5 temsirolimus plus interferon alpha 4.7	Interferon alpha 7.3 temsirolimus 10.9 temsirolimus plus interferon alpha 8.4
Escudier et al.: sorafenib in advanced clear cell renal cell carcinoma [23]	Sorafenib versus placebo	903	First line	Sorafenib 5.5 placebo 2.8 HR 0.44 $P < 0.01$	Sorafenib not reached placebo not reached HR 0.72 $P < 0.001$
Rini et al.: comparative effectiveness of axitinib versus sorafenib in advanced renal cell carcinoma (AXIS): a randomised phase 3 trial [24]	Axitinib versus sorafenib	723	Second line	Axitinib 6.7 Sorafenib 4.7	Not available
Choueiri et al.: cabozantinib versus everolimus in advanced renal cell carcinoma (METEOR): final results from a randomised, open-label, phase 3 trial [25]	Cabozantinib versus everolimus	658	Second line or subsequent	Cabozantinib 7.4 everolimus 3.9 HR 0.051 $p < 0.0001$	Cabozantinib 18.8 everolimus 16.5 HR 0.66 $p = 0.00026$

Trial	Drug	Number of patients (n)	Line of treatment	Disease-free survival (DFS) (months)	Overall survival (OS) (months)
Armstrong et al.: everolimus versus sunitinib for patients with metastatic non-clear cell renal cell carcinoma (ASPEN): a multicentre, open-label, randomised phase 2 trial [26]	Everolimus versus sunitinib	108 (non-clear cell histology)	First line	Everolimus 5.6 Sunitinib 8.3 HR 1.41 p = 0.16	Everolimus 13.2 Sunitinib 31.5 HR1.12 p = 0.60

Table 2. Trials of tyrosine kinase inhibitors in the metastatic renal cancer setting.

who wish for a fuller explanation, the cellular mechanism of the immunotherapy agents is now outlined. In the tumour microenvironment, tumour neoantigens are released by cancer cells. These are captured by antigen presenting cells (APCs). These neoantigens cause the expression of major histocompatibility complexes (MHC) and T-cell receptors (TCRs) on the surface of CD8+ cytotoxic T cells. PD-1 expression is induced. Tumour cells can highly express PD-L1 and PD-L2, which can bind with PD-1 on the T cell and ultimately lead to T-cell exhaustion. Drugs such as nivolumab and pembrolizumab inhibit the interaction of PD-1 with PD-L1 and PD-L2, which results in enhanced T-cell cytotoxicity, increased cytokine, and tumour-associated macrophage activity. Anti-PD-L1 antibody therapies such as atezolizumab, durvalumab and avelumab, specifically target the interaction between PD-L1 and PD-1. Tumour neoantigens also cause peptides bound to MHC II molecules to be presented to CD4+ T helper cells. Through a series of co-stimulatory signals transmitted via CD28 T cells, CTLA-4 is upregulated. The upregulated CTLA-4 competes with CD28 to bind with CD80 and/or CD86 on the APC. The interaction of CTLA-4 with CD80 or CD86 results in inhibitory signalling, which in turn promotes tumour growth. Ipilimumab is an anti-CTLA-4 antibody; thus, it blocks CTLA-4, allowing an enhanced immune response [34]. A pictorial explanation of the mechanism of both CTLA-4 and PD-1 immunotherapy targeted agents is available in **Image 2.**

Immunotherapy has a different safety profile from targeted TKI therapies or standard chemotherapies. Typically, autoimmune reactions are seen that can be varying and at times severe. The most common is diarrhoea and colitis, but pneumonitis and endocrine problems are also observed.

There has also been some investigation in using the combinations of immunotherapy with targeted agents. Nivolumab was paired with pazopanib or sunitinib in the CheckMate 014 trial; however, toxicity was very high with 70% of patients experiencing a grade 3 or 4 toxicity and 25% discontinuing the treatment due to toxicity. This trial has led to caution in combining immunotherapy and TKIs [35] (**Table 3**).

4.4. Sequencing of agents

The natural history of targeted agents in all cancers, and reflected here in RCC, is developing ultimate resistance. Therefore, a patient may undertake several lines of treatment. Both the European Society of Medical Oncology (ESMO) and National Comprehensive Cancer

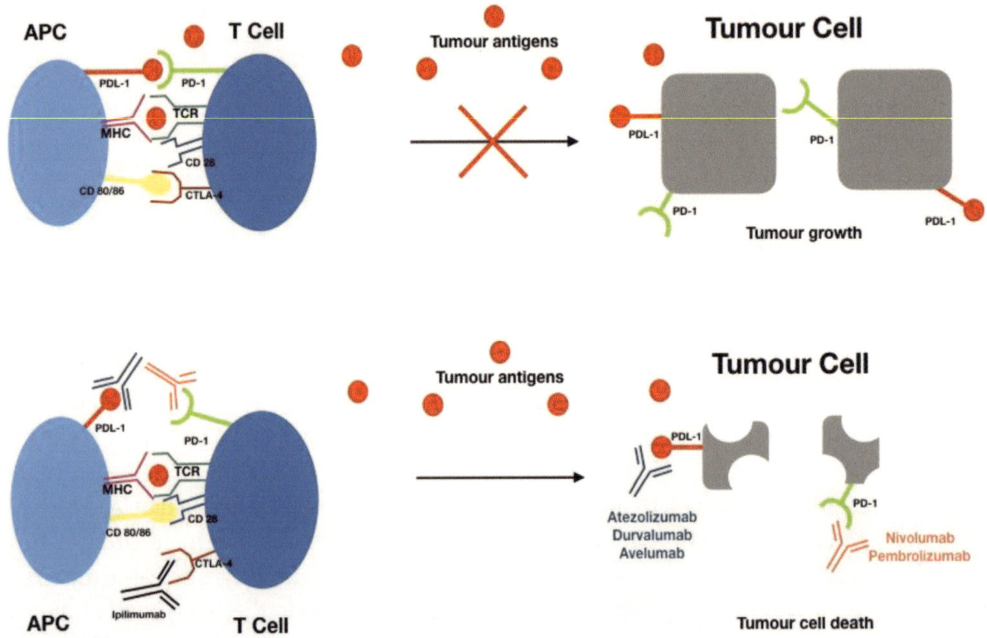

Image 2. Pictorial representation of the mechanism of action of immunotherapy agents.

Trial	Drug	Number of patients (n)	Line of treatment	Progression-free survival (PFS) (months)	Overall survival (OS) (months)
CheckMate 025 Motzer et al. [33]	Nivolumab versus everolimus	823	Second or subsequent	Nivolumab 4.6 Everolimus 4.4 HR 0.88 p = 0.11	Nivolumab 25.0 Everolimus 19.6 HR 0.73 p = 0.002
CheckMate 214 Motzer et al. [16]	Nivolumab plus ipilimumab (nivo+ipi) versus sunitinib	1096	First line	Nivo+ipi 11.6 Sunitinib 8.4	Nivo+ipi-not reached Sunitinib 26.0 18 months of OS rate Nivo+ipi 75% sunitinib 60%
CheckMate 016 Amin et al. [35]	Nivolumab in combination with sunitinib or pazopanib	55	First line	Nivolumab plus sunitinib 12.7 Nivolumab plus pazopanib 7.2	Nivolumab plus sunitinib not reached Nivolumab plus pazopanib 27.9

Table 3. Immunotherapy trials in metastatic renal cell carcinoma.

Network (NCCN) provide up-to-date guidelines advising oncologists of the latest evidence to help determine the most advantageous sequence of agents [36, 37]. At the time of publication, we would suggest a suitable sequence of therapies to be followed: first-line sunitinib or pazopanib (in poor-risk patients temsirolimus), second-line axitinib or nivolumab, with a preference to nivolumab in poor-risk patients, and third-line cabozantinib [36]. In non-cell histology, sunitinib is recommended first line, although few trials have specifically recruited non-clear cell histological subtypes for investigation [26, 36].

We recognise that as new agents are developed and further research is conducted in this field, the advice may change. Another strategy that has been investigated is active surveillance. Patients with indolent metastatic disease may safely remain on surveillance until their disease begins to progress. A cohort study of patients with metastatic RCC on surveillance demonstrated a median time to starting systemic therapy of 14.9 months [38].

5. Cytoreductive nephrectomy in the age of TKI

Historically, cytoreductive nephrectomy has been used in metastatic disease in a selected number of patients. It has been especially used in fit patients with asymptomatic, low burden of metastatic disease and troublesome local symptoms such as bleeding and pain [39]. However, publication of the CARMENA trial in 2018, where sunitinib versus cytoreductive nephrectomy plus sunitinib was evaluated, demonstrated non-inferiority of sunitinib alone [40]. The trial was designed to demonstrate non-inferiority and non-superiority of one investigational arm; however, it was noted that the median OS of sunitinib alone was 18.4 months versus 13.9 months as compared to sunitinib with nephrectomy [40]. Although further evaluation is required, and for symptomatic management, cytoreductive nephrectomy may still be beneficial in the metastatic setting, this new evidence has called into question the validity of this approach routinely used for patients in the contemporary systemic treatment setting.

6. Oligometastatic disease in kidney cancer

An interesting development across oncology in all tumour groups has been the change in approach to the management of oligometastatic disease [41]. Oligometastatic disease is a term used to describe a patient with a small number of metastatic lesions; in most studies, this is defined as 1–3 or 1–5 lesions [41]. Aggressive resection of the metastasis can be attempted surgically or an increasing number of patients can be treated with high doses of radiotherapy using stereotactic ablative body radiotherapy (SABR) [41, 42]. Traditionally, RCC has been thought to be a radio-resistant disease; however, large ablative doses of radiotherapy used in an SABR technique induce different pathways of apoptosis and as such good long-term control can be achieved in certain patients. Metastasis in bone, lungs, brain, lymph nodes, and adrenal glands are all potentially treatable with SABR [43–45].

Metastasectomy can be employed for metastatic disease in a number of sites including bone, lungs and brain. Good long-term outcomes have been observed, especially with careful patient selection [46, 47].

A combination of metastasectomy and post-operative SABR for brain metastasis has been employed with excellent results and has been shown to have less side effects than post-operative treatment with whole brain radiotherapy [48].

7. Adjuvant treatment

Adjuvant therapy in oncology describes the use of additional treatment alongside the primary, definitive, usually surgical, treatment, in an attempt to achieve higher rates of progression-free and overall survival. In RCC, this has not been widely employed as many trials have shown adjuvant treatment in early stage renal cancer not to translate into an overall survival benefit [49, 50]. However, it is also recognised that many patients with early stage disease will also go on to relapse, and therefore, interest in this area has remained high and guidelines recommend that for intermediate- and high-risk patients, adjuvant treatment, as part of a clinical trial, should be considered [36, 49]. In ASSURE trial, sunitinib or sorafenib failed to demonstrate an improvement in disease-free survival (DFS) compared to placebo [51]. In S-TRAC trial, sunitinib did increase 5-year DFS, but not overall survival data, although the overall survival data have not yet improved [52]. In the PROTECT trial, pazopanib failed to

Trial	Drug	Number of patients (n)	Disease-free survival (DFS)	Overall survival (OS)
ASSURE Haas et al. [50]	Sorafenib/Sunitinib versus placebo	1943	Sorafenib 6.1 years (HR 0.97 P = 0.718) Sunitinib 5.8 years (HR 1.02 P = 0.804) Placebo 6.6 years	At 5 years Sorafenib 80.5% Sunitinib 77.9% Placebo 80.3% *No significant difference between groups*
S-TRAC Ravaud et al. [51]	Sunitinib versus placebo	615	Sunitinib 6.8 years Placebo 5.6 years (HR 0.76 P = 0.03)	Mature data not available.
PROTECT Motzer et al. [52]	Pazopanib versus placebo	1538	HR 0.86 P = 0.165	Not available
ATLAS Gross-Goupil et al. [53]	Axitinib versus placebo	724	HR 0.870 P = 0.3211	Not available

Table 4. Trials of tyrosine kinase inhibitors in the adjuvant renal cancer setting post-nephrectomy.

show a statistically significant improvement in DFS [53]. In the ATLAS trial, using axitinib in the adjuvant setting, the primary end point was not reached and the study was abandoned due to futility at the interim assessment point [54]. It is also worth noting that the majority of patients in these adjuvant trials had ccRCC histology. A summary of the reported trials is shown in **Table 4**.

Several trials are still ongoing using targeted therapies in high-risk patients post-nephrectomy including: SORCE trial (NCT00492258) assessing sorafenib and EVEREST trial (NCT01120249) investigating everolimus [50]. Further trials are underway to assess the use of immunotherapy in the adjuvant setting using a variety of checkpoint inhibitors. These include the IMmotion101 trial (NCT03024996) with atezolizumab, PROSPER trial (NCT03055013) comparing neoadjuvant and adjuvant nivolumab versus observation, KEYNOTE-564 trial (NCT03142334) evaluating pembrolizumab versus placebo and CheckMate 914 trial (NCT03138512) comparing nivolumab with ipilimumab versus placebo [50]. The results of these trials are likely to be reported in the coming years; however, the standard of care at present is not to prescribe adjuvant therapy, of any kind, post-nephrectomy in renal cell carcinoma.

8. Emerging treatments and trends

An area of particular interest for oncologist is the search for reliable biomarkers, which will guide us into targeting our treatments to the patients who will benefit from them the most. Renal cell carcinoma is no exception and the hunt for a biomarker is of high interest to academics and drug companies alike. Biomarkers are being investigated in the areas of imaging serum, histology, and urine, both to determine treatment strategies and to differentiate between benign and malignant processes [55]. One biomarker of particular interest is carbonic anhydrase IX, which has demonstrated excellent specificity and ability to predict treatment response [56]. Researchers are also keen to identify reliable biomarkers for use with immune checkpoint inhibitors in the treatment of RCC, especially to help differentiate between the progression and pseudoprogression on treatment [57].

Research has been conducted on the use of vaccine therapy in RCC. Vaccines are designed to induce a specific immune response in the patient; however, this is yet to translate into an overall survival benefit [58, 59]. In the new era of targeted medicine and next-generation immunotherapy, the role of vaccines remains uncertain and only further research in this area, with associated success in randomised trials, will confirm vaccine therapy as a viable treatment strategy for the future.

Interesting evidence has been published on the use of SABR in patients who are not fit for partial nephrectomy. High doses of highly targeted radiotherapy are given to the tumour patients with the hope of ablation of the tumour. The treatment was well tolerated with low toxicity and good local control rates in 2 years [60]. Further ongoing evaluation of this technique is needed, but it is likely that use of SABR in this format will increase in the future.

9. Summary

The take-home points are as follows:

- prognostic risk stratification is used to guide treatment decisions in metastatic renal cell carcinoma patients;
- the mainstay of treatment for metastatic renal cell carcinoma is TKI therapy;
- immunotherapy has been shown to be effective in metastatic renal cell carcinoma and is now routinely used;
- cytoreductive nephrectomy should not be used routinely in metastatic renal cell carcinoma patients;
- adjuvant systemic treatment lacks robust evidence for routine use in renal cell carcinoma patients outside of the clinical trial setting.

The medical treatment of renal cell carcinoma is rapidly evolving with the introduction of new treatments entering the market on a regular basis. Whilst this is challenging for the physician treating renal cell carcinoma, it is excellent news for our patients who will benefit from the greater arsenal of treatments available.

Author details

Jennifer Turner[1], Adrian Simoes[2], Albert Edwards[1] and Rakesh Raman[1]*

*Address all correspondence to: rakeshraman@nhs.net

1 Kent Oncology Centre, East Kent Hospitals University NHS Foundation Trust,
Kent and Canterbury Hospital, Canterbury, United Kingdom

2 Department of Urology, East Kent Hospitals University NHS Foundation Trust,
Kent and Canterbury Hospital, Canterbury, United Kingdom

References

[1] Bray F, Ferlay J, Soerjomataram I, Siegel RL, Torre LA, Jemal A. Global cancer statistics 2018: GLOBOCAN estimates of incidence and mortality worldwide for 36 cancers in 185 countries. CA: A Cancer Journal for Clinicians. 2018;**68**(6):394-424

[2] Siegel RL, Miller KD, Jemal A. Cancer statistics, 2017. CA: A Cancer Journal for Clinicians. 2017;**67**:7-30

[3] UK CR. 2018. Available from: https://www.cancerresearchuk.org/health-professional/cancer-statistics/statistics-by-cancer-type/kidney-cancer#heading-Two

[4] Ridge CA, Pua BB, Madoff DC. Epidemiology and staging of renal cell carcinoma. Seminars in Interventional Radiology. 2014;**31**(1):3-8

[5] Research. WCRFAIfC. Continuous Update Project Expert Report 2018. Diet, Nutrition, Physical Activity and Kidney Cancer. 2018

[6] Sánchez-Gastaldo A, Kempf E, González del Alba A, Duran I. Systemic treatment of renal cell cancer: A comprehensive review. Cancer Treatment Reviews. 2017;**60**:77-89

[7] Muglia VF, Prando A. Renal cell carcinoma: Histological classification and correlation with imaging findings. Radiologia Brasileira. 2015;**48**(3):166-174

[8] Amin MB, Edge SB, Greene FL, et al. AJCC Cancer Staging Manual. 8th ed. Switzerland: Springer; 2017

[9] Graham J, Dudani S, Heng DYC. Prognostication in kidney cancer: Recent advances and future directions. Journal of Clinical Oncology. 2018;**79**:0147

[10] Heng DY, Xie W, Regan MM, Warren MA, Golshayan AR, Sahi C, et al. Prognostic factors for overall survival in patients with metastatic renal cell carcinoma treated with vascular endothelial growth factor-targeted agents: Results from a large, multicenter study. Journal of Clinical Oncology: Official Journal of the American Society of Clinical Oncology. 2009;**27**(34):5794-5799

[11] Heng DY, Xie W, Regan MM, Harshman LC, Bjarnason GA, Vaishampayan UN, et al. External validation and comparison with other models of the international metastatic renal-cell carcinoma database consortium prognostic model: A population-based study. The Lancet Oncology. 2013;**14**(2):141-148

[12] Ko JJ, Xie W, Kroeger N, Lee JL, Rini BI, Knox JJ, et al. The international metastatic renal cell carcinoma database consortium model as a prognostic tool in patients with metastatic renal cell carcinoma previously treated with first-line targeted therapy: A population-based study. The Lancet Oncology. 2015;**16**(3):293-300

[13] Connor Wells J, Donskov F, Fraccon AP, Pasini F, Bjarnason GA, Beuselinck B, et al. Characterizing the outcomes of metastatic papillary renal cell carcinoma. Cancer Medicine. 2017;**6**(5):902-909

[14] Wells JC, Stukalin I, Norton C, Srinivas S, Lee JL, Donskov F, et al. Third-line targeted therapy in metastatic renal cell carcinoma: Results from the international metastatic renal cell carcinoma database consortium. European Urology. 2017;**71**(2):204-209

[15] Spain L, Turajlic S. Current management of renal cell cancer. Trends in Urology & Men's Health. 2017;**8**(2):21-25

[16] Motzer RJ, Tannir NM, McDermott DF, Arén Frontera O, Melichar B, Choueiri TK, et al. Nivolumab plus Ipilimumab versus Sunitinib in advanced renal-cell carcinoma. New England Journal of Medicine. 2018;**378**(14):1277-1290

[17] Ochoa CE, Joseph RW. Nivolumab in renal cell carcinoma: Current trends and future perspectives. Journal of Kidney Cancer and VHL. 2018;**5**(1):15-18

[18] Cowey CL, Rathmell WK. VHL gene mutations in renal cell carcinoma: Role as a biomarker of disease outcome and drug efficacy. Current Oncology Reports. 2009;**11**(2):94-101

[19] Motzer RJ, Hutson TE, Tomczak P, Michaelson MD, Bukowski RM, Rixe O, et al. Sunitinib versus interferon alfa in metastatic renal-cell carcinoma. The New England Journal of Medicine. 2007;**356**(2):115-124

[20] Sternberg CN, Davis ID, Mardiak J, Szczylik C, Lee E, Wagstaff J, et al. Pazopanib in locally advanced or metastatic renal cell carcinoma: Results of a randomized phase III trial. Journal of Clinical Oncology: Official Journal of the American Society of Clinical Oncology. 2010;**28**(6):1061-1068

[21] Motzer RJ, Hutson TE, Cella D, Reeves J, Hawkins R, Guo J, et al. Pazopanib versus sunitinib in metastatic renal-cell carcinoma. The New England Journal of Medicine. 2013; **369**(8):722-731

[22] Hudes G, Carducci M, Tomczak P, Dutcher J, Figlin R, Kapoor A, et al. Temsirolimus, interferon alfa, or both for advanced renal-cell carcinoma. The New England journal of medicine. 2007;**356**(22):2271-2281

[23] Escudier B, Eisen T, Stadler WM, Szczylik C, Oudard S, Siebels M, et al. Sorafenib in advanced clear-cell renal-cell carcinoma. The New England Journal of Medicine. 2007; **356**(2):125-134

[24] Rini BI, Escudier B, Tomczak P, Kaprin A, Szczylik C, Hutson TE, et al. Comparative effectiveness of axitinib versus sorafenib in advanced renal cell carcinoma (AXIS): A randomised phase 3 trial. Lancet (London, England). 2011;**378**(9807):1931-1939

[25] Choueiri TK, Escudier B, Powles T, Tannir NM, Mainwaring PN, Rini BI, et al. Cabozantinib versus everolimus in advanced renal cell carcinoma (METEOR): Final results from a randomised, open-label, phase 3 trial. The Lancet Oncology. 2016;**17**(7):917-927

[26] Armstrong AJ, Halabi S, Eisen T, Broderick S, Stadler WM, Jones RJ, et al. Everolimus versus sunitinib for patients with metastatic non-clear cell renal cell carcinoma (ASPEN): A multicentre, open-label, randomised phase 2 trial. The Lancet Oncology. 2016;**17**(3):378-388

[27] Escudier B, Bellmunt J, Negrier S, Bajetta E, Melichar B, Bracarda S, et al. Phase III trial of bevacizumab plus interferon alfa-2a in patients with metastatic renal cell carcinoma (AVOREN): Final analysis of overall survival. Journal of Clinical Oncology: Official Journal of the American Society of Clinical Oncology. 2010;**28**(13):2144-2150

[28] Hainsworth JD, Spigel DR, Burris HA 3rd, Waterhouse D, Clark BL, Whorf R. Phase II trial of bevacizumab and everolimus in patients with advanced renal cell carcinoma. Journal of Clinical Oncology: Official Journal of the American Society of Clinical Oncology. 2010;**28**(13):2131-2136

[29] Negrier S, Gravis G, Perol D, Chevreau C, Delva R, Bay JO, et al. Temsirolimus and bevacizumab, or sunitinib, or interferon alfa and bevacizumab for patients with advanced renal cell carcinoma (TORAVA): A randomised phase 2 trial. The Lancet Oncology. 2011;**12**(7):673-680

[30] Harshman LC, Barbeau S, McMillian A, Srinivas S. A phase II study of bevacizumab and everolimus as treatment for refractory metastatic renal cell carcinoma. Clinical Genitourinary Cancer. 2013;**11**(2):100-106

[31] Rini BI, Bellmunt J, Clancy J, Wang K, Niethammer AG, Hariharan S, et al. Randomized phase III trial of temsirolimus and bevacizumab versus interferon alfa and bevacizumab in metastatic renal cell carcinoma: INTORACT trial. Journal of Clinical Oncology: Official Journal of the American Society of Clinical Oncology. 2014;**32**(8):752-759

[32] Brahmer JR, Hammers H, Lipson EJ. Nivolumab: Targeting PD-1 to bolster antitumor immunity. Future Oncology (London, England). 2015;**11**(9):1307-1326

[33] Motzer RJ, Escudier B, McDermott DF, George S, Hammers HJ, Srinivas S, et al. Nivolumab versus Everolimus in advanced renal-cell carcinoma. New England Journal of Medicine. 2015;**373**(19):1803-1813

[34] Varricchi G, Galdiero MR, Marone G, Criscuolo G, Triassi M, Bonaduce D, et al. Cardiotoxicity of immune checkpoint inhibitors. ESMO Open. 2017;**2**(4):e000247

[35] Amin A, Plimack ER, Ernstoff MS, Lewis LD, Bauer TM, McDermott DF, et al. Safety and efficacy of nivolumab in combination with sunitinib or pazopanib in advanced or metastatic renal cell carcinoma: The CheckMate 016 study. Journal for ImmunoTherapy of Cancer. 2018;**6**(1):109

[36] Escudier B, Porta C, Schmidinger M, Rioux-Leclercq N, Bex A, Khoo V, et al. Renal cell carcinoma: ESMO clinical practice guidelines for diagnosis, treatment and follow-up. Annals of Oncology: Official Journal of the European Society for Medical Oncology. 2016;**27**(suppl 5):v58-v68

[37] Motzer RJ, Jonasch E, Agarwal N, Bhayani S, Bro WP, Chang SS, et al. Kidney cancer, version 2.2017, NCCN clinical practice guidelines in oncology. Journal of the National Comprehensive Cancer Network: JNCCN. 2017;**15**(6):804-834

[38] Rini BI, Dorff TB, Elson P, Rodriguez CS, Shepard D, Wood L, et al. Active surveillance in metastatic renal-cell carcinoma: A prospective, phase 2 trial. The Lancet Oncology. 2016;**17**(9):1317-1324

[39] Heng DY, Wells JC, Rini BI, Beuselinck B, Lee JL, Knox JJ, et al. Cytoreductive nephrectomy in patients with synchronous metastases from renal cell carcinoma: Results from the international metastatic renal cell carcinoma database consortium. European Urology. 2014;**66**(4):704-710

[40] Méjean A, Ravaud A, Thezenas S, Colas S, Beauval J-B, Bensalah K, et al. Sunitinib alone or after nephrectomy in metastatic renal-cell carcinoma. New England Journal of Medicine. 2018;**379**(5):417-427

[41] Palma DA, Salama JK, Lo SS, Senan S, Treasure T, Govindan R, et al. The oligometastatic state—Separating truth from wishful thinking. Nature Reviews. Clinical Oncology. 2014;**11**(9):549-557

[42] Franzese C, Franceschini D, Di Brina L, D'Agostino GR, Navarria P, Comito T, et al. Role of stereotactic body radiation therapy in the management of oligometastatic renal cell carcinoma. The Journal of Urology. Jan 2019;**201**(1):70-76

[43] Lippitz B, Lindquist C, Paddick I, Peterson D, O'Neill K, Beaney R. Stereotactic radiosurgery in the treatment of brain metastases: The current evidence. Cancer Treatment Reviews. 2014;**40**(1):48-59

[44] Kothari G, Louie AV, Pryor D, Vela I, Lo SS, Teh BS, et al. Stereotactic body radiotherapy for primary renal cell carcinoma and adrenal metastases. Chinese Clinical Oncology. 2017;**6**(Suppl 2):S17

[45] Wang CJ, Christie A, Lin MH, Jung M, Weix D, Huelsmann L, et al. Safety and efficacy of stereotactic ablative radiation therapy for renal cell carcinoma extracranial metastases. International Journal of Radiation Oncology, Biology, Physics. 2017;**98**(1):91-100

[46] van der Poel HG, Roukema JA, Horenblas S, van Geel AN, Debruyne FM. Metastasectomy in renal cell carcinoma: A multicenter retrospective analysis. European Urology. 1999; **35**(3):197-203

[47] Ljungberg B. The role of metastasectomy in renal cell carcinoma in the era of targeted therapy. Current Urology Reports. 2013;**14**(1):19-25

[48] Scheitler-Ring K, Ge B, Petroski G, Biedermann G, Litofsky NS. Radiosurgery to the postoperative tumor bed for metastatic carcinoma versus whole brain radiation after surgery. Cureus. 2016;8(11):e885-e.

[49] Janowitz T, Welsh SJ, Zaki K, Mulders P, Eisen T. Adjuvant therapy in renal cell carcinoma-past, present, and future. Seminars in Oncology. 2013;**40**(4):482-491

[50] Figlin RA, Leibovich BC, Stewart GD, Negrier S. Adjuvant therapy in renal cell carcinoma: Does higher risk for recurrence improve the chance for success? Annals of Oncology: Official Journal of the European Society for Medical Oncology. 2018;**29**(2):324-331

[51] Haas NB, Manola J, Uzzo RG, Flaherty KT, Wood CG, Kane C, et al. Adjuvant sunitinib or sorafenib for high-risk, non-metastatic renal-cell carcinoma (ECOG-ACRIN E2805): A double-blind, placebo-controlled, randomised, phase 3 trial. Lancet (London, England). 2016;**387**(10032):2008-2016

[52] Ravaud A, Motzer RJ, Pandha HS, George DJ, Pantuck AJ, Patel A, et al. Adjuvant sunitinib in high-risk renal-cell carcinoma after nephrectomy. New England Journal of Medicine. 2016;**375**(23):2246-2254

[53] Motzer RJ, Haas NB, Donskov F, Gross-Goupil M, Varlamov S, Kopyltsov E, et al. Randomized phase III trial of adjuvant pazopanib versus placebo after nephrectomy in patients with locally advanced renal cell carcinoma (RCC) (PROTECT). Journal of Clinical Oncology. 2017;**35**(15_suppl):4507

[54] Gross-Goupil M, Kwon TG, Eto M, Ye D, Miyake H, Seo SI, et al. Axitinib versus placebo as an adjuvant treatment for renal cell carcinoma: Results from the phase III, randomized ATLAS trial. Annals of Oncology. 1 Dec 2018;**29**(12):2371-2378

[55] Farber NJ, Kim CJ, Modi PK, Hon JD, Sadimin ET, Singer EA. Renal cell carcinoma: The search for a reliable biomarker. Translational Cancer Research. 2017;**6**(3):620-632

[56] McGuire BB, Fitzpatrick JM. Biomarkers in renal cell carcinoma. Current Opinion in Urology. 2009;**19**(5):441-446

[57] Flynn M, Pickering L, Larkin J, Turajlic S. Immune-checkpoint inhibitors in melanoma and kidney cancer: From sequencing to rational selection. Therapeutic Advances in Medical Oncology. 2018;**10**:1758835918777427

[58] Amato RJ, Hawkins RE, Kaufman HL, Thompson JA, Tomczak P, Szczylik C, et al. Vaccination of metastatic renal cancer patients with MVA-5T4: A randomized, double-blind, placebo-controlled phase III study. Clinical Cancer Research: An Official Journal of the American Association for Cancer Research. 2010;**16**(22):5539-5547

[59] Rini BI, Stenzl A, Zdrojowy R, Kogan M, Shkolnik M, Oudard S, et al. IMA901, a multipeptide cancer vaccine, plus sunitinib versus sunitinib alone, as first-line therapy for advanced or metastatic renal cell carcinoma (IMPRINT): A multicentre, open-label, randomised, controlled, phase 3 trial. The Lancet Oncology. 2016;**17**(11):1599-1611

[60] Siva S, Louie AV, Warner A, Muacevic A, Gandhidasan S, Ponsky L, et al. Pooled analysis of stereotactic ablative radiotherapy for primary renal cell carcinoma: A report from the international radiosurgery oncology consortium for kidney (IROCK). Cancer. 2018;**124**(5):934-942

Chapter 10

Current Role of Adjuvant Therapy in High Risk for Recurrence Resected Kidney Cancer

Fadil Hassan, Shahid Lambe, Kiran Sharma and Anil Kapoor

Additional information is available at the end of the chapter

http://dx.doi.org/10.5772/intechopen.78684

Abstract

Renal cell carcinoma accounts for about 2% of all adult malignancies. More than 300,000 individuals are affected each year. Unfortunately, around 30% of cases are discovered in advanced stages. Surgical resection remains the mainstay of treatment for localized disease and relapses can reach up to 40% in some cases. The effective treatment of metastatic RCC with systemic targeted therapy gives a strong rationale for its use as adjuvant treatment in high-risk patients. This chapter reviews different modalities that have been used as an adjuvant therapy for nonmetastatic renal cancer. Clinical trials using targeted therapy are discussed in detail, as they are becoming options for treatment in high-risk patients. While the current set of completed adjuvant clinical trials have provided conflicting results, there are additional large-scale trials that are still in progress. Future directions include—incorporating a genetic recurrence score to evaluate risk of relapse in patients, developing an adequate and an objective standardized adjuvant trial design, identifying novel biomarkers, and evaluating novel drug targets. Based upon current clinical trial evidence, motivated high-risk patients should have a discussion with the urology oncology team regarding the benefits of adjuvant TKI sunitinib or consider enrollment in current ongoing immuno-oncology (IO) adjuvant clinical trials.

Keywords: renal cell carcinoma, adjuvant treatment for RCC, treatment of high-risk RCC, targeted therapy as adjuvant

1. Introduction

Every year, approximately 338,000 individuals are diagnosed with kidney cancer globally, representing about 2% of all cancers [1]. Renal cell carcinoma (RCC) accounts for approximately 90% of all kidney cancers—affecting an estimated 300,000 people each year [2, 3]. Approximately 30% of kidney cancer patients represent an advanced disease stage at diagnosis, with an average 5-year survival rate of approximately 16% [4, 5].

The management of RCC, regardless of its histological subtype or stage, involves surgical resection of the tumor through either a radical or partial nephrectomy [6]. While surgery is not curative in cases involving metastatic disease, with localized RCC, surgical intervention is considered the optimal standard of care [6, 7].

But despite that, postsurgical recurrence of cancer is a prevalent issue in cases of localized RCC (stage 2 or 3 disease) with a 5-year relapse rate of 30–40% and, as such, surgery is insufficient for long-term disease free survival [8, 9]. Hence, even though the current standard for postoperative care continues to be radiographic surveillance, the need for effective adjuvant therapy for localized high risk for recurrence RCC would be helpful and desired by the surgical community [8–10].

In view of these findings and the effective treatment of metastatic RCC with Immunotherapy in the 1990s or more recently with targeted therapy, a strong rationale for systemic adjuvant therapy exists in high risk for recurrence patients.

In this chapter, we review different treatment modalities have been used as an adjuvant therapy for nonmetastatic renal cancer postsurgical resection with emphasis on targeted therapy as becoming an option to offer patients.

2. Stratifying risk of recurrence

A critical element in both the testing and effective clinical use of adjuvant therapy involves determining whether there is a high risk of disease recurrence post nephrectomy and accordingly identifying patients that are most likely to benefit from the therapy. As discussed earlier, the determination of recurrence risk is currently nonstandardized in adjuvant therapy testing. Several models and clinical nomograms have been developed to predict the risk of disease recurrence and progression, as well as evaluate additional oncological endpoints [11–19]. Examples of some validated models include the Cindolo Recurrence Risk Formula, Leibovich scoring system, Karakiewicz scoring system, Kattan nomogram, Mayo Clinic stage, size, grade, and necrosis scoring system (SSIGN), and the University of California Los Angeles Integrated Staging System (UISS) [11–19] (**Tables 1** and **2**). These systems usually incorporate information regarding different variables and various prognostic signs and indictors such as tumor size, stage and characteristics, clinical risk factors, and various other pathological features and signs for a relatively robust evaluation [11–21]. Among these models, the UISS, Kattan and SSIGN nomograms have shown relatively better discriminative accuracy in some comparative studies and hence are most commonly utilized [13, 22, 23].

In terms of a general approximation, recurrence risk can be segregated into three broad categories based on the UISS nomogram: low, intermediate and high risk [18]. These three risk groups

Characteristics		Points
Tumor	pT1a	0
	pT1b	2
	pT2	3
	pT3-pT4	4
Dimension	<10 cm	0
	>10 cm	1
Fuhrman	1–2	0
	3	1
	4	3
Tumor necrosis	Absent	0
	Present	1
Lymph nodes	pNx/pN0	0
	pN1-pN2	2

Table 1. Leibovich prognosis score.

T stage	1				2	3				4
Furman grade	1–2		3–4		1–4	1		2–4		1–4
ECOG PS	0	>1	any	>1	any	0	>1	0	>1	any
Risk group	Low	Intermediate							High	

Table 2. UISS prognosis score.

are differentiated based on the probability of survival and disease recurrence and patients, in a clinical setting, can be stratified through an independent clinical assessment of UISS components, such as tumor stage, grade, and other pathophysiological characteristics [18, 19]. While the UISS components have not been formally validated as independent recurrence risk prediction models, they are important prognostic indicators for various oncological outcomes and endpoints that are invariably linked with the risk of disease relapse [18, 19]. As such, an evaluation of tumor characteristics—particularly tumor stage—can serve as a rough guide for preliminary differentiation between high, intermediate and low risk categories in the clinical setting. [24–27] This correlation has been supported by independent studies which have reported higher recurrence free survival (RFS) rates for smaller, T1a-T1b stage tumors and lower RFS rates for larger, T3-T4 stage tumors [24–27]. Thus, patients with T1a-T2a tumors can be estimated to have lower recurrence risk while those with T3b-T4 tumors can be placed into the high-risk category [24–27]. Among these varying risk levels, currently only those who present a high risk of disease recurrence can potentially benefit from adjuvant therapy postsurgical resection of the tumor.

The incorporation of biotechnology and an improved understanding of genetic and molecular markers may potentially lead to the next major advancement in improving the predictive accuracy of relapse risk. Recent studies have reported the development of novel gene assays and have further elucidated several new biomarkers [28–31]. Nonetheless, further investigation, testing and development is required before molecular approaches can be incorporated for clinical application in an efficient and economically viable manner.

3. Immunotherapy IL2,IFα

Two trials that used adjuvant IFN-α [32, 33] and one study that used adjuvant high-dose IL-2 (82) were negative for any benefit. The latter study was designed and powered to show an improvement in predicted 2-year DFS from 40% for the observation group to 70% for the treatment group. Despite full accrual 30% improvement in 2-year DFS could not be achieved which lead to early study closure.

Combination treatment with IFN-α and IL2 also failed to improve DFS in one trial [34].

The combination of cytokines with 5-fluorouracil (5-FU) also failed to improve DFS in the adjuvant setting [35, 36].

In one randomized adjuvant trial, triple combination therapy using IL-2, IFN-α, and5-FU was associated with significant toxicity which leads to 35% of the patients did not complete the study and also resulted in no benefit in DFS or OS [37].

4. Tumor vaccines

Autologous irradiated tumor cells mixed with bacillus Calmette-Guérin (BCG) were tested in two randomized trials and did not result in prolonged DFS [38–40].

Similarly, autologous, tumor-derived heat-shock protein (glycoprotein 96)-peptide complex (HSPPC-96; vitespen) did not result in a statistically significant improvement of DFS [41].

A trial with an autologous renal tumor cell vaccine only reported improved DFS in the vaccine group [42], but the number of patients lost after the randomization step, the imbalance of this loss, and the absence of tabulation of OS led to criticism of the results [43].

This therapy has not been implemented in routine clinical practice.

5. Hormonal therapy

The occasional response of patients with metastatic RCC to hormonal therapy with medroxyprogestrone acetate (MPA) provided a rationale in trying it in adjuvant sitting.

In a prospective randomized trial of adjuvant MPA after radical nephrectomy, 136 patients received either MPA 500 g (three times a week) for 1 year or observation. With a median follow up of 5 years. There were no significant differences in relapses between the adjuvant group and the observation group (32.7 vs. 33.9%, respectively) [44].

6. Radiotherapy

Radiotherapy has been used for symptoms palliation in metastatic RCC like hematuria and painful bone metastasis. Also, long-term PFS has been reported for in a subset of patients following radiotherapy for solitary bone metastases [31].

One prospective, randomized study in 72 patients comparing administration of radiation of the kidney bed, and ipsilateral and contralateral lymph nodes for stages II and III RCC versus observation reported relapse rates of 48% in both groups. Forty-four percent of patients in the radiotherapy arm had significant complications that contributed to the death of 19% of patients [45–47].

7. Adjuvant therapy in the era of the new targeted therapy

7.1. Targeted therapy

Systemic therapy for mRCC has particularly changed over the last decade with the introduction of targeted therapy and the evolvement of tyrosine kinase inhibitors (TKI) [7, 49–53]. This development has directly resulted from an improved understanding of the pathogenesis and molecular biology of RCC [49–54]. TKIs have provided a novel therapeutic approach for better managing the pathology through the inhibition of targets such as the mammalian target of rapamycin (mTOR) pathway and the vascular endothelial growth factor receptor (VEGFR), which consequently help inhibit processes that are critical for cancer progression [7, 49–53]. Particularly in cases of metastatic RCC, these inhibitors have been effective in increasing the overall survival and response rates than previously used immunotherapy and chemotherapy agents [7, 49–53].

Seven drugs are now approved for targeted therapy, and several others are being evaluated in clinical trials [50–53, 55]. At the molecular level, the mechanism of these drugs involves interrupting the molecular signal transduction of various signaling pathways which then ultimately affects pathogenic factors like tumor vascularity, growth and progression [50–53, 55]. Sunitinib and Pazopanib are currently the accepted standard of care for the management of metastatic RCC and are the most widely used first line agent due to their robust clinical efficacy and established toxicity profile [50–53, 55]. The current set of therapeutic agents used in targeted therapy exploit the Von Hippel-Lindau (VHL) and hypoxia-inducible factor (HIF) pathway associated with clear cell RCC pathogenesis [56, 57].

7.2. VHL-HIF pathway

Clear Cell RCC (ccRCC) normally entails a biallelic inactivation of the VHL tumor suppressor gene at the 3p25-26 locus. VHL inactivation, which occurs due to factors such as mutation, hyper-methylation, or deletions, results in the formation of defective pVHL protein—ultimately leading to the activation and upregulation of HIF-1α [56, 57]. Activated HIF protein serves as a transcription factor for various pro-tumorigenic target genes such as vascular endothelial growth factor (VEGF), transforming growth factor-α and platelet-derived growth factor (PDGF) that are involved in pathogenic processes like angiogenesis, tumor cell proliferation and cell survival. [56, 57] Apart from this central pathway, the mTOR pathway also intersects with HIF pathway upstream of the VHL gene and hence also plays a critical role in influencing HIF process and function. [56, 57] Thus, inhibiting different targets in this pathway has yielded favorable results in mRCC cases [50–53, 55–57]. Given the success of targeted therapy agents in the metastatic setting, recent efforts have been focused into translating this into the adjuvant setting.

7.3. Clinical trials: targeted therapy in adjuvant setting

The contemporary endeavors to transpose targeted therapy in the adjuvant setting have been inspired by the increased clinical knowledge gained through the development and evaluation of interventions for stage IV disease [9, 10, 58, 59]. There are currently seven multicenter, double-blind, placebo-controlled, randomized adjuvant clinical trials, involving targeted therapy agents [9, 10, 58, 59]. Five of these trials involve tyrosine kinase inhibitors, while one involves an mTOR inhibitor and the other a monoclonal chimeric antibody [9, 10, 58–63]. So far, four of these trials have been completed including the, ARISER, ASSURE, S-TRAC and PROTECT trials while the other ones are still in progress [60–63].

7.3.1. ARISER trial

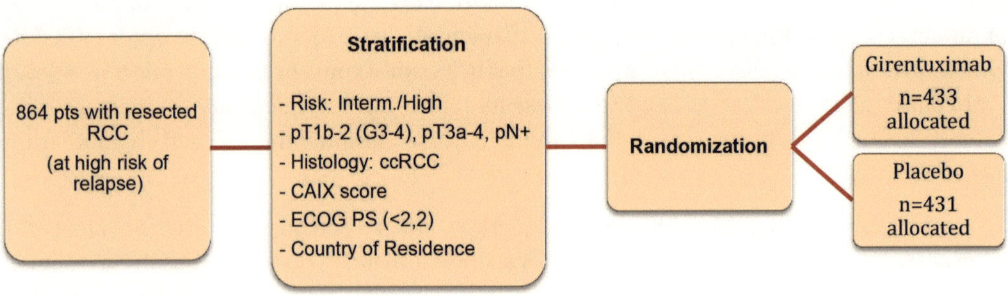

This ARISER trial, completed in 2014, evaluated the efficacy of girentuximab [60], a monoclonal antibody to carbonic anhydrase IX (a HIF downstream target gene), in the adjuvant setting for intermediate to high risk for recurrence patients. This multicenter, phase III trial involved 864 patients with resected clear cell tumors, who were randomized to receive either girentuximab or placebo, once a week, for 24 weeks. Girentuximab recipients received a 50 mg dose during the first week followed by a weekly dose of 20 mg for the next 23 weeks. The median disease free survival (DFS) duration for the participants in the intervention arm was 71.4 months (HR: 0.97; 95% CI, 0.79–1.18) while the endpoint was never reached for the placebo group. As such, the study indicated no interventional advantage but it recommended further investigation of adjuvant girentuximab in patients with high levels of CAIX in affected renal tissue.

7.3.2. ASSURE trial

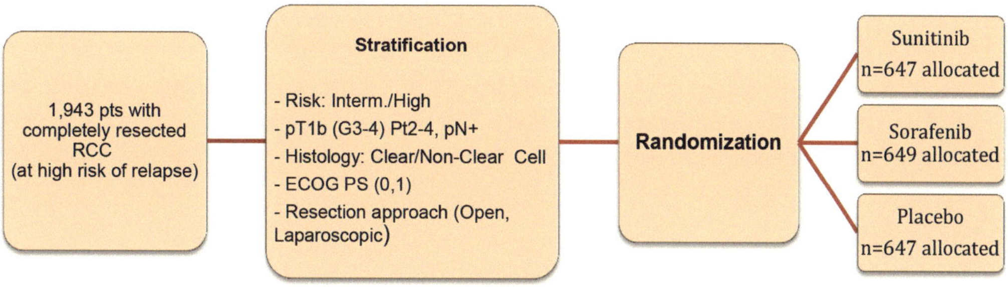

The ASSURE trial, completed in 2016, was a randomized, double-blind, placebo-controlled, phase 3 clinical trial in which 1943 patients from 226 study centers in North America were assigned to one of three intervention arms—sunitinib, sorafenib or placebo in intermediate to high-risk patients [61]. Sunitinib patients received 50 mg for 54 weeks on a 4 of 6 week cycle; sorafenib recipients received 400 mg twice per day throughout each cycle, and placebo recipients were randomly assigned either the sunitinib placebo or the sorafenib placebo. The interventions were evaluated using DFS as the primary endpoint. Trial results indicated that the median DFS duration was approximately 5.8 years for sunitinib [HR: 1.02; 97.5% CI: 0.85–1.23; P = 0.8038], 6.1 years for sorafenib (HR: 0.97; 97.5% CI: 0.80–1.17; P = 0.7184), and 6.6 years for placebo—hence suggesting no survival benefit from the interventions relative to the placebo. Instead, the results further reported detrimental effects due to the increased toxicity of the treatment despite the dose reductions—suggesting no benefit of the particular TKI in the adjuvant setting. Of note, this trial had a higher number of TKI dose reductions (potentially suggesting suboptimal drug dosing) and more intermediate risk for recurrence patients than other trials.

7.3.3. S-TRAC trial

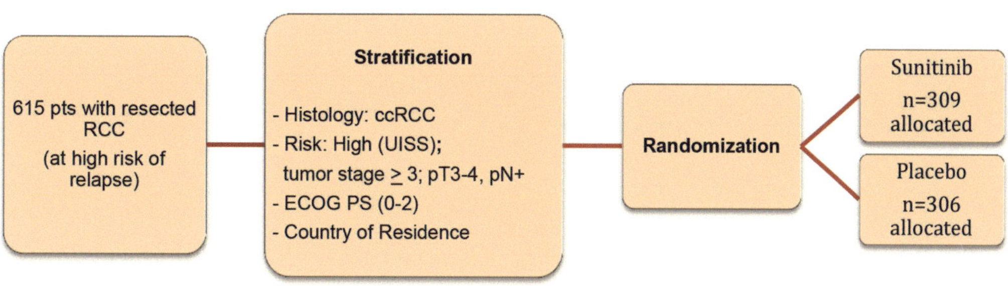

The S-TRAC study, also completed in 2016, was a prospective, randomized, double-blind, phase 3 clinical trial involving 615 patients from 21 countries [62]. Of the 615 patients who underwent randomization, 309 were assigned to the sunitinib arm and 306 to the placebo arm. These patients were all "high risk of recurrence." Sunitinib recipients received 50 mg for a year on a 4 of 6 week cycle. The interventions were evaluated by comparing DFS, the primary endpoint of the study, between the two trial arms. The study results indicated that the median DFS duration was 6.8 years (95% CI: 5.8 to not reached) in the sunitinib group and 5.6 years (95% CI: 3.8–6.6) in the placebo group (HR: 0.76; 95% CI: 0.59–0.98; P = 0.03). The adverse effects observed in sunitinib recipients were consistent with its known toxicity profile. As such, the results from this trial support the potential for sunitinib as a treatment option in the adjuvant setting with a DFS advantage. However, overall survival endpoints have not yet been reported.

7.3.4. PROTECT trial

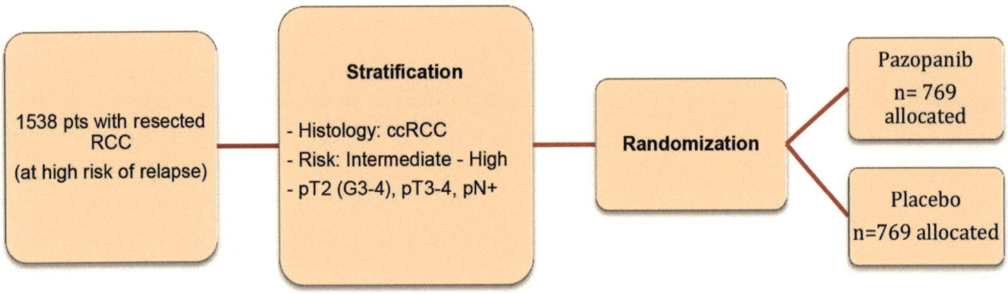

The PROTECT study, completed recently in 2017, was a phase 3 randomized clinical trial that evaluated the efficacy of adjuvant pazopanib as compared to placebo in preventing RCC recurrence in intermediate to high-risk patients [63]. The trial enrolled 1538 participants and the majority of the pazopanib recipients received a revised dosage of 600 mg, daily for a year, following a dose reduction from 800 mg which caused severe side effects. The interventions were evaluated by comparing DFS as the primary endpoint measure between the two trial arms. The study did not meet its primary endpoint and indicated no significant benefit of pazopanib-600 mg in prolonging DFS as compared to placebo (HR: 0.86; 95% CI, 0.70–1.06; P = 0.165). However, a subgroup analysis of pazopanib-800 mg recipients indicated a 31% decline in DFS (HR, 0.69; 95% CI, 0.51–0.94; *P* = 0.02). While the DFS results were conflicting between the 600 mg and 800 mg groups, the study reported similar adverse event profiles between both the groups.

7.3.5. Comparison of current adjuvant trial design

The differing outcomes that have been indicated in the current set of completed trials may be accounted for by the distinct sample groups, dose regimens, risk assessment criteria and trial methods [60–63]. This collectively represents a fundamental limitation that underscores all current adjuvant clinical trials. First, the patient inclusion criteria characteristically differ, in multiple ways, across all adjuvant trials [60–63]. For example, in the S-TRAC trial, the selected sample exclusively included patients with late-stage, loco-regional, clear-cell RCC while other trials such as the ASSURE, ARTISER and PROTECT trials used a less restricted criteria and included patients with stage 1 or stage 2 tumors and non-clear-cell histologies [60–63]. In addition, another major cause of heterogeneity lies in the risk assessment and stratification criteria as the scoring system used in the current set of adjuvant trials are not standardized, and hence this invariably contributes to a varied assessment of recurrence risk [60–63]. With respect to the conflicting sunitinib trials (S-TRAC vs. ASSURE), additional sources of variation that might have led to inconsistent outcomes include varying dose regimens, specifically with respect to the midtrial dose reductions for sunitinib, as well as differing trial criteria for establishing disease status and assessing primary end point status [61, 62, 64].

7.4. Targeted immunomodulatory therapy

The development of therapy that targets oncogenic signaling pathways has advanced the treatment landscape for patients with advanced renal cell carcinoma. While nonspecific immunotherapy with IL-2 and IFN-α was the former mainstay in the management of metastatic disease, there was a shift away from it with the advent of targeted therapy which yielded relatively better response rates [32–34, 48–54, 65–68]. However, over the last couple of years, cancer immunotherapy has been revisited and, as a result, targeted immunomodulatory therapy, involving novel immunomodulating agents, has been reincorporated in combination therapy regimes for mRCC management—hence allowing for an induced immuonologic effect in addition to the inhibitory effect on tumor biology and microenvironment [69, 70]. This has been inspired in part by disease resistance that is progressively manifesting itself against standard targeted therapy in the landscape of metastatic disease management [69, 70].

Given that multiple mechanisms are employed by tumors to evade and suppress the immune system, research toward better understanding those mechanisms of immunomodulation has been critical in informing the therapeutic landscape [69, 71]. Particularly, an improved understanding of the factors regulating the antitumor immune response has led to the development a novel form of cancer immunotherapy involving checkpoint inhibitors and other immune therapies such as T-cell agonists, adoptive T-cell therapies and novel vaccines which are being evaluated across different trials for metastatic RCC [69, 71].

7.5. Immune checkpoint inhibitors

Immune checkpoints serve a critical protective function of preventing immune response against host cells through a series of complex interactions [71–73]. However, investigation into the pathogenic mechanisms of RCC revealed that cancer cells can induce similar interactions with host checkpoint receptors and can hence suppress the human immune response [71–73]. Immune checkpoint inhibitors counter these molecular mechanisms through which tumor cells evade immune recognition [71–73].

Programmed cell death protein 1 (PD-1) and cytotoxic T-lymphocyte-associated antigen 4 (CTLA-4) are currently the most well understood inhibitory checkpoint receptors [71–73]. The PD-1/PD-L1 axis involves an inhibitory interaction between a T-cell inhibitory ligand PD-L1, expressed on tumor cell surface, and a PD-1 receptor on the lymphocyte [71–73]. Hence, mimicking this interaction ultimately allows tumor cells to evade the adaptive immune response through suppression of T-cell function. The CTLA-4 pathway is similarly exploited by tumor cells [71–73]. During an adaptive immune response, immune activation occurs through an interaction between the T-cell receptor (TCR) and the antigen-presenting cell (APC) along with the co-stimulation of CD28 on the T cell [71–73]. This activation is negatively regulated by an inhibitory interaction between CTLA-4 and its ligands—CD80 or CD86 [71–73]. Thus, the targeted inhibition of these checkpoint receptors through targeted antibodies, in both the pathways mentioned above, could allow for T-cell activation and effective immune function [71–73].

The first checkpoint inhibitor which demonstrated a survival benefit in patients with metastatic RCC was nivolumab—an anti-PD1 monoclonal antibody [74]. The inhibitor, which received FDA approval in 2015 based on the results from a trial evaluating nivolumab versus everolimus, is effective in yielding positive response rates when used for treatment of advanced RCC in patients who have undergone prior anti-angiogenic therapy [74]. Apart from nivolumab, multiple other checkpoint inhibitors are being currently evaluated in different trials against advanced RCC [71–73].

7.6. Immunomodulatory therapy in the adjuvant setting

Given their recent development, many immune checkpoint inhibitors are still being evaluated for their efficacy and toxicity against metastatic RCC, and hence investigation of these inhibitors in the adjuvant setting has been limited. Currently, there are a few ongoing clinical trials that are evaluating different checkpoint inhibitors in both the adjuvant setting as well as the neo-adjuvant (presurgery) setting (**Table 3**) [75–78].

The *IMmotion*, *KEYNOTE-564*, and *CheckMate 914* are phase III trials evaluating the efficacy and safety of adjuvant atezolizumab, pembrolizumab, and nivolumab/ipilimumab (combinational regimen) respectively in prolonging the DFS of RCC patients who are at high risk of disease recurrence post nephrectomy [75, 77, 78]. In addition to the adjuvant trials, an ongoing study in the neo-adjuvant setting includes the PROSPER trial which is evaluating the efficacy of pre-nephrectomy nivolumab [75]. These trials, which have either started already or are expected to begin later this year, are currently in their recruitment or pre-recruitment phases and are anticipated to be completed by 2022–2024. [75, 77, 78] Apart from these clinical

Adjuvant clinical trials in RCC using immune therapies

Authors	Intervention	Patient population	Design	No. of patients	Outcome
Pizzocarro et al. [32]	IFN-α2b vs. placebo	Robson stages II and III (T3aN0M0 and T3bN0M0 or T2/3N1-3M0)	Multicenter, randomized, controlled trial	247	5-year OS: 0.665 (control) vs. 0.660 (treatment) (HR 1.040; 95% CI, 0.671–1.613, P ¼ _0.861)
					5-year DFS: 0.671 (control) vs. 0.567 (treatment) (HR 1.412; 95% CI, 0.927–2.149, P ¼ _0.107)
Passalacqua et al. [34]	IL-2 and IFN-α _v observation	pT1, T2, T3 a-b-c; pN0-pN3,M0M	Multicenter, randomized, controlled trial	310	5-year DFS: 0.73 (control) vs. 0.73 (treatment)
					10-year DFS: 0.60 (control) vs. 0.73 (treatment) (HR 0.84; 95% CI, 0.54–1.33, P ¼ _0.47)

Adjuvant clinical trials in RCC using immune therapies

Authors	Intervention	Patient population	Design	No. of patients	Outcome
Clark et al. [48]	IL-2 vs. observation	T3b-4 or N1-3 (LA) or M1	Multicenter, randomized, controlled trial	69 total; 44 LA, 25M1 disease	2-year DFS: 48% (control in LA patients) vs. 53% (treatment in LA patients) (P ¼ _0.73) 2-year OS: 77% (control in LA patients) vs. 86%
Messing et al. [33]	IFN-α-NL vs. observation	pT3–4a and/or node-positive	Multicenter, randomized, controlled trial	283	At 10.4 years median follow-up: Median survival: 7.4 years (control) vs. 5.1 years (treatment) (P ¼ _0.09). DFS: 3.0 years (control) vs. 2.2 years (treatment) (P ¼ _0.33)
Atzpodien et al. [35]	IL-2 and IFN-α2a and intravenous 5 vs. fluorouracil	pT3b/c pN0 or pT4pN0), pN, complete resection of tumor relapse or solitary metastasis (R0)	Multicenter, randomized, controlled trial	203	At median follow-up of 4.3 years: 2-year OS: 91% (control) vs. 81% (treatment) 5-year OS: 76% (control) vs. 58% (treatment) 8-year OS: 66% (control) vs. 58% (treatment) (P ¼ _0.0278) 2-year DFS: 62% (control) vs. 54% (treatment) 5-year DFS: 49% (control) vs. 42% (treatment) 8-year DFS: 49% (control) vs. 39% (treatment) (P ¼ _0.2398)
Aitchison et al. [36]	IL-2 and IFN-α2a and intravenous 5-fluorouracil	T3b-c,T4 or any pT and pN1 or pN2 or positive microscopic margins or microscopic vascular invasion	Multicenter, randomized, controlled trial	309	3-year DFS: 50% (control) vs. 60% (treatment) (HR 0.87; 95% CI, 0.63–1.20) 5-year OS: 60% (control) vs. 68% (treatment) (HR 0.91; 95% CI, 0.60–1.38)

Adjuvant clinical trials in RCC using immune therapies					
Authors	**Intervention**	**Patient population**	**Design**	**No. of patients**	**Outcome**
Galligioni et al. [39]	Autologous irradiated tumor cells and BCG vs. observation	Stages I, II, and III	Prospective, randomized, controlled trial	120	At 61 months median follow-up: 5-year OS: 78% (control) vs. 69% (treatment) 5-year DFS: 72% (control) vs. 63% (treatment)
Adler et al. [40]	Autologous irradiated tumor cells & BCG & hormone vs. hormone	All stages	Prospective, randomized, controlled trial	43	Trend for prolongation of DFS for stage I, II, and III (P o.1)
Wood et al. [41]	Autologous, tumor-derived heat-shock protein (glycoprotein 96)-peptide complex (HSPPC-96; vitespen) vs. observation	cT1b–T4 N0 M0, or cTanyN1-2M0Multicenter	Multicenter, randomized, controlled trial	819	At 1.9 years median follow-up: recurrence: 39.8% (control) vs. 37.7% (treatment) (HR 0.923; 95% CI, 0.729–1.169, P ¼ _0.506) OS not mature
Jocham et al. [42]	Autologous renal tumor cells (Reniale)	pT2–3b pN0–3	Multicenter, randomized, controlled trial	558	At 5-year follow-up: DFS: 67.8% (control) vs. 77.4% (treatment) (P ¼ _0.0204). At 70-month follow-up: DFS: 59.3% (control) vs. 72% (treatment). HR for tumor progression: 1.58 (95% CI 1.05–2.37) and 1.59 (1.07–2.36) (P ¼ _0.0204)

IFN, interferon; IL, interleukin; NL, neutral lymphoblastoid; LA, locally advanced; BCG, bacillus Calmette-Guérin; CI, confidence interval; LA, locally advanced; HR, hazard ratio; M, metastatic; OS, overall survival; DFS, disease-free survival.

Table 3. Adjuvant clinical trials in RCC using immune therapies.

studies, there are several checkpoint inhibitors that are in development as well as others that are currently being evaluated in trials for mRCC and would subsequently be assessed in the adjuvant setting [71–73] (**Tables 4–6**).

7.7. Change of practice

The European Association of Urology Renal Cell Cancer Guidelines Panel, which includes patient representatives and clinicians, considered a number of different scenarios to determine what would be required from S-TRAC to change practice. The decision on practice change

http://dx.doi.org/10.5772/intechopen.78684

Trial name.	Trial ID	Intervention	Sample size	Inclusion criteria (histology; stage/ grade)	Primary endpoint measure	Completion date
ARISER	NCT00087022	Girentuximab	864	**ccRCC**; T1b,N0, NX,MO, T2,N0, NX,MO (grade ≥ 3) (risk: intermediate-High)	DFS,OS	2014
ASSURE	NCT00326898	Sorafenib or Sunitinib	1943	**Any**; pT1bN0M0 (grades 3–4), pT2-4N1-3M0 (risk: intermediate-high)	DFS	2016
S-TRAC	NCT00375674	Sunitinib	615	**ccRCC**; pT2N0M0 (grades 3–4) or pT3-4N0M0 or pTxN1M0 (risk: High)	DFS	2016
PROTECT	NCT01235962	Pazopanib	1500	**ccRCC**; pT2N0M0 (grades 3–4) or pT3-4N0M0 or pTxN1M0 (risk: intermediate-high)	DFS	2017

Table 4. RCC adjuvant clinical trials that have been completed.

was taken in the context of the data from ASSURE. Results showed that only 1 out of 15 (6%) of the panel would change their standard of care when considering the DFS and OS closest to S-TRAC (DFS: HR 0.75, $p < 0.05$; OS: HR 1.0, $p > 0.05$). Standard practice would only be significantly influenced by a significant survival benefit. In addition, kidney cancer patients from the International Kidney Cancer Coalition (IKCC) participated in a questionnaire about

Trial name.	Trial ID	Intervention	Sample size	Inclusion criteria (histology; stage/ grade)	Primary endpoint measure	Estimated completion date
SORCE	NCT00492258	Sorafenib	1420	**Any**; pT1a N0M0 (grade 4), pT1b N0M0 (grades 3–4), pT2-4N0M0, pT1b-4N1M (risk: intermediate-high)	DFS	2019
ATLAS	NCT01599754	Axitinib	592	**ccRCC**; pT2-4N0M0 or pTxN1M0 (risk: high)	DFS	2019
EVEREST	NCT01120249	Everolimus	1218	**Any**; pT1bN0M0 (grades 3–4) or pT2-4N1-3M0 (risk: intermediate-high)	DFS	2021

Table 5. Current set of adjuvant clinical trials that are still in progress.

Trial name	Trial ID	Intervention	Estimated enrollment	Primary endpoint measure	Start date	Completion date
PROSPER	NCT03055013	Nivolumab (pre-Nx)	766	DFS	February 2, 2017	2022
KEYNOTE-564	NCT03142334	Pembrolizumab	950	DFS	June 9, 2017	2022
CheckMate 914	NCT03138512	Nivolumab, ipilimumab	800	DFS	July 3, 2017	2023
IMmotion010	NCT03024996	Atezolizumab	664	DFS	January 3, 2017	2024

Table 6. Ongoing adjuvant and neo-adjuvant clinical trials.

the implications for STRAC. The results lacked clarity. Twenty-two patient representatives from the IKCC network were asked what degree of PFS advantage would be needed to justify taking sunitinib for 1 year. Approximately one-third of patients favored not taking sunitinib when faced with the S-TRAC results [79].

Recently, on November 2017, the FDA approved the use sunitinib for the adjuvant treatment of adult patients at high risk of recurrent renal cell carcinoma following nephrectomy. The approval was based on (S-TRAC) trail.

8. Conclusions and future directions

Targeted therapy has become the current mainstay in the management of metastatic RCC and its success with advanced stage disease has been the driving force behind the increasing number of targeted therapy trials in the adjuvant setting. The emergence of immune checkpoint inhibitors in the last couple of years has further led to important advances in our understanding and management of mRCC. However, many ongoing trials are yet to be completed in both cases and there is ample potential for further investigation—especially with respect to combinational therapy regimes. This includes the combination of TKIs with immune therapies (e.g., NCT01513187: Pazopanib with Interferon Alfa 2-A), combination of TKIs with chemotherapeutics (e.g., NCT00556049: Sunitinib with Gemcitabine), and the combination of anti-VEGF antibodies and mTOR inhibitors (e.g., NCT01399918: bevacizumab and everolimus). All of these treatments may be of interest for future adjuvant trials in RCC if they are found to be effective in stage IV disease. However, they may have more side effects, making them less suitable in particular for adjuvant treatment. Nonetheless, the current information, which has resulted from all the progress in the field, remains incongruent. While the current set of completed adjuvant clinical trials have provided negative or conflicting results (ARISER, PROTECT, S-TRAC vs. ASSURE), there are additional large-scale trials that are still in progress. The existing trial design has several limitations, the key one being the overall lack of standardization seen across various assessment criteria. Future directions include incorporating a genetic recurrence score to evaluate risk of relapse in patients, developing an adequate and an objectively standardized adjuvant trial design, identifying novel biomarkers and evaluating novel drug targets.

That based on results from current trials, the "high risk for recurrence" RCC patient population (T3-T4, grade 3-4) may benefit from adjuvant sunitinib providing DFS advantage but pending OS results. Patients, in this category, interested in adjuvant therapy would benefit from a discussion with an oncologist regarding the potential benefits and risks of adjuvant treatment post kidney cancer surgery. Overall, the landscape of adjuvant treatment in nonmetastatic high-risk RCC is expected to expand and to further develop in the coming years.

Author details

Fadil Hassan[1], Shahid Lambe[1], Kiran Sharma[1] and Anil Kapoor[2]*

*Address all correspondence to: akapoor@mcmaster.ca

1 McMaster University, Hamilton, ON, Canada

2 Division of Urology, McMaster University, Hamilton, ON, Canada

References

[1] Ferlay J, Shin HR, Bray F, Forman D, Mathers C, Parkin DM. GLOBOCAN 2008 v1.2, Cancer Incidence and Mortality Worldwide. Lyon, France: International Agency for Research on Cancer; 2010

[2] Canadian Cancer Society's Advisory Committee on Cancer Statistics. Canadian Cancer Statistics 2015. Toronto, ON: Canadian Cancer Society; 2015

[3] Renal Cell Carcinoma. Cleveland Clinic. 2013. Available from: http://www.clevelandclinicmeded.com/medicalpubs/diseasemanagement/nephrology/renal-cell-carcinoma/

[4] Kidney Cancer Association. About Kidney Cancer. October, 2016. Available from: http://www.kidneycancer.org/knowledge/learn/about-kidney-cancer/

[5] National Cancer Institute: SEER Stat Fact Sheets: Kidney and Renal Pelvis. Key Fact Available from: http://seer.cancer.gov/statfacts/html/kidrp.html (link is external)

[6] Kidney Cancer—Mayo Clinic [Internet]. Mayoclinic.org. Available from: http://www.mayoclinic.org/diseases-conditions/kidney-cancer/basics/definition/con-20024753

[7] Abe H, Kamai T. Recent advances in the treatment of metastatic renal cell carcinoma. International Journal of Urology. Oct 2013;**20**:944-955

[8] Janzen NK, Kim HL, Figlin RA, Belldegrun AS. Surveillance after radical or partial nephrectomy for localized renal cell carcinoma and management of recurrent disease. The Urologic Clinics of North America. 2003;**30**:843-852

[9] Janowitz T, Welsh SJ, Zaki K, Mulders P, Eisen T. Adjuvant therapy in renal cell carcinoma—Past, present, and future. Seminars in Oncology. 2013;**40**:482-491

[10] Pal SK, Haas NB. Adjuvant therapy for renal cell carcinoma: Past, present, and future. The Oncologist. 2014;**19**(8):851-859. DOI: 10.1634/theoncologist.2014-0105

[11] Cindolo L et al. A preoperative clinical prognostic model for non-metastatic renal cell carcinoma. BJU International. 2003;**92**:901-905

[12] Leibovich BC, Blute ML, Cheville JC, et al. Prediction of progression after radical nephrectomy for patients with clear cell renal cell carcinoma: A stratification tool for prospective clinical trials. Cancer. 2003;**97**(7):1663-1671

[13] Sorbellini M et al. A postoperative prognostic nomogram predicting recurrence for patients with conventional clear cell renal cell carcinoma. The Journal of Urology. 2005;**173**(1): 48-51

[14] Kattan M et al. A postoperative predictive nomogram for renal cell carcinoma. The Journal of Urology. 2001;**166**:63-67

[15] Frank I et al. An outcome prediction model for patients with clear cell renal cell carcinoma treated with radical nephrectomy based on tumor stage, size, grade and necrosis: The SSIGN score. The Journal of Urology. 2002;**168**(6):2395-2400

[16] Zisman A et al. Improved prognostication of renal cell carcinoma using an integrated staging system. Journal of Clinical Oncology. 2001;**19**(6):1649-1657

[17] Karakiewicz PI et al. Multi-institutional validation of a new renal cancer-specific survival nomogram. Journal of Clinical Oncology. 2007;**25**(11):1316-1322

[18] Patard JJ, Kim HL, Lam JS, et al. Use of the University of California, Los Angeles integrated staging system to predict survival in renal cell carcinoma: An international multicenter study. Journal of Clinical Oncology. 2004;**22**(16):3316-3322

[19] Yaycioglu O, Roberts WW, Chan T, Epstein JI, Marshall FF, Kavoussi LR. Prognostic assessment of nonmetastatic renal cell carcinoma: A clinically based model. Urology. 2001;**58**(2):141-145

[20] Patard JJ, Dorey FJ, Cindolo L, et al. Symptoms as well as tumor size provide prognostic information on patients with localized renal tumors. The Journal of Urology. 2004;**172** (6 pt 1):2167-2171

[21] Motzer RJ, Mazumdar M, Bacik J, Berg W, Amsterdam A, Ferrara J. Survival and prognostic stratification of 670 patients with advanced renal cell carcinoma. Journal of Clinical Oncology. 1999;**17**(8):2530-2540

[22] Cindolo L et al. Comparison of predictive accuracy of four prognostic models for nonmetastatic renal cell carcinoma after nephrectomy: A multicenter European study. Cancer. 2005;**104**(7):1362-1371

[23] Parker WP et al. Application of the stage, size, grade, and necrosis (SSIGN) score for clear cell renal cell carcinoma in contemporary patients. European Urology. 2017 Apr;**71**(4):665-673

[24] Crispen PL et al. Outcomes following partial nephrectomy by tumor size. The Journal of Urology. 2008;**180**(5):1912-1917

[25] Lam JS et al. Postoperative surveillance protocol for patients with localized and locally advanced renal cell carcinoma based on a validated prognostic nomogram and risk group stratification system. The Journal of Urology. 2005;**174**(2):466-472. discussion 472; quiz 801

[26] Adamy A et al. Clinical characteristics and outcomes of patients with recurrence 5 years after nephrectomy for localized renal cell carcinoma. The Journal of Urology. 2011;**185**(2):433-438

[27] Du Y, Grüllich C, Hadaschik B, Hatiboglu G, Hohenfellner M, Pahernik S. Local recurrence after curative surgical treatment of renal cell cancer: A study of 91 patients. Clinical Genitourinary Cancer. 2016;**14**(4):e379-e385

[28] Cancer Genome Atlas Research Network. Comprehensive molecular characterization of clear cell renal cell carcinoma. Nature. 2013;**499**(7456):43-49

[29] Klatte T, Seligson DB, LaRochelle J, et al. Molecular signatures of localized clear cell renal cell carcinoma to predict disease-free survival after nephrectomy. Cancer Epidemiology, Biomarkers & Prevention. 2009;**18**:894

[30] Rini B, Goddard A, Knezevic D, et al. A 16-gene assay to predict recurrence after surgeryin localised renal cell carcinoma: Development and validation studies. The Lancet Oncology. 2015;**16**:676

[31] Speed J, Trinh Q, Choueiri T, Sun M. Recurrence in localized renal cell carcinoma: A systematic review of contemporary data. Current Urology Reports. 2017;**18**(2)

[32] Giorgio P et al. Interferon adjuvant to radical nephrectomy in Robson stages II and III renal cell carcinoma: A multicentric randomized study. Journal of Clinical Oncology. 2001;**19**(2):425-431

[33] Messing EM et al. Phase III study of interferon alfa-NL as adjuvant treatment for resectable renal cell carcinoma: An Eastern Cooperative Oncology Group/Intergroup Trial. Journal of Clinical Oncology. 2003;**21**(7):1214-1222

[34] Passalacqua R, Buzio C, Buti S, et al. Adjuvant low-dose interleukin-2 (IL2) plus interferon-alpha (IFN) in operable renal cell cancer (RCC). A phase III, randomized, multicenter, independent trial of the Italian Oncology Group for Clinical Research (GOIRC). Journal of Clinical Oncology. 2007;**25**:18S. 2007 ASCO Annual Meeting Proceedings Part I

[35] Atzpodien J et al. Interleukin-2-and interferon alfa-2a-based immunochemotherapy in advanced renal cell carcinoma: A prospectively randomized trial of the German Cooperative Renal Carcinoma Chemoimmunotherapy Group (DGCIN). Journal of Clinical Oncology. 2004;**22**(7):1188-1194

[36] Aitchison M, Bray C, Van Poppel H, Sylvester R, Graham J, Innes C, McMahon LVP. Preliminary results from a randomized phase III trial of adjuvant interleu- kin-2, interferon alpha and 5-fluorouracil in patients with a high risk of relapse after nephrectomy for renal cell carcinoma (RCC). Journal of Clinical Oncology. 2008;**26**(suppl)

[37] Ahmedin J et al. Global cancer statistics. CA: A Cancer Journal for Clinicians. 2011;**61**(2): 69-90

[38] Poppel V, Hein SJ, Van Gool SW. Vaccine therapy in patients with renal cell carcinoma. European Urology. 2009;**55**(6):1333-1344

[39] Galligioni E et al. Adjuvant immunotherapy treatment of renal carcinoma patients with autologous tumor cells and Bacillus Calmette-Guèrin: Five-year results of a prospective randomized study. Cancer. 1996;**77**(12):2560-2566

[40] Adler A et al. Active specific immunotherapy of renal cell carcinoma patients: A prospective randomized study of hormono-immuno-versus hormonotherapy. Preliminary report of immunological and clinical aspects. Journal of Immunotherapy. 1987;**6**(6):610

[41] Wood C et al. An adjuvant autologous therapeutic vaccine (HSPPC-96; vitespen) versus observation alone for patients at high risk of recurrence after nephrectomy for renal cell carcinoma: A multicentre, open-label, randomised phase III trial. The Lancet. 2008;**372**(9633):145-154

[42] Jocham D et al. Adjuvant autologous renal tumour cell vaccine and risk of tumour progression in patients with renal-cell carcinoma after radical nephrectomy: Phase III, randomised controlled trial. The Lancet. 2004;**363**(9409):594-599

[43] Fishman M, Antonia S. Specific antitumour vaccine for renal cancer. The Lancet. 2004; **363**(9409):583-584

[44] Maxwell PH et al. The tumour suppressor protein VHL targets hypoxia-inducible factors for oxygen-dependent proteolysis. Nature. 1999;**399**(6733):271-275

[45] Dorothea FS, Kjølseth I, Lund G. Radiotherapy of metastases from renal cancer. European Urology. 1982;**8**:340-342

[46] Mogens K, Frederiksen PL, Engelholm S. Postoperative radiotherapy in stage II and III renal adenocarcinoma. A randomized trial by the Copenhagen renal cancer study group. International Journal of Radiation Oncology Biology Physics. 1987;**13**(5):665-672

[47] Mogens K et al. A randomized trial of postoperative radiotherapy versus observation in stage II and III renal adenocarcinoma: A study by the Copenhagen Renal Cancer Study Group. Scandinavian Journal of Urology and Nephrology. 1987;**21**(4):285-289

[48] Clark JI et al. Adjuvant high-dose bolus interleukin-2 for patients with high-risk renal cell carcinoma: A cytokine working group randomized trial. Journal of Clinical Oncology. 2003;**21**(16):3133-3140

[49] Escudier B, Albiges L, Sonpavde G. Optimal management of metastatic renal cell carcinoma: Current status. Drugs. 2013;**73**(5):427-438

[50] Motzer RJ, Hutson TE, Tomczak P, Michaelson MD, Bukowski RM, Rixe O, Oudard S, Negrier S, Szczylik C, Kim ST, Chen I. Sunitinib versus interferon alfa in metastatic renal-cell carcinoma. The New England Journal of Medicine. 2007;**356**(2):115-124

[51] Motzer R, Hutson T, Tomczak P, Michaelson M, Bukowski R, Oudard S, et al. Overall survival and updated results for sunitinib compared with interferon alfa in patients with metastatic renal cell carcinoma. Journal of Clinical Oncology. 2009;**27**(22):3584-3590

[52] Powles T, Chowdhury S, Jones R, Mantle M, Nathan P, Bex A, et al. Sunitinib and other targeted therapies for renal cell carcinoma. British Journal of Cancer. 2011;**104**(5):741-745

[53] Coppin C, Kollmannsberger C, Le L, Porzsolt F, Wilt T. Targeted therapy for advanced renal cell cancer (RCC): A cochrane systematic review of published randomised trials. BJU International. 2011;**108**(10):1556-1563

[54] Pal SK, Williams S, Josephson DY, et al. Novel therapies for metastatic renal cell carcinoma: Efforts to expand beyond the VEGF/mTOR signaling paradigm. Molecular Cancer Therapeutics. 2012;**11**:526-537

[55] Ljunberg et al. Guidelines on Renal Cell Carcinoma. European Association of Urology. 2015. Available from: http://uroweb.org/wp-content/uploads/10-Renal-Cell-Carcinoma_LR1.pdf

[56] Ellis L, Hicklin D. VEGF-targeted therapy: Mechanisms of anti-tumour activity. Nature Reviews. Cancer. 2008;**8**(8):579-591

[57] Baldewijns M, van Vlodrop I, Vermeulen P, Soetekouw P, van Engeland M, de Bruïne A. VHL and HIF signalling in renal cell carcinogenesis. The Journal of Pathology. 2010;**221**(2):125-138

[58] Pal SK, Bergerot P, Figlin RA. Renal cell carcinoma: An update for the practicing urologist. Asian Journal of Urology. 2015;**2**(1):19-25

[59] Patel D, Figlin R, Kim H. Adjuvant treatment for renal cell carcinoma: Do we finally have a major breakthrough? Clinical Advances in Hematology & Oncology. 2016;**14**(11)

[60] Chamie K, Donin NM, Klöpfer P, Bevan P, Fall B, Wilhelm O, Störkel S, Said J, Gambla M, Hawkins RE, Jankilevich G, Kapoor A, Kopyltsov E, Staehler M, Taari K, Wainstein AJA, Pantuck AJ, Belldegrun AS. Phase III ARISER data for the adjuvant treatment of clear cell renal cancer with RENCAREX® including retrospective subgroup analysis. Presented at ASCO; 1-3 June, 2013

[61] Haas NB, Manola J, Uzzo RG, et al. Adjuvant sunitinib or sorafenib for high-risk, non-metastatic renal-cell carcinoma (ECOG-ACRIN E2805): A double-blind, placebo-controlled, randomised, phase 3 trial. Lancet. 2016;**387**:2008-2016

[62] Ravaud A, Motzer RJ, Pandha HS, et al. Adjuvant sunitinib in high-risk renal-cell carcinoma after nephrectomy. The New England Journal of Medicine. 2016;**375**:2246-2254. DOI: 10.1056/NEJMoa1611406

[63] RJM M, Naomi HB, et al. Randomized phase III trial of adjuvant pazopanib versus placebo after nephrectomy in patients with locally advanced renal cell carcinoma (RCC) (PROTECT). Journal of Clinical Oncology. 2017;**35**(15_suppl):4507-4507

[64] Porta C, Chiellino S. ASSURE vs. S-TRAC: Conflicting results of adjuvant treatments for kidney cancer in the era of targeted agents and genomics. Annals of Translational Medicine. 2016;**4**(Suppl 1)

[65] Atzpodien J, Kirchner H, Illiger HJ. IL-2 in combination with IFN- alpha and 5-FU versus tamoxifen in metastatic renal cell carcinoma: Long-term results of a controlled randomized clinical trial. British Journal of Cancer. 2001;**85**(8):1130-1136

[66] Atzpodien J, Kirchner H, Jonas U. Interleukin-2- and interferon alfa-2a-based immunochemotherapy in advanced renal cell carcinoma: A prospectively randomized trial of the German Cooperative Renal Carcinoma Chemoimmunotherapy Group (DGCIN). Journal of Clinical Oncology. 2004;**22**(7):1188-1194

[67] Atzpodien J, Schmitt E, Gertenbach U. Adjuvant treatment with interleukin-2- and interferon-alpha2a-based chemoimmunotherapy in renal cell carcinoma post tumour nephrectomy: Results of a prospectively randomised trial of the German Cooperative Renal Carcinoma Chemoimmunotherapy Group (DGCIN). British Journal of Cancer. 2005;**92**(5):843-846

[68] Aitchison M, Bray C, Van Poppel H, Sylvester R, Graham J, Innes C, McMahon LVP. Preliminary results from a randomized phase III trial of adjuvant interleukin-2, interferon alpha and 5-fluorouracil in patients with a high risk of relapse after nephrectomy for renal cell carcinoma (RCC). Journal of Clinical Oncology. 2008;**26**(suppl):5040. abstr

[69] De Maeseneer D, Delafontaine B, Rottey S. Checkpoint inhibition: New treatment options in urologic cancer. Acta Clinica Belgica. 2017;**72**(1):24-28

[70] Kuusk T, Albiges L, Escudier B, Grivas N, Haanen J, Powles T, et al. Antiangiogenic therapy combined with immune checkpoint blockade in renal cancer. Angiogenesis. 2017

[71] Mellman I, Coukos G, Dranoff G. Cancer immunotherapy comes of age. Nature. 2011;**480**: 480-489

[72] Pardoll DM. The blockade of immune checkpoints in cancer immunotherapy. Nature Reviews. Cancer. 2012;**12**:252-264

[73] Carlo M, Voss M, Motzer R. Checkpoint inhibitors and other novel immunotherapies for advanced renal cell carcinoma. Nature Reviews. Urology. 2016;**13**(7):420-431

[74] Motzer R, Escudier B, McDermott D, George S, Hammers H, Srinivas S, et al. Nivolumab versus Everolimus in advanced renal-cell carcinoma. The New England Journal of Medicine. 2015 Nov 5;**373**(19):1803-1813. DOI: 10.1056/NEJMoa1510665. Epub 2015 Sep 25

[75] US National Library of Medicine. ClinicalTrials.gov. 2017. https://clinicaltrials.gov/ct2/show/NCT03055013

[76] US National Library of Medicine. ClinicalTrials.gov. 2017. https://clinicaltrials.gov/ct2/show/NCT03142334

[77] US National Library of Medicine. ClinicalTrials.gov. 2017. https://clinicaltrials.gov/ct2/show/NCT03138512

[78] US National Library of Medicine. ClinicalTrials.gov. 2017. https://clinicaltrials.gov/ct2/show/NCT03024996

[79] Bex A, Albiges L, Ljungberg B, Bensalah K, Dabestani S, Giles RH, Hofmann F, Hora M, Kuczyk MA, Lam TB, Marconi L, Merseburger AS, Staehler M, Volpe A, Powles T. Updated European Association of Urology Guidelines regarding adjuvant therapy for renal cell carcinoma. European Urology. May 2017;**71**(5):719-722. DOI: 10.1016/j.eururo.2016.11.034

Section 4

Surgical Approach to Kidney Cancer

Chapter 11

Surgical Strategy for the Management of Renal Cell Carcinoma with Inferior Vena Cava Tumor Thrombus

Cheng Peng, Liangyou Gu, Luojia Yang,
Baojun Wang, Qingbo Huang, Dan Shen,
Songliang Du, Xu Zhang and Xin Ma

Additional information is available at the end of the chapter

http://dx.doi.org/10.5772/intechopen.73294

Abstract

The hallmark of renal cell carcinoma is its biological characteristic of invading the renal vein and/or inferior vena cava (IVC), which occurs in 4–10% of patients. Radical nephrectomy (RN) with tumor thrombectomy is the standard approach for treating such challenging cases. Except tumor thrombus height, several factors can determine the surgical strategy, including the effect of targeted molecular therapy (TMT), invasion of the IVC wall, venous occlusion, establishment of collateral circulation, IVC thromboembolism, and primary tumor location. The surgical strategy for patients with retrohepatic vena cava tumor thrombi depends on the upper extent of the tumor thrombus. In addition, the first porta hepatis and hepatic veins are important anatomical boundaries. Based on previous studies, the effect of pre-surgical TMT is limited. The safety of IVC venography, an imaging modality that can observe congestion of the tumor thrombus and show the collateral circulation, has considerably improved. IVC interruption plays an important role in tumor thrombectomy for patients with invasion of the venous walls, complete occlusion of the vena cava, and the presence of distal thrombus. A series of retrospective and prospective studies are needed to be conducted, which will provide our clinical work with more powerful reference and basis.

Keywords: renal cell carcinoma, tumor thrombus, targeted molecular therapy, inferior vena cava venography, vascular resection, surgical strategy

1. Introduction

The Chinese Cancer Registry Annual Report of 2015 indicates that renal cell carcinoma (RCC) represents approximately 2–3% of new cases of malignant tumor in China annually and the trend in the morbidity of RCC has been increasing [1]. The hallmark of RCC is its biological characteristic of invading the renal vein and/or inferior vena cava (IVC), which occurs in 4–10% of patients [2]. Past clinical decision making mostly adopts conservative treatment, in terms of high morbidity and mortality rates during this kind of procedures. Radical nephrectomy (RN) with tumor thrombectomy is the standard approach for treating such challenging cases [3]. These patients were able to obtain, as literature reported, better long-term survival, and the tumor-specific survival rate is in up to 50% [4–7].

With the development of laparoscopy and robotic technology and the accumulation of practical experience in surgery, we noted that the height of IVC thrombus could not sufficiently guide the choice of surgical strategy, considering that only the thrombus height was assessed. Several factors, such as the effect of neoadjuvant targeted molecular therapy (TMT), invasion of the IVC wall, venous occlusion, establishment of collateral circulation, IVC thromboembolism, and primary tumor location, can determine the surgical strategy. The present comprehensive review describes how those factors influence surgical strategy and patient outcomes.

2. Technological innovations and classifications

RCC tends to invade the renal venous system, forming a thrombus that invades the IVC and even involving the right atrium [2]. RN with tumor thrombectomy is the standard approach for treating such challenging cases. The grading system based on tumor thrombus height was created to determine surgical strategies. As early as 1987, the Mayo Clinic had adopted the "NEVES grading." Level I is defined as a tumor thrombus that is <2 cm apart from the orificium of the renal vein. Level II is defined as a tumor thrombus extending to the IVC >2 cm above the renal vein but below the hepatic veins. Level III is defined as a tumor thrombus that extends above the hepatic veins but below the diaphragm. Level IV is defined as a tumor thrombus located above the diaphragm. Surgical strategies are varied in corresponding levels. Traction of the liver is required in levels I to II. Turning-up the liver, blocking-up vessels located below the diaphragm, and clamping the portal vein are required in levels II to III. The establishment of an extracorporeal circulation is necessary in levels III and IV [8]. In 2002, the University of Miami divided level III tumor thrombus into four categories ulteriorly, which corresponded to diverse surgical strategies [9]. However, the most classic guideline is the "5-level classification" of a tumor thrombus, which was proposed by the Mayo Clinic in 2004 [10]. Idiographic grading standards and surgical strategies are shown in **Table 1**.

Nevertheless, these grading systems are completely based on the experience of open surgery. Since Skinner first reported the open surgery of IVC tumor thrombectomy in 1972 [11], the technique of IVC tumor thrombectomy has been improving continuously. Some scholars had attempted to accomplish these surgeries with laparoscope in 2002 [12, 13]. In 2011, Abaza first reported on robot-assisted IVC tumor thrombus extraction [14]. In recent years, several medical centers have investigated the safety and feasibility of robot-assisted laparoscopic IVC thrombectomy (RAL-IVCTE) [15–18]. Based on the anatomic characteristics of RCC, we

Tumor thrombus level	Definition	Surgical strategy
0	Tumor thrombus is limited to the renal vein	Radical nephrectomy of renal cell carcinoma
I	Tumor thrombus extend into IVC with <2 cm above the renal vein	Tumor thrombus could be extruded to renal vein and then radical nephrectomy
II	Tumor thrombus extends in to IVC >2 cm above the renal vein but below the hepatic veins	The traction of liver is required; blocking-up the section of IVC underneath hepatic vein
III	Tumor thrombus which extends above the hepatic veins but below diaphragm	The mobilization of the liver; vena-venous bypass is required
IV	Tumor thrombus is above diaphragm	Intraoperative extracorporeal circulation is requisite

IVC = inferior vena cava.

Table 1. The grading standards and surgical strategies tumor thrombus.

reported the particular steps of robot-assisted surgery and concluded that RAL-IVCTE is safe, and different sides require different techniques [18]. Gu and colleagues performed a retrospective comparison between open and robotic surgeries in IVC thrombus. The study indicated that level I–II IVC tumor thrombectomy performed with robot-assisted surgery resulted in better perioperative periodical outcomes and analogous oncological outcomes compared with open surgery, marking that such surgery has entered the era of mini-traumatic surgery [19].

3. Surgical procedure

3.1. Anesthesia and patient position

After general anesthesia induction and Foley catheter placement, the patients were positioned in a left lateral decubitus position with a 60–70° bump (**Figure 1A** and **B**). For right RCC, R-IVCTE and RN can be both completed with this position. For left RCC, R-IVCTE can be completed with this position. After R-IVCTE, the placement of patients was converted to a right lateral decubitus position with a 60–70° bump, and left RN was performed.

3.2. Right RN and IVC thrombectomy

The hepatocolic, hepatorenal, and chain ligaments were incised. The liver required to be up-retracted. The anterior layer of the perirenal fascia was opened, the duodenum was dissected and retracted inside, and the IVC was exposed. Full dissection of the IVC, left renal vein, and part of the lumbar vein were required at the location of the tumor thrombus (**Figure 1C**). For level II IVC thrombus, the hepatic short vein, and even right central vein of the adrenal gland, was also clipped and divided (**Figure 1D**). Sequential clamping of the caudal IVC, left renal vein, and cephalic IVC were performed using vessel loops (**Figure 1E**). After the vessels were clamped, the IVC wall was cut, and the thrombus was removed (**Figure 1F**). After the IVC

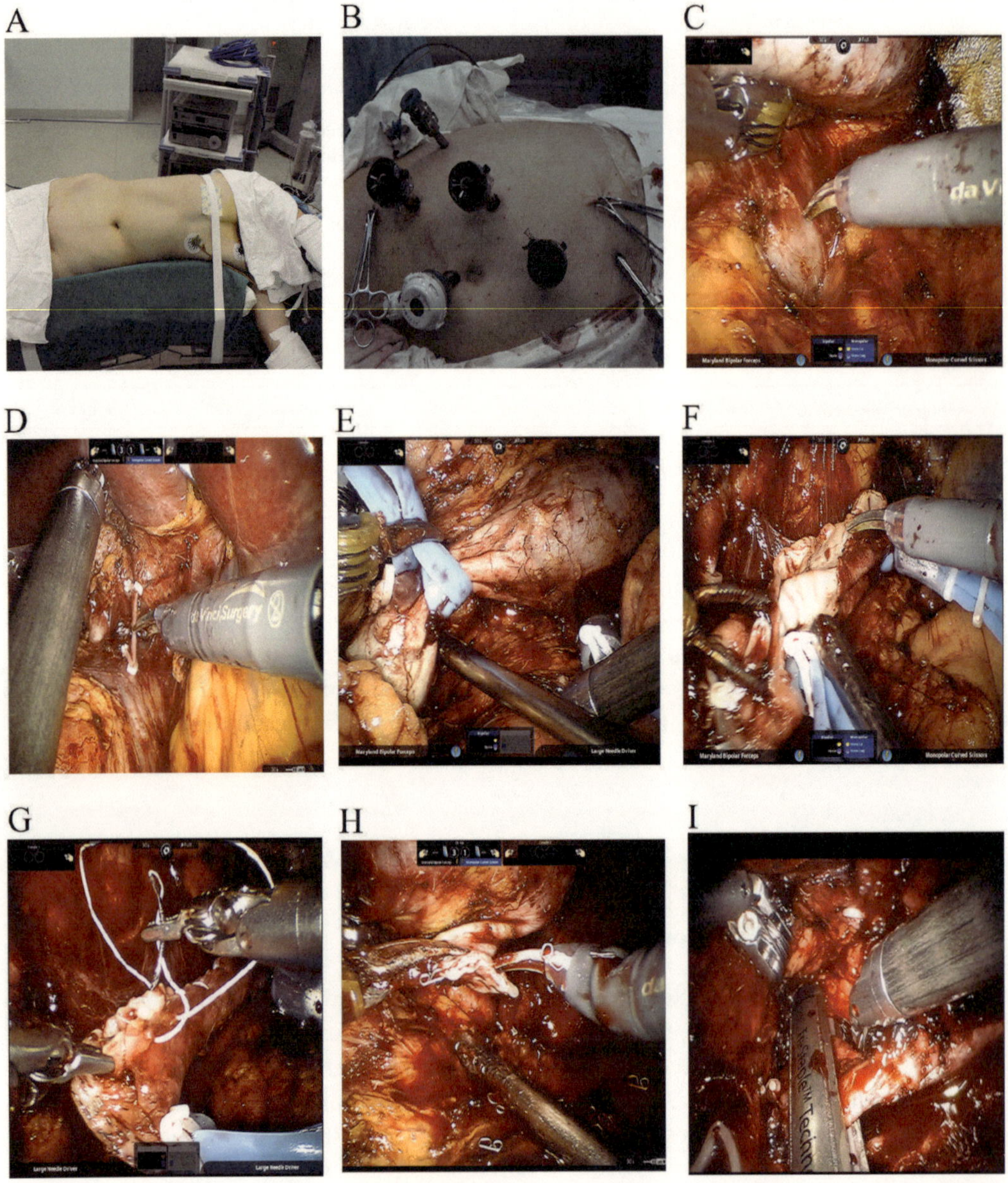

Figure 1. Surgical procedure for robot-assisted laparoscopic inferior vena cava thrombectomy. Patient position and port placement is shown, with three assistant ports used. (A and B). The inferior vena cava and left renal vein was exposed (C). The hepatic short vein was clipped and divided (D). Sequential clamping caudal IVC, left renal vein, and cephalic IVC were performed by vessel loops (E). The thrombus was removed (F). The IVC was closed with 5-0 polypropylene suture (G). Ligation and division of the left renal vein for the left RCC (H). Intraoperative IVC interruption in selected cases (I). IVC = inferior vena cava; RCC = renal cell carcinoma.

lumen was irrigated with heparinized saline, 5-0 polypropylene suture was used to close the IVC (**Figure 1G**). The tourniquets of the caudal IVC, left renal vein, and cephalic IVC were sequentially loosened. In the same position, right RN was completed.

http://dx.doi.org/10.5772/intechopen.73294

3.3. Left RN and IVC thrombectomy

The patient position and port placement were the same as those for the right RCC. However, we suggest that left renal artery embolization must be performed 1–2 h preoperatively. The steps were similar in dissecting the IVC. Subsequently, we ligated and divided the left renal vein, which included the thrombus, with Endo-GIA (**Figure 1H**). The clamping sequence was the caudal IVC first, followed by the right renal artery, right renal vein, and cephalic IVC. After thrombus removal, the placement of the patients was converted to a right lateral decubitus position, with a 60–70°bump, and left RN was performed.

3.4. Surgical technique for retro- or superohepatic IVC thrombus

Recently, the latest research completed by our team investigated the surgical method of robot-assisted retro- or superohepatic vena caval tumor thrombectomy and its influence factor. We found that the surgical strategy for patients with retrohepatic vena caval tumor thrombi depends on the upper extent of the tumor thrombus [20]. In addition, the first porta hepatis and hepatic veins are important anatomical boundaries. The surgical technique was described as follows. If the retrohepatic thrombus was located inferior to the first porta hepatis (**Figure 2A**), some short hepatic veins should be ligated, but the liver should not be mobilized. If the retrohepatic thrombus was located between the first porta hepatis and hepatic veins (**Figure 2B**), mobilization of the right lobe of the liver is an important step. For retrohepatic thrombus located closer or above the second porta hepatis (liver vein) but below the infra-diaphragm (**Figure 2C**), mobilization both the right and left lobes of the liver can facilitate high proximal control of the superohepatic IVC. In addition, the first porta hepatis should be clamped. For superohepatic (level IV) thrombus, thoracoscope-assisted open atriotomy was performed to cut the atrial part of the thrombus, and vena caval tumor thrombectomy was subsequently performed by clamping the superodiaphragm IVC after cardiopulmonary bypass was established (**Table 2**).

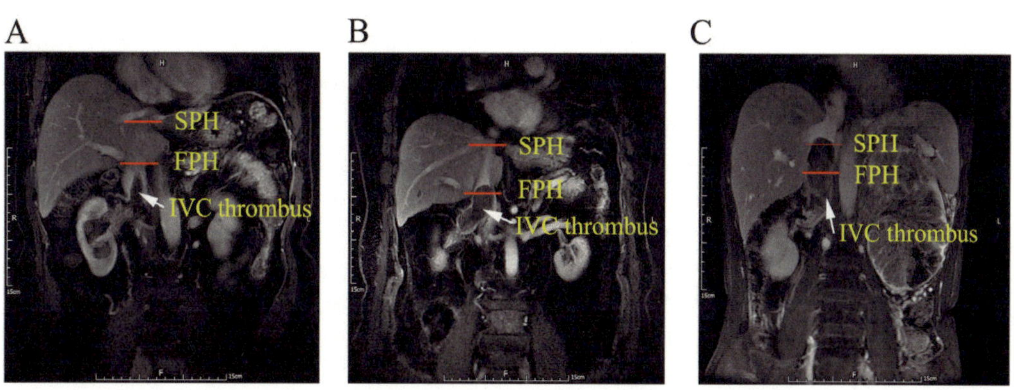

Figure 2. The first porta hepatis and hepatic veins are important anatomical boundaries on representative images of radiography. The retrohepatic thrombus inferior to the first porta hepatis (A). The retrohepatic thrombus inferior to the first porta hepatis (B). The retrohepatic thrombus closer or above the second porta hepatis (liver vein) but blew infra-diaphragm (C). FPH = first porta hepatis; SPH = second porta hepatis; IVC = inferior vena cava tumor.

Location of IVC thrombus	Surgical strategy
Retrohepatic but inferior to the FPH	1. Ligating some SHV 2. Retracting but not liver mobilization
Retrohepatic and between the FPH and hepatic veins	1. Ligating more SHV 2. Mobilizing the right lobe of the liver. 3. Not clamping FPH
Retrohepatic and closer (level II) or above (level III) the second porta hepatis (liver vein) yet infra-diaphragm	1. Mobilizing both the right and left lobes of the liver 2. High proximal control of superohepatic IVC 3. Clamping of the FPH Simultaneously
Superohepatic (level IV)	1. Thoracoscopic atriotomy for cutting atrial part of the thrombus 2. Establishing cardiopulmonary bypass 3. Performing IVC tumor thrombectomy after Clamping the superodiaphragm IVC

IVC = inferior vena cava; SHV = short hepatic vein; FPH = first porta hepatis.

Table 2. Changes of techniques for robot-assisted retro- or supero-hepatic vena caval tumor thrombectomy in our method.

4. Preoperative targeted therapy

Although mini-traumatic surgery has been applied in patients with RCC and tumor thrombus, level III and IV tumor thrombus might have lethal complications, including hemorrhage, thrombotic shedding, etc. The operative mortality and overall morbidity rates of postoperative complication of patients with tumor thrombus patients have been reported up to 5–10% and 38%, respectively [21]. Moreover, as tumor thrombus level advanced, the morbidity of perioperative periodical complications is higher accordingly. With regard to patients with level III and IV tumor thrombus, surgical strategies usually involve thoracotomy, dealing with retro- or superohepatic IVC, and establishing extracorporeal circulation, which can be achieved with the assistance of hepatobiliary and cardiovascular surgeons.

With the targeted molecular therapy (TMT) of rising, TMT has been widely acknowledged as the most effective treatment for advanced RCC, particularly for patients with metastatic RCC. In recent years, targeted drugs have been reported to be applied in preoperative adjunctive therapy for tumor thrombus because of its high success rate in the treatment of advanced RCC [22, 23]. The purpose of administering target drugs was to lessen the height of tumor thrombus or shrink the primary lesions or metastases, which may enhance the safety and feasibility of surgical intervention. The results of some retrospective observations with a small sample present diversities [24–26]. After preoperative TMT, 44–76% of the patients' IVC tumor thrombus had shrinkage in different degrees, with tumor thrombus degradation averaging approximately 20%. Cost and colleagues reported a retrospective outcome from a sample of 25 patients, wherein three patients (12%) had a reduction in the thrombus degradation, and one patient (4%) had an increase [25]. As a result of first-class evidence deficiency, this therapeutic regimen has not been recommended by the guidelines. Thus, further prospective investigations with a larger number of patients are needed to overcome the limitations.

5. Postoperative targeted therapy in patients without metastasis

For patients with non-metastatic RCC and tumor thrombus, the recurrence rate of the tumor is approximately 50% at 3 years preoperatively, despite performing RN [27]. Thus, for these patients, only operative treatment may not be sufficient. Adjuvant IL-2/IFN applied in prophase postoperatively, chemotherapy, and hormone therapy are all negative for high-recurrence risk RCC [28]. Small molecules targeting the vascular endothelial growth factor pathway prolong the progression-free survival of patients with advanced RCC [29, 30]. Based on these, the postoperative application of antiangiogenic medicine for patients with high-relapse risk RCC will play a positive role. Three randomized controlled trials, currently, have reported the outcomes of adopting targeted therapy for high-recurrence risk RCC. Although a study found that sunitinib treatment 1-year postoperatively prolonged relapse-free survival for 1–2 years. Two other studies did not find a survival benefit [31–33]. Therefore, the European Association of Urological Surgeons does not recommend targeted drugs for postoperative RCC with high risk of relapse [34].

For patients with non-metastatic RCC and tumor thrombus, a cohort study designed by the Chinese PLA General Hospital analyzed the efficacy and safety of the postoperative administration of sorafenib or sunitinib. The results showed that no survival benefit was observed for patients with tumor thrombus or IVC tumor thrombus who were administered postoperative adjuvant sorafenib or sunitinib [19].

6. Strategies and indications of IVC venography

Sufficient preoperative imaging data is requisite for successful thrombectomy. However, several problems in the imaging diagnosis of IVC tumor thrombus still exist: Type-B ultrasound has difficulty in accurately diagnosing abnormal changes owing to numerous interferences. Magnetic resonance imaging (MRI) and computed tomography cannot effectively reflect the collateral circulation, and cannot define the degree of occlusion [35]. Therefore, more effective means are required to supplement these three routine examinations. IVC venography can observe the thrombus occlusion through the lateral position, which enables to maximize a rich data of tumor thrombus preoperatively and to make a more accurate surgical plan.

IVC venography has been widely used in the diagnosis of Budd-Chiari syndrome and other diseases [36]. There are still more applications in renal cancer with IVC tumor thrombus yet. Some studies reported that <15% of cases of patients with cancer thrombus would use IVC venography, and some researchers previously thought that the inspection might have false-positive or false-negative results. Meanwhile, there is a risk of emboli-induced pulmonary embolism or tumor embolus exfoliate diffusion. Therefore, performing IVC venography routinely is not recommended [37, 38].

However, with the improvement of radiographic technique in recent years, the safety of IVC venography has been observably improved, and this method may define the formation of collateral circulation of the vena cava and help develop a thrombectomy strategy, which has unique diagnostic advantages. Hence, conducting a new study for IVC venography is necessary. Based on our experience, we speculate that the following patients may be a candidate for IVC venography: (1) RCC with IVC tumor thrombus; (2) clearance of the tumor thrombus plane; (3) definition of the degree of occlusion; (4) existence of collateral circulation, which may affect intraoperative vascular resection; (5) detection of the variation of the communicating branches of vena cava, such as the variation communicating between IVC and vena azygos, which might interfere with the surgery.

7. Indications and strategies of intraoperative IVC interruption

With regard to dealing with the IVC intraoperatively is one of the difficulties of IVC thrombectomy. There necessity of reconstruction after IVC resection is still controversial.

Indications for vena caval interruption include invasion of the venous walls, severe adhesion of the tumor to the vascular endothelium, complete occlusion of the vena cava, and the presence of distal thrombus [21, 39, 40]. In addition, the texture of the cancer thrombus is one of the influencing factors. With regard to preoperative imaging, the IVC in line with the indications of interruption and accompanied by sufficient collateral circulation, meanwhile, without serious cardiac, hepatic, and renal insufficiencies can be completely cut off. IVC venography and intraoperative ultrasound can help determine the disjointed lumina, which enables protection of the established collateral circulation trunk. IVC interruptions include complete and partial vena caval resections with reconstruction. Based on our experience, for right tumors, the height of the tumor thrombus, which is below the secondary hepatic portal, linear cutters are used to successively cut off the proximal, distal, and left renal veins of the tumor thrombus (**Figure 1I**). With regard to right tumor thrombus above the secondary hepatic portal, or left tumor thrombus above the level of the right renal vein and combined with distal thrombus, the vena cava can be resected partially. Methods for right thrombectomy include cutting off the lumina of the IVC below the secondary hepatic portal and reconstructing the lumina of the IVC above the secondary hepatic portal. The left thrombectomy procedure is resecting the lumina of the IVC below the level of the right renal vein and reconstructing the lumina of the IVC above the level of the renal vein.

Meanwhile, IVC interruption is safe and feasible during vena caval thrombectomy [39, 40], and the establishment of collateral circulation can avoid severe hemodynamic disorders. Different strategies of interruption ought to be generated preoperatively based on the height of tumor thrombus, tumor side, degree of vena caval obstruction and invasion, and establishment of collateral circulation.

8. IVC tumor thrombus with thrombosis and treatment recommendations

Vena cava tumor thrombus with thrombosis is common. The prevalence of thrombosis gathered by the Urological Department of Chinese PLA General Hospital is 19.2%. Thrombosis, at the same time, is not found within the renal venous tumor thrombus; all thrombosis occurred in the vena cava tumor thrombus. Among them, vena caval thrombi were all located on the right, the thrombus was located in the distal end of the tumor thrombus, and the distal thrombus could reach the bifurcation of the iliac vessel. Preoperative MRI can help determine the location and length of the thrombus.

Preoperative anticoagulation therapy is recommended for patients with thrombosis, and medication should be administered from the diagnosis of tumor thrombus and thrombus. Low-molecular heparin is recommended for anticoagulation therapy, withdrawing drugs 24 h preoperatively, maintaining the international normalized ratio of 2–3, and anticoagulation therapy is continued for 48 h postoperatively and maintained for 6 months, except for the following: patients with tumor or tumor thrombus who did not undergo complete resection; those with metastasis; needs for systemic treatment; and patients with pulmonary embolism. Pre- and postoperative placement of the vena cava stent is not recommended only if the patient has pulmonary embolism and contraindications of anticoagulation therapy [41, 42]. Preoperative imaging examinations are required for patients with extensive thrombosis at the distal end of the tumor thrombus [43]. IVC interruption is recommended, which prevents embolization caused by thrombus shedding, for patients who meet the indications and possess sufficient collateral circulation.

9. Other developments and issues

Besides the previously mentioned issues, some problems need to be solved in the field of RCC with tumor thrombus. First, whether the tumor thrombus is invading the venous walls is an important issue in diagnosis and treatment process to decide on the preoperative surgical strategies. Furthermore, it may also relate to postoperative survival. However, because the diagnostic criteria of imaging and pathology are currently insufficient, further studies should be conducted.

Second, the survival of patients with RCC and venous thrombus postoperatively was significantly worse than those with localized RCC, particularly in patients with preoperative distant metastases. For IVC tumor thrombus, particularly patients with level III–IV tumor thrombus, the perioperative risk and mortality are higher. At the same time, although some patients completed the radical resection of tumor, survival after surgery is still less than 6 months. Therefore, for patients with high surgical risk or short life expectancy, the necessity for surgery deserves further discussions. The prognosis of patients with RCC and venous tumor thrombus, at present, lacks the preoperative predicting models particularly related to imaging features. The study of preoperative imaging characteristics of tumor thrombus and biological behavior of the tumor and the prognosis of patients may provide some guidance for preoperative choice of treatment.

Augmented reality (AR) is a real-time technology to calculate the location and angle of the camera images and add corresponding images. The goal of this technology is to set the virtual world in the real world and interact with it on screen [44]. Based on individual anatomy, the AR and computer system have been used in partial nephrectomy as a new technology *in vivo* and *in vitro* [45–47]. To overcome the problem of soft tissue and organ shift, Teber and colleagues reported a new navigation approach added to endoscope that was used in laparoscopic partial nephrectomy [47]. The study showed that the new AR tracking system proved to be effective, with a reasonable margin of error and a time to match each other. In addition, combining pre- or intraoperative imaging features with real-time endoscopy will simplify and increase the accuracy of laparoscopic surgery [47]. Thus, AR combined with three-dimensional vision has a great application value in robotic surgery in the future.

Finally, although RCC invades the venous system to form tumor thrombus, the tissue components between the primary tumor of the kidney and the tumor thrombus has a large difference. Meanwhile, heterogeneity exists in primary RCC and tumor thrombus, which may be the reason why primary tumor and tumor thrombus response to preoperative targeted therapy was asynchronous, and drugs among different patients respond differently. Therefore, the research of heterogeneity between primary RCC and venous tumor thrombus may find a more effective therapeutic target and drug for the reduction of tumor thrombus level, which can provide the basis for selecting appropriate patients for neoadjuvant targeted therapy preoperatively.

10. Future perspectives

Open IVCTE is still a standard surgery for RCC with IVC thrombus. With the development of laparoscopy and robotic technology in recent years, the safety and feasibility of robot-assisted laparoscopic IVC thrombectomy have been investigated at several centers. Those successful experiences mark that such surgery tends to enter the era of mini-traumatic surgery. Considering the complexity of the patient and the high complication rates, multidisciplinary cooperation and detailed preoperative assessment will play an important role in surgical decisions in future. Some new or mature techniques will also provide a basis for the surgical strategies, including artificial blood vessel, augmented reality, transesophageal echocardiography, IVC venography, and so on. From a safety perspective, IVCTE is still a challenging technology. Only a hospital with skilled laparoscopic and mature surgical team is recommended. Preoperative TMT is expected to shrink the IVC thrombus and reduce the complexity of the surgery. However, prospective investigations are required in the future.

11. Conclusions

RCC tends to invade the venous system and form venous tumor thrombus in 4–10% of patients. Surgical treatment is the standard therapy for these patients; however, postoperative complications include hemorrhage, thrombotic shedding, and other risks. Because of the huge population and relatively backward treatment concepts, the proportion and number of patients with advanced RCC in China are significantly higher than those in developed countries, such as Europe and the United States. With regard to patients with RCC and tumor thrombus, the strategies for diagnosis and treatment are mostly based on open surgery. Several clinic-related strategies are no longer suitable for current laparoscopic and robot-assisted mini-traumatic surgeries owing to the development of surgical techniques and improvement of auxiliary equipment. With regard to the tumor thrombus, a series of retrospective and prospective studies are needed to be conducted, which would enable to solve some difficulties and issues in the course of diagnosis and treatment, to improve the clinical strategies of diagnosis and treatment of patients with RCC and tumor thrombus ulteriorly, and to provide our clinical work with more powerful reference and basis.

http://dx.doi.org/10.5772/intechopen.73294

Acknowledgements

This work was supported by the People's Republic of China and the National High Technology Research and Development Program ("863" Program) of China: the screening and clinical validation of characteristic protein biomarkers in renal cancer based on a large-scale biobank (2014AA020607).

Conflict of interest

The authors have declared that they have no conflict of interest.

Author details

Cheng Peng†, Liangyou Gu†, Luojia Yang, Baojun Wang, Qingbo Huang, Dan Shen, Songliang Du, Xu Zhang* and Xin Ma*

*Address all correspondence to: urologist@foxmail.com and xzhang@foxmail.com

Department of Urology/State Key Laboratory of Kidney Diseases, Chinese PLA General Hospital/Chinese PLA Medical Academy, Beijing, P. R. China

† These authors contributed equally to this work.

References

[1] Chen WQ et al. Cancer statistics in China. CA: A Cancer Journal for Clinicians. 2016;**66**(2): 115-132

[2] Hatcher PA et al. Surgical management and prognosis of renal cell carcinoma invading the vena cava. Journal of Urology. 2002;**3**(1):37-43

[3] Parra J et al. Oncological outcomes in patients undergoing radical nephrectomy and vena cava thrombectomy for renal cell carcinoma with venous extension: A single-centre experience. European Journal of Surgical Oncology. The Journal of the European Society of Surgical Oncology & the British Association of Surgical Oncology. 2011;**37**(5):422-428

[4] Haferkamp A et al. Renal cell carcinoma with tumor thrombus extension into the vena cava: Prospective long-term followup. Journal of Urology. 2007;**177**(5):1703

[5] Kaushik D et al. The impact of histology on clinicopathologic outcomes for patients with renal cell carcinoma and venous tumor thrombus: A matched cohort analysis. Urology. 2013;**82**(1):136-141

[6] Tilki D et al. Impact of histologic subtype on cancer-specific survival in patients with renal cell carcinoma and tumor thrombus. European Urology. 2014;**66**(3):577-583

[7] Liangyou Gu MD et al. A proposal of post-operative nomogram for overall survival in patients with renal cell carcinoma and venous tumor thrombus. Journal of Surgical Oncology. 2017;**115**(7):905-912

[8] Neves RJ, Zincke H. Surgical treatment of renal cancer with vena cava extension. BJU International. 1987;**59**(5):390

[9] Ciancio G et al. Management of renal cell carcinoma with level III thrombus in the inferior vena cava. Journal of Urology. 2002;**168**(1):1374-1377

[10] Blute ML et al. The Mayo Clinic experience with surgical management, complications and outcome for patients with renal cell carcinoma and venous tumour thrombus. BJU International. 2004;**94**(1):33

[11] Skinner DG, Pfister RF, Colvin R. Extension of renal cell carcinoma into the vena cava: The rationale for aggressive surgical management. Journal of Urology. 1972;**107**(5):711-716

[12] Fergany AF et al. Laparoscopic radical nephrectomy with level II vena caval thrombectomy: Survival porcine study. Journal of Urology. 2002;**168**(6):2629-2631

[13] Sundaram CP et al. Hand assisted laparoscopic radical nephrectomy for renal cell carcinoma with inferior vena caval thrombus. Journal of Urology. 2002;**168**(1):176

[14] Abaza R. Initial series of robotic radical nephrectomy with vena caval tumor thrombectomy. European Urology. 2011;**59**(4):652

[15] Bansal RK et al. Laparoscopic management of advanced renal cell carcinoma with renal vein and inferior vena cava thrombus. Urology. 2014;**83**(4):812-817

[16] Abaza R et al. Multi-institutional experience with robotic nephrectomy with IVC tumor thrombectomy. Journal of Urology. 2015;**195**(4):865-871

[17] Shao P et al. Laparoscopic radical nephrectomy and inferior vena cava thrombectomy in the treatment of renal cell carcinoma. European Urology. 2014;**68**(1):115-122

[18] Wang B et al. Robot-assisted laparoscopic inferior vena cava thrombectomy: Different sides require different techniques. European Urology. 2016;**69**(6):1112

[19] Gu L et al. Postoperative adjuvant sorafenib or sunitinib for nonmetastatic renal cell carcinoma with venous tumor thrombus: A prospective cohort study. Translational Oncology. 2017;**10**(6):949

[20] Wang B et al. Robot-assisted retrohepatic inferior vena cava thrombectomy: First or second porta hepatis as an important boundary landmark. European Urology. 2017;**17**(12):9-18

[21] Psutka SP, Leibovich BC. Management of inferior vena cava tumor thrombus in locally advanced renal cell carcinoma. Therapeutic Advances in Urology. 2015;**7**(4):216

[22] Powles T et al. Safety and efficacy of pazopanib therapy prior to planned nephrectomy in metastatic clear cell renal cancer. JAMA Oncology. 2016;**2**(10):1303

[23] Peters I et al. Neoadjuvant targeted therapy in a primary metastasized renal cell cancer patient leads to down-staging of inferior vena cava thrombus (IVC) enabling a cardio-pulmonary bypass-free tumor nephrectomy: A case report. World Journal of Urology. 2014;**32**(1):245-248

[24] Bigot P et al. Neoadjuvant targeted molecular therapies in patients undergoing nephrectomy and inferior vena cava thrombectomy: Is it useful? World Journal of Urology. 2014;**32**(1):109

[25] Cost NG et al. The impact of targeted molecular therapies on the level of renal cell carcinoma vena caval tumor thrombus. European Urology. 2011;**59**(6):912-918

[26] Fukuda H et al. Limited benefit of targeted molecular therapy for inferior vena cava thrombus associated with renal cell carcinoma. International Journal of Clinical Oncology. 2017;**6**:1-7

[27] Thomas AA et al. Surgical resection of renal cell carcinoma after targeted therapy. Journal of Urology. 2009;**182**(3):881-886

[28] Janowitz T et al. Adjuvant therapy in renal cell carcinoma-past, present, and future. Seminars in Oncology. 2013;**40**(4):482-491

[29] Motzer RJ et al. Sunitinib versus interferon alfa in metastatic renal-cell carcinoma. New England Journal of Medicine. 2007;**356**(2):115

[30] Negrier S. Sorafenib in advanced clear-cell renal-cell carcinoma—NEJM. New England Journal of Medicine. 2007;**356**(2):125

[31] Ravaud A et al. Adjuvant sunitinib in high-risk renal-cell carcinoma after nephrectomy. New England Journal of Medicine. 2016;**375**(23):2246

[32] Haas NB et al. Adjuvant sunitinib or sorafenib for high-risk, non-metastatic renal-cell carcinoma (ECOG-ACRIN E2805): A double-blind, placebo-controlled, randomised, phase 3 trial. Lancet. 2016;**387**(10032):2008-2016

[33] Motzer RJ et al. Randomized phase III trial of adjuvant pazopanib versus placebo after nephrectomy in patients with localized or locally advanced renal cell carcinoma. Journal of Clinical Oncology. 2017;**35**(35):3916-3923

[34] Bex A et al. Updated European Association of Urology guidelines regarding adjuvant therapy for renal cell carcinoma. European Urology. 2017;**71**(5):719-722

[35] Hallscheidt PJ et al. Preoperative staging of renal cell carcinoma with inferior vena cava thrombus using multidetector CT and MRI: Prospective study with histopathological correlation. Journal of Computer Assisted Tomography. 2005;**29**(1):64

[36] Erden A. Budd-Chiari syndrome: A review of imaging findings. European Journal of Radiology. 2007;**61**(1):44-56

[37] Goldfarb DA et al. Magnetic resonance imaging for assessment of vena caval tumor thrombi: A comparative study with venacavography and computerized tomography scanning. Journal of Urology. 1990;**144**(5):1100-1103

[38] Jr SJ et al. Inferior vena caval invasion by renal cell carcinoma: False positive diagnosis by venacavography. Journal of Urology. 1990;**143**(3):464-467

[39] Blute ML et al. Results of inferior vena caval interruption by greenfield filter, ligation or resection during radical nephrectomy and tumor thrombectomy. Journal of Urology. 2007;**178**(2):440

[40] Caso J et al. Circumferential resection of the inferior vena cava for primary and recurrent malignant tumors. The Journal of Urology. 2009;**182**(3):887-893

[41] Lyman GH et al. American Society of Clinical Oncology Guideline: Recommendations for venous thromboembolism prophylaxis and treatment in patients with cancer. Journal of Clinical Oncology. 2007;**25**(34):5490-5505

[42] Woodruff DY et al. The perioperative management of an inferior vena caval tumor thrombus in patients with renal cell carcinoma. Urologic Oncology. 2013;**31**(5):517

[43] Greenfield LJ, Proctor MC. Vena caval filters for the prevention of pulmonary embolism. New England Journal of Medicine. 1998;**338**(7):463-464

[44] Mch H et al. Intraoperative imaging techniques to support complete tumor resection in partial nephrectomy. European Urology Focus. 2017;**3**(3):112-124

[45] Drewniak T et al. Augmented reality for image guided therapy (ARIGT) of kidney tumor during nephron sparing surgery (NSS): animal model and clinical approach. Folia Medica Cracoviensia. 2011;**51**(1-4):77

[46] Su L-M et al. Augmented reality during robot-assisted laparoscopic partial nephrectomy: Toward real-time 3D-CT to stereoscopic video registration. Urology. 2009;**73**(4):896-900

[47] Teber D et al. Augmented reality a new tool to improve surgical accuracy during laparoscopic partial nephrectomy. European Urology. 2009;**56**(2):332

Chapter 12

Focal Therapy in Kidney Cancer

Manar Malki and Amr Emara

Additional information is available at the end of the chapter

http://dx.doi.org/10.5772/intechopen.85819

Abstract

The widespread use of imaging has led to an unprecedented increase in the diagnosis of small renal masses. Incidence rate has increased worldwide and most notable in older population (more than 75 years). There has been an evident revolution in the management of patients with small renal masses. Treatment strategies include active surveillance, partial nephrectomy, radical nephrectomy and focal ablative therapies. Nephron sparing surgery for small renal tumours offers comparable cancer-specific survival and better overall survival when compared to radical nephrectomy. Nevertheless, complications related to extirpative surgery must be taken into consideration. Thermal ablative therapies were developed in an attempt to provide a reproducible treatment option with low risk of complications. Energy based renal ablation therapy offers treatment flexibility, technically less challenging procedure with acceptable oncological outcomes.

Keywords: small renal tumours, kidney cancer, cryoablation, radiofrequency ablation, microwave ablation

1. Introduction

A number of population based studies reported an increase in the incidence of diagnosed small renal masses ≤4 cm [1–2]. Nephron sparing treatment remains the recommended treatment for cT1a renal masses, especially in young healthy patients. Partial nephrectomy carries the same oncological outcomes to radical nephrectomy in treating patients with cT1a renal masses [3–6].

Over the last 2 decades, thermal ablation has emerged as alternative treatment option for the management of patients with renal masses <3 cm in size. Focal ablative treatment is associated with fewer complications and less morbidity. It offers a viable treatment alternative especially in patients whom might not be medically suitable for extirpative surgery.

Focal ablative treatment offers flexibility with treatment's approach. Tumours could be treated laparoscopically, percutaneously or less often open approach. The American Urological Association recommends percutaneous access over surgical approach whenever is feasible [8].

Focal ablative therapy is well tolerated and technically less challenging. Hilar dissection and clamping is not a prerequisite in focal ablative therapy. Renal parenchymal loss is minimal following ablative therapy.

2. Cryoablation

2.1. Mode of action

The therapeutic principle of cryotherapy treatment is selective destruction of tumour cells with minimal injury to the surrounding tissue. Argon and helium are the most commonly used freezing agents. New cryotherapy systems use the Joule-Thomson principle to generate lethal temperature down to −187.5°C. Very low temperature causes direct cellular damage during freezing phase and indirect reperfusion injury during the thawing phase.

Cellular changes secondary to cryotherapy treatment could be summarised in four main stages:

- Formation of extracellular ice crystals leading to hyperosmolar extracellular environment and cells shrinkage
- Formation if intracellular ice crystals causing cells damage
- Metabolic activity stops at −40°C
- Thrombosis and micro capillary damage leading to necrosis

To achieve the described cellular changes, it is essential to achieve the following aspects of the cryotherapy treatment [7].

2.1.1. Target treatment temperature

It is understood that irreversible tissue damage is achieved when cells are exposed to temperature between −20 and −50°C. Different structures of the kidney react differently to freezing temperatures. This behaviour is largely related to collagen and elastin content. Renal collecting system and renal vasculature tolerate cryoablation without real long term injuries. However, renal parenchyma is usually destroyed at −19.4°C. It is recommended to achieve temperature of −40°C or below to ensure killing tumour cells. Thermosensors are usually placed at the edge of the tumour to ensure adequate treatment temperature for the area of interest.

2.1.2. Double freeze-thaw cycle

The standard of care during renal tumour cryoablation is double freeze-thaw cycle. This concept has been established after an experiment on 16 female dogs. More adequate area of treatment and liquefaction was achieved following two freeze-thaw cycles compared to dogs who had only one treatment cycle.

2.1.3. Satisfactory ablation area

It is recommended to perform cryoablation treatment for renal tumours under real-time imaging. The operator should aim for treatment area of 10 mm beyond the margin of tumour to ensure adequate treatment temperatures.

2.1.4. Duration of treatment

The duration of treatment should be balanced against risk of suboptimal treatment with short cycles or risk of tissue fracture and bleeding with long treatment. The optimal duration of freezing cycles is not well described in the literature. Two active cycles with initial freeze cycle of 8–10 min and a second freeze cycle of 6–8 min is considered the optimal.

2.2. Guidelines

The European Association of Urology guidelines state that, due to lack of high quality data, no recommendation can be made on cryoablation and radiofrequency ablation [9]. The American Urological Association (AUA) recently released its guidelines for management of patients diagnosed with small renal masses [8]. Focal ablative therapy should be offered as an option rather than standard treatment in high risk patients [8, 9].

Cryotherapy treatment offers a viable alternative to surgery especially in following clinical circumstances:

- Patients with multiple comorbidities
- Elderly patients
- Patients with multiple/bilateral renal tumours
- Patients with impaired renal function

Cryotherapy is usually recommended for small renal tumours (<3 cm in size). Cystic renal masses and hilar masses represent relative contraindications for cryotherapy treatment. Untreated coagulopathy is an absolute contraindication for cryotherapy treatment.

2.3. Modality of treatment

Cryotherapy treatment can be delivered percutaneously, laparoscopically or less often with open surgical approach.

Laparoscopic mobilisation of the kidney and accurate dissection of the tumour might provide an excellent exposure of the tumour. It allows treating anteriorly located tumours safely, thus avoiding injury to surrounding structures. Laparoscopic approach allows real time monitoring of ice-ball formation in cryotherapy treatment and confirmation of probes positioning.

Location of the tumour and surgical expertise would normally mandate the approach of laparoscopic cryoablation (transperitoneal or retroperitoneal). Standard three ports technique is used. Gerota fascia is incised. The kidney is mobilised and tumour is identified. The overlaying and surrounding fat might be excised to allow accurate assessment during the treatment. Histological confirmation with 18-gauge biopsy needle is advocated if no prior biopsies have been taken.

Cryoprobes are inserted percutaneously under direct vision. Laparoscopic ultrasonography is used to confirm the location of the probes and the margins of the tumour. Treatment is delivered with double freeze-thaw cycle. Cryoprobes are removed. Low pressure check is performed to check for any post-interventional bleeding.

Percutaneous cryotherapy can be performed as an outpatient procedure under conscious sedation or general anaesthesia. It might offer an advantage to laparoscopic approach especially patients requiring multiple procedures as in Von Hippel-Lindau (VHL) disease. The American Urological Association (AUA) recommends a renal biopsy prior to ablation to provide pathological diagnosis and minimise over treatment of benign conditions [8].

Following anaesthetic induction patient is positioned in the prone or flank position. Lesion is characterised following the administration of intravenous contrast depending on imaging technique (iodinated or gadolinium contrast). Tumour is localised with finder needle (20-gauge). A representative biopsy is taken with 18-gauge Try-Cut core biopsy needle under CT/MRI guidance. Positioning of cryoprobes and prongs are confirmed with repeat imaging. Cryotherapy treatment is carried out achieving the standard of care principles. Once treatment is completed; cryoprobes are removed. Post treatment imaging is performed to check treatment adequacy and evaluate for potential bleeding.

2.4. Follow-up and oncological outcomes

The absence of histological evidence for treatment success remains an inherent criticism for focal ablative therapy. The interpretation of a routine biopsy following cryotherapy treatment is highly controversial. Therefore, the determination of treatment success is solely reliant on radiological evaluation. Radiological evaluation of treatment success is interpreted by complete loss of contrast enactment of follow-up CT or MRI scan. Treated renal lesion is expected to shrink by >50% in size within the first year following cryotherapy treatment. Most of urological institutions recommend first CT scan or MRI scan with 3–6 months post cryotherapy treatment. Currently, there is no consensus on surveillance after RCC treatment. A six monthly CT scan is usually recommended within the first year of follow-up. Annual CT scan is recommended thereafter if favourable response to treatment has been established.

Selective post cryotherapy treatment biopsy should be sought in the following situations:

- If a lesion demonstrates persistent contrast enhancement following treatment (Incomplete treatment).
- If a lesion demonstrates enlargement following cryotherapy treatment and or new contrast enhancement (Local tumour recurrence or progression).

2.5. Treatment outcomes

Currently, there are no RCTs comparing treatment outcomes of PN with focal ablative therapies for small renal masses. The CONSERVE trial was a feasibility multicentre RCT attempted to compare PN with CA and RFA. The study was however unable to recruit the desired number of patients [10].

Rai and colleagues [11] performed recent meta-analysis in which they compared outcomes of partial nephrectomy and cryoablation. This study highlighted significantly lower recurrences rates following RAPN. The overall recurrence rates in the CA cohort were 11.5% compared with 0% in the RAPN cohort. Similar results were concluded from met analysis of 13 studies comparing laparoscopic and RAPN with LCA; 9.4 vs. 0.4% respectively [12]. The analysis suggested LCA might be associated with improved peri-operative outcomes. These meta-analyses found that impact on oncological survival and mortality outcomes was profound. These results should be carefully evaluated, as it might reflect the short oncological follow-up [11, 12]. A retrospective review of more than 800 patients reviewed the intermediate oncological outcomes of LCA. The 5 and 10 year disease survival was reported at 90.4 and 80.0% respectively; however the 5- and 10-year overall survival in the study was 83.2 and 64.4% [13].

2.6. Complications

Cryotherapy is relatively safe procedure with low risk profile. Percutaneous and laparoscopic cryotherapy have similar overall complication rates [14, 15]. As one might expect, the length of in hospital stay following percutaneous cryoablation is shorter when compared to laparoscopic cryoablation [15, 16]. A recent systematic review reported the overall rates of complications following cryoablation therapy range from 7.8 to 20%. Zargar and colleagues [17] found that complications rate for percutaneous cryoablation are lower than laparoscopic cryoablation (2.8–12.9% vs. 15–20% respectively). The incidence of major urological complications following cryotherapy is 4.9% (3.3–7.4%).

Post-operative haemorrhage is the common reported complication. Other reported complications are ureteric injury and obstruction, peri-renal abscess and haematuria. Other minor non-urological complications include pain and paraesthesia at the probe site, urinary tract infections and self-limited haematuria. Reintervention following cryoablation therapy is reported at 2.6%.

3. High temperature ablative techniques

Cancer cells are very sensitive to both very high and low temperature. Radiofrequency and microwave energies use the concept of high temperature (above 55°C). Thermal ablation causes denaturation of cellular proteins and vascular necrosis of tumour cells resulting in instantaneous cellular death.

3.1. Radiofrequency ablation

3.1.1. Mode of action

Electric current passes through radiofrequency ablation (RFA) probe/electrode into tumour creating closed loop circuit with a generator and grounding pads. The current triggers disruption of intracellular ions and friction between molecules producing heat. The electromagnetic field generates high temperature typically above 55°C. The generated heat results in cytotoxic effect and instantaneous cell death occurring with temperature reaching 60°C [18].

3.1.2. Technique

Small renal masses (≤3 cm) can be treated with single cycle of RFA. However, larger tumours (up to 5 cm) might be suitable for treatment using overlapping cycles technique. RFA achieves excellent results in treating exophytic and endophytic tumours.

RFA is carried out under general anaesthetic or conscious sedation. Different types of RFA electrodes could be used including; single tip, multi-tined expandable electrodes, or a cluster tip electrode. RFA electrodes are inserted into the tumour under CT/MRI or ultrasound guidance. Hydro-dissection can be used if the tumour is adjacent to bowel segment.

Once electrodes are positioned; a 12 min cycle is delivered. Some RFA systems use internal cooled electrodes to avoid adjacent tissue carbonization. This method might have an impact on heat distribution to distant area of the tumour and subsequently might affect the efficacy of treatment [19, 20].

3.2. Microwave ablation

3.2.1. Mode of action

Microwave ablation uses the same concept of thermal ablation as RFA technique. Thermal ablation results in coagulative necrosis of tumour cells. Microwave ablation uses different energy source. It produces an electromagnetic spectrum with frequency of 900–2450 MHz. The oscillating microwave field causes polarisation of molecules resulting in increased kinetic energy producing heat.

Microwave ablation has several advantages over radiofrequency ablation. It is possible to treat larger tumours without the need of overlapping treatments. Microwave ablation does not cause charring effect. Skin pads are not required during microwave ablation treatment; therefore the risk of skin burns is minimal.

3.2.2. Technique

Two microwave antennae are inserted under CT or ultrasound guidance. A fibre-optic thermal sensor inserted at the periphery of the tumour to provide continuous temperature monitoring. It is recommended to delivers 3 cycles achieving temperature of 60°C. Each cycle lasts for 20 min [21].

3.3. Possible side effects of high thermal ablative techniques

- Heat sink effect: kidney is well perfused organ. this may result in unequal distribution of the heat particularly close to the larger vessels.
- Thermal injury to neighbouring structures such as bowels, ureter, genitofemoral nerve and psoas major muscle.
- Post-ablation syndrome: the syndrome is usually self-limiting. Patients might suffer symptoms of low-grade fever (37.5–38.5°C), delayed pain, nausea, vomiting, malaise, and myalgia.
- Haematuria and peri-nephric haematoma are usually self-limiting.
- Hyper adrenal crisis is very rare. This might be secondary to adrenal thermal injury.
- Skin burns (mainly with radio-frequency ablation).
- Calyceocutaneous fistulae.
- Infection and abscess formation.
- Acute tubular necrosis and decreases overall renal function [22].

3.4. Oncological efficacy

Few studies have evaluated the short and intermediate oncological outcomes. The technical success rate has been reported to be 95.5–98.5%. The average need for repeat treatment is thought to be around 3%. Small renal tumours (<3 cm) and exophytic location were independent factors for successful treatment. The overall 5 year survival rate was reported between 65–85% and cancer specific survival rate of 88–97.9% [23–25].

3.5. Monitoring and follow up

Most urological institutions recommend contrast enhanced CT scan at 3 months to evaluate treatment success. Follow-up CT scan is suggested every 6 months for the first 2 years. Annual CT scan is suggested thereafter for a period up to 7 years.

4. Investigational and experimental treatments

4.1. Laser interstitial thermal therapy (LITT)

This treatment modality is currently being evaluated for treatment of solid tumours including brain, pancreatic, breast, thyroid and prostate cancer. LITT utilizes image guided low voltage laser probes to deliver heat and destroy target tissue. Optical fibres are inserted directly to the target tissue. Laser light delivers heat that is converted to heat. The emitted light energy from laser fibres is absorbed and converted to heat. This would result in thermal destruction of the cancer cells [26]. Neodymium: yttrium-aluminium-garnet (Nd:YAG) laser has been used to treat small renal tumours. All reports are based on small number of treated patients with short follow up [27, 28]. LITT remains an experimental treatment.

4.2. Extracorporeal high-intensity focused ultrasonography (HIFU)

The therapeutic use of the ultrasound to treat cancer was established in the 1970s. The mechanism of HIFU involves mechanical and thermal effects. Some of the acoustic wave is converted to heat once absorbed by the tissue. The thermal phenomenon causes cell death by coagulation necrosis once tissue temperature exceeded the 65°C. The mechanical effect causes micro-streaming, cavitation and radiation force [29].

HIFU offers completely trackless non-invasive ablative technology. Treatment session can be lengthy. Several studies reported incomplete treatment when renal tumours were excised following HIFU treatment. Skin burns were reported up to 10% of the patients. Respiratory movement and acoustic interference could impede on delivering treatment accurately. Other limitations to HIFU treatment include limited focal zone depth and inability to monitor treatment progression in real life [30–32]. Recent studies investigated the role of magnetic resonance-guided high intensity focused ultrasound. The results are promising, however it remains experimental [33, 34].

Laparoscopic HIFU has recently evolved to overcome the challenges related to respiratory movements, targeting tumours and acoustic interference.

HIFU is considered to be experimental treatment. It could be considered in some selected cases.

5. Conclusion

In conclusion, ablative therapies have emerged as an alternative option to extirpative surgical treatment. Percutaneous focal ablative therapies represent a valid treatment option especially for high risk patients. Randomised controlled trials are needed to compare treatment outcomes of PN with focal ablative therapies for small renal masses.

Conflict of interest

None declared.

Notes/thanks/other declarations

None.

http://dx.doi.org/10.5772/intechopen.85819

Author details

Manar Malki[1]* and Amr Emara[2]

*Address all correspondence to: manar.malki@nhs.net

1 Frimley Park Hospital, Frimley, UK

2 Basingstoke and North Hampshire Hospital, Basingstoke, UK

References

[1] Ries LAG, Melbert D, Krapcho M, Stinchcomb DG, Howlader N, Horner MJ, et al. editors. SEER Cancer Statistics Review, 1975-2005. Bethesda, MD: National Cancer Institute; 2008

[2] Hollingsworth JM, Miller DC, Daignault S, et al. Rising incidence of small renal masses: A need to reassess treatment effect. Journal of the National Cancer Institute. 2006;**98**:1331

[3] Butler BP, Novick AC, Miller DP, et al. Management of small unilateral renal cell carcinomas: Radical versus nephronsparing surgery. Urology. 1995;**45**:34

[4] Gratzke C, Seitz M, Bayrle F, et al. Quality of life and perioperative outcomes after retroperitoneoscopic radical nephrectomy (RN), open RN and nephron-sparing surgery in patients with renal cell carcinoma. BJU International. 2009;**104**:470

[5] D'Armiento M, Damiano R, Feleppa B, et al. Elective conservative surgery for renal carcinoma versus radical nephrectomy: A prospective study. British Journal of Urology. 1997;**79**:15

[6] Van Poppel H, Da Pozzo L, Albrecht W, et al. A prospective, randomised EORTC intergroup phase 3 study comparing the oncologic outcome of elective nephron-sparing surgery and radical nephrectomy for low-stage renal cell carcinoma. European Urology. 2011;**59**:543

[7] White WM, Kaouk J. Ablative therapy for renal tumours. In: Walsh PC, Retik AB, Stamey TA, Vaughan ED, editors. Campbell's Urology. 10th ed. Philadephia, PA: WB Saunders Co; 2012

[8] Campbell S, Uzzo RG, Allaf ME, et al. Renal mass and localized renal cancer: AUA guideline. The Journal of Urology. 2017;**198**(3):520-529

[9] Ljungberg B, Albiges L, Bensalah K, et al. EAU Guidelines on Renal Cell Carcinoma. 2018. Available from: https://uroweb.org/wp-content/uploads/EAU-RCC-Guidelines-2018-large-text.pdf

[10] A feasibility study for a multicentre randomised controlled trial to compare Surgery (partial nephrectomy) with needle ablation techniques (radiofrequency ablation/

cryotherapy) for the treatment of people with small renal masses (4 cm), CONSERVE study. Available from: http://www.isrctn.com/ISRCTN23852951

[11] Rai BP, Jones P, Tait C, et al. Is cryotherapy a genuine rival to robotic-assisted partial nephrectomy in the management of suspected renal malignancy? A systematic review and meta-analysis. Urology. 2018;**118**:6-11

[12] Klatte T, Shariat SF, Remzi M. Systematic review and meta-analysis of perioperative and oncologic outcomes of laparoscopic cryoablation versus laparoscopic partial nephrectomy for the treatment of small renal tumours. The Journal of Urology. 2014;**191**(5):1209-1217

[13] Nielsen TK, Lagerveld BW, Keeley F, et al. Oncologic outcomes and complication rates after laparoscopic-assisted cryoablation: A European registry for renal cryoablation (EuRECA) multi-institutional study. BJU International. 2017;**119**(3):390-395

[14] Sisul DM, Liss MA, Palazzi KL, et al. RENAL nephrometry score is associated with complications after renal cryoablation: A multicenter analysis. Urology. 2013;**81**(4):775-780

[15] Kim EH, Tanagho YS, Bhayani SB, et al. Outcomes of laparoscopic and percutaneous cryoablation for renal masses. The Journal of Urology. 2013;**189**:e492

[16] Goyal J, Verma P, Sidana A, et al. Single-center comparative oncologic outcomes of surgical and percutaneous cryoablation for treatment of renal tumors. Journal of Endourology. 2012;**26**:1413

[17] Zargar H, Atwell TD, Cadeddu JA, de la Rosette JJ, et al. Cryoablation for small renal masses: Selection criteria, complications, and functional and oncologic results. European Urology. 2016;**69**:116

[18] Hong K, Georgiades C. Radiofrequency ablation: Mechanism of action and devices. Journal of Vascular and Interventional Radiology. 2010;**21**(8, Suppl):S179-S186

[19] Gunn AJ, Gervais DA. Percutaneous ablation of the small renal mass—Techniques and outcomes. Seminars in Interventional Radiology. 2014;**31**(1):33-34

[20] McCarthy CJ, Gervais DA. Decision making: Thermal ablation options for small renal masses. Seminars in Interventional Radiology. 2017;**34**(2):167-175

[21] Hinshaw JL, Lubner MG, Ziemlewicz TJ, et al. Percutaneous tumor ablation tools: Microwave, radiofrequency, or cryoablation—What should you use and why? Radiographics. 2014;**34**(5):1344-1362

[22] Wah TM, Irving HC, Gregory W, et al. Radiofrequency ablation (RFA) of renal cell carcinoma (RCC): Experience in 200 tumours. BJU International. 2014;**113**:416-428

[23] Tracy CR, Raman JD, Donnally C, et al. Durable oncologic outcomes after radiofrequency ablation: Experience from treating 243 small renal masses over 7.5 years. Cancer. 2010;**116**:3135-3142

[24] Zagoria RJ, Pettus JA, Rogers M, et al. Long-term outcomes after percutaneous radiofrequency ablation for renal cell carcinoma. Urology. 2011;**77**:1393-1397

[25] Aron M, Kamoi K, Haber GP et al. Laparoscopic renal cryoablation: long-term oncologic outcomes with minimum 5 year follow up. The Journal of Urology. 2008;179(Suppl): 209-210

[26] Stafford RJ, Fuentes D, Elliott AA, et al. Laser-induced thermal therapy for tumor ablation. Critical Reviews in Biomedical Engineering. 2010;**38**(1):79-100

[27] Gettman MT, Lotan Y, Lindberg G, et al. Laparoscopic interstitial laser coagulation of renal tissue with and without hilar occlusion in the porcine model. Journal of Endourology. 2002;**16**(8):565-570

[28] Williams JC, Swischuk PN, Morrison PM, et al. Laser-induced thermotherapy of renal cell carcinoma in man: Dosimetry, ultrasound, and histopathologic correlation. Proceedings of SPIE. Vol. 3907. 2000. pp. 230-239

[29] Vallancien G, Chartier-Kastler E, Harouni M, et al. Focused extracorporeal pyrotherapy: Experimental study and feasibility in man. Seminars in Urology. 1999;**11**(1):7-9

[30] Kohrmann KU, Michel MS, Gaa J, et al. High intensity focused ultrasound as noninvasive therapy for multilocal renal cell carcinoma: Case study and review of the literature. The Journal of Urology. 2002;**167**(6):2397-2403

[31] Marberger M, Schatzl G, Cranston D, et al. Extracorporeal ablation of renal tumours with high-intensity focused ultrasound. BJU International. 2005;**95**(Suppl 2):52

[32] Hacker A, Michel MS, Marlinghaus E, et al. Extracorporeally induced ablation of renal tissue by high-intensity focused ultrasound. BJU International. 2006;**97**(4):779-785

[33] de Senneville BD, Moonen C, Ries M. MRI-guided HIFU methods for the ablation of liver and renal cancers. Advances in Experimental Medicine and Biology. 2016;**880**:43-63

[34] van Breugel JMM, de Greef M, Wijlemans JW. Thermal ablation of a confluent lesion in the porcine kidney with a clinically available MR-HIFU system. Physics in Medicine and Biology. 2017;**62**(13):5312-5326

Chapter 13

Robotic Surgery and Successful Set-Up: A Stepwise Approach

Christopher J. Anderson and Hiten R.H. Patel

Additional information is available at the end of the chapter

http://dx.doi.org/10.5772/intechopen.86026

Abstract

Robot purchase, implementation, and sustainability require a number of key challenges to overcome. We provide our experience of managing a potentially daunting task, summarizing the key steps to help deliver such an exciting project. We will take you through team approach options for purchase and safe implementation in the current financial climate.

Keywords: robotics, financial planning, sustainability, patient safety, implementation, training

1. Introduction

Minimally invasive surgery has well-established advantages: shorter length of hospital stay, markedly reduced postoperative pain, fast return to preoperative state of activity, lowered postoperative ileus, and a preservation of immune function [1]. Importantly, laparoscopic urology has been superseded by the robot-assisted laparoscopic surgery [2]. The main reasons for this significant change from pure laparoscopic urology to robot-assisted laparoscopy are mainly surgeon factors such as shorter learning curve and less surgeon fatigue [2]. In our opinion, the patient factors as described above are similar.

Importantly, robotic assistance allows all surgeons (open and minimally invasive) to perform advanced laparoscopic surgery. Dual video cameras provide an adjustable magnification within the surgical field, which is 3D. Robotic instruments allow 6 degrees of freedom of movement, which is similar to the human hand. Laparoscopic instruments allow 4 degrees of freedom of movement. The robot removes surgeon tremor, by motion scaling, which allows incredible dexterity and precision during the surgery.

Allowing robotic technologies into the operating room can provide significant advantages. For example, the robot can provide a precise translation of the surgeon hand movements, through the robotic instruments during the actual surgery. Importantly, the robot facilitates surgeons without advanced laparoscopic skills to perform complex surgeries with short/limited training. In addition, the robotic technology has increased the types of surgeries undertaken. The endo-wristed tools with motion scaling (avoids tremor) and 3D zoomed operative fields promote the ability of the surgeon to undertake microdissection and intra-abdominal suturing with great accuracy [3].

The rapid rise of robotic technologies has allowed more complex reconstructive surgeries to be performed even in children [4]. Instruments such as 3–5 mm trocars have aided robotic surgery in children. Importantly, single-port and multi-arm (non-central) platforms are becoming commercially accessible.

As this advancement continues, the financial and clinical issues surrounding the employment of a robotic system within any hospital require planning. This planning starts from identifying the finances (business planning) through to purchase, and identifying key members of the team who will provide training to the team as a whole and oversee clinical and financial governance of the system.

2. Clinical to hospital administration collaboration

Surgical outcomes are determined by high levels of competence of the team and optimal team working. Therefore, surgeons rely on the team. Robotic surgery is no exception, particularly as the surgeon works at a console and therefore relies on the team which includes the bedside assistant who performs important tasks at the patient bedside. Educating the robotic (or other) operating room team of nurses, anesthesia staff, and bedside assistant is crucial for patient outcome success. It is crucial that the team and team leader communicate with other staff and mentors to provide the support and guidance needed during the training stage.

Administrators and surgeons must work together to define the needs of the hospital, when developing a robotic programme. A surgeon with administrator can develop a programme which is often more patient-centric and deployable. Interestingly, robotic use can improve patient referrals, which is often the reason the administrators are supportive. The best situation is for the surgical teams and administrators to co-plan and co-deliver robotics within a hospital or strategic health partnership.

In a teaching hospital, teams generally work cohesively, allowing intellectual debate, particularly around new technologies such as robotics. They usually find funding through academic pathways or sizeable donors. This is important for training the next generation of surgeons, and improving our understanding of where robotic surgery can take us. As robotics develop in this way through research and resident training, these programmes can be delivered into more peripheral centres. Once this occurs, a close "hub-and-spoke" relationship between the teaching centre and the peripheral hospital is important if the latter wishes to improve robotic programmes and assist with the financial planning of such programmes.

Business plan and timeline development require robust data collection, concerning business planning. A reduction in length of stay with faster recovery has cost benefits as well as an increase in patient volume from increased referrals. Part of this calculation will of course be the recurring costs (disposables, instruments, maintenance) of robotics in addition to the capital outlay. As with any negotiation, one should show non-clinical administrators that robotics will benefit patient care and improve hospital income, plus reputation.

3. Financial implications

Currently, the average cost of the da Vinci robotic system is $1.4–1.9 million, and the annual maintenance is approximately $240,000. Link et al. [5] suggest an increase in robotic surgery volume which can counter for the depreciation and maintenance costs. They showed that robotic pyeloplasty (RLP) is more expensive than laparoscopic pyeloplasty, if performed by a surgeon competent in intracorporeal suturing. The study also concluded that the combined longer operative time and substantial expense for robot depreciation and consumables made RLP a much more expensive procedure (2.7 times more than laparoscopic pyeloplasty). Importantly, increasing the number of robotic procedures can neutralize the cost imbalance, such as performing 10 robotic prostate surgeries per week (cost neutral compared to open prostate surgery) [6].

These debates are important to be aware of, but the main issues are the steep learning curve for the average surgeon using pure laparoscopy and thus greater risk to the patient. The robotic platform offers a truncated learning curve, and therefore the financial burden becomes more acceptable. A further point is that, as the robotic surgeons gain more experience, the robotic

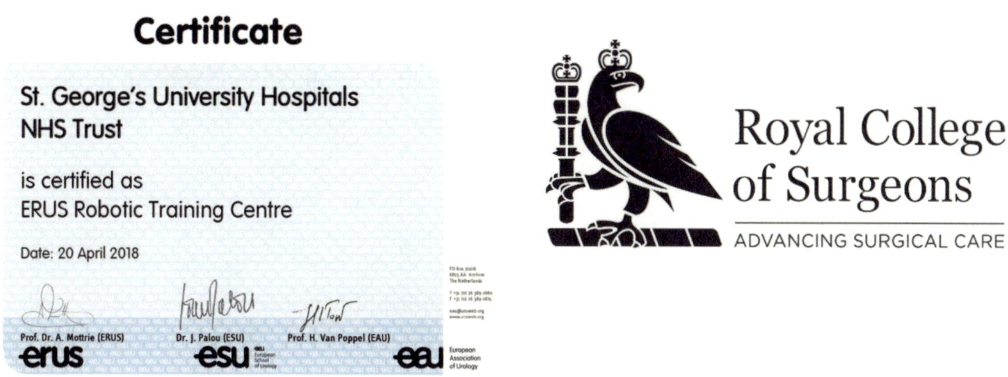
Certificate
St. George's University Hospitals
NHS Trust
is certified as
ERUS Robotic Training Centre
Date: 20 April 2018
Prof. Dr. A. Mottrie (ERUS)
Dr. J. Palou (ESU)
Prof. H. Van Poppel (EAU)
erus
esu
eau
European Association of Urology
Royal College
of Surgeons
ADVANCING SURGICAL CARE

Figure 1. Robotic Urology Surgery Training Centre Accreditation (European) and Royal College of Surgeons of England.

operative times diminish considerably and in many institutions may be quicker than the equivalent operation performed laparoscopically. The economic arguments are not therefore constant or static but an ever-changing field.

Importantly, once the hospital has agreed that a budget is available and a sensible financial plan is in place, the early adopters of the robotic technology need to be identified and offered a curriculum-based training programme [7] (**Figure 1**).

4. Robotic surgeon training

Robot-assisted surgery is rapidly gaining popularity among urologists and is becoming subspecialised. Generally the three main categories that need fellowship or hands-on training are prostatectomy, partial nephrectomy, and radical cystectomy. It is not acceptable to begin robotic surgery without the appropriate training [7]. Currently, robot-assisted radical prostatectomy is the most commonly performed robotic procedure worldwide. There is mounting evidence that the robot assistance provides significant benefits to the patient and surgeon, especially shortening operating time and surgeon fatigue [2]. There has been a major shift of treatment of prostate cancer by surgery in wealthier countries from open to a laparoscopic approach, and now robotic. A modern comparison is with radical nephrectomy in the 1990s.

The learning curve to deliver laparoscopic radical prostatectomy (LRP) is estimated at 40–60 cases with skilled surgeons and 80–100 cases, with inexperienced surgeons. The robot shortens the prostatectomy learning curve for all surgeons, particularly experienced open prostatectomists. Interestingly, a surgeon skilled in open surgery was able to transfer his open skills to robotic surgery in 8–12 cases [8]. However, currently we recommend fellowship training such as the ERUS-approved programmes (**Figure 1**).

A fellowship-trained laparoscopic surgeon has a similar, short learning curve for robotic prostatectomy compared to an experienced open surgeon. The data showed a safe and reproducible surgery, interestingly even during the learning curve. Importantly, the outcomes were the same for early robotic surgery and a large cohort of open prostate surgery [8]. There was an emphasis on having a good mentor, experienced in robotics being present during the initiation of the programme.

5. Animal model and training

Animal model training in robotics, prior to human application, is effective. Most of all robotic surgeries were initially tested in an animal model. Sung et al. [9] in 1995 performed a porcine robotic pyeloplasty. As the learning curve associated with surgical robotic use is unknown, a safe and modular training programme in an animal model would result in measurable improvement in robotic surgical skills.

http://dx.doi.org/10.5772/intechopen.86026

Robotic (ZEUS; Computer Motion) and laparoscopic instrument learning curves were compared within inanimate models and showed a greater learning curve with robotics [10]. Another animal study showed that multiple surgical disciplines in a "near hospital operating room" environment with same-member healthcare teams improved their average set-up times by 30%, each time they prepared the robot [11]. In addition, the console operators improved their operation times by over 20% each time they practiced. They showed that in-house training saved them significant monies (approximately $52,895) and improved operative and set-up times by 40–50%.

6. Training the robotic surgical team

Curiosity and commitment to robotics are helpful when motivating a team. However, it helps to have the support and enthusiasm of your hospital, including the management through your clinical colleagues and team leaders (**Figure 2**).

The primary group to get on board are the surgeons committed to robotics. Importantly, robotic surgery programmes develop purposefully and often slowly. Each step requires audit cycles, critically analysing the robotic team performance and not simply the surgeon. Team leaders in the operating room should be empowered to feedback performance values at each step of the process for safe and effective outcomes. Once the team engages in this process, it is the most rewarding experience.

Training within a team is an early and crucial step. Using a standard learning tool such as an objective-based curriculum, which is visual and live, allows for the best results. This should allow foundation building from experiences, in a stepwise manner (modular). For the more specialized team member requiring understanding of specific operative nuances, a more specialized skill set is needed [12].

The generic robotic team should begin the process by understanding the set-up, draping, and both electrical and mechanical troubleshooting. These basic steps would suffice to then return

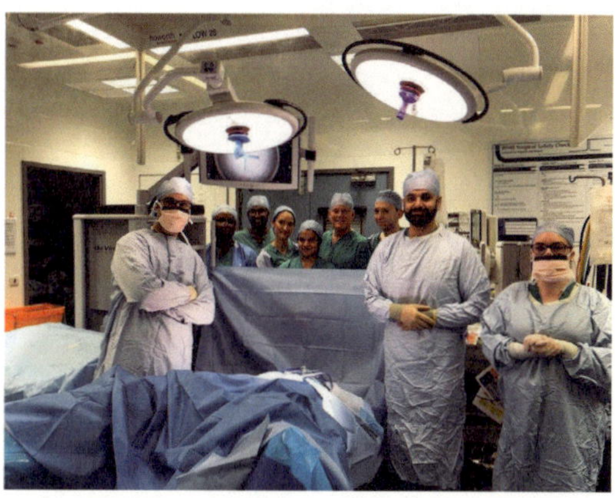

Figure 2. A happy and supportive robotic team is essential!

to the host hospital and apply the knowledge to the local robot surgery. Most teams learn the advanced objectives in their host institution.

Training programmes are now cross-specialty [13], with real surgery observation, didactic sessions, video-based modular training, dry laboratories, and cadaveric training access [14].

Non-technical skills are vitally important to develop as part of the team training programme [15]. These human factors are crucial to running a seamless patient journey through a robotic-assisted surgery (or any other surgery).

7. Resident training

While surgical educators in resident training centres in which robotic surgery has been adopted are still charged with the responsibility of teaching residents the surgical management (see **Figure 3a** and **b**), they now face a new challenge in how to teach a resident to assist at and perform a surgery when not physically standing at the operating room table [16].

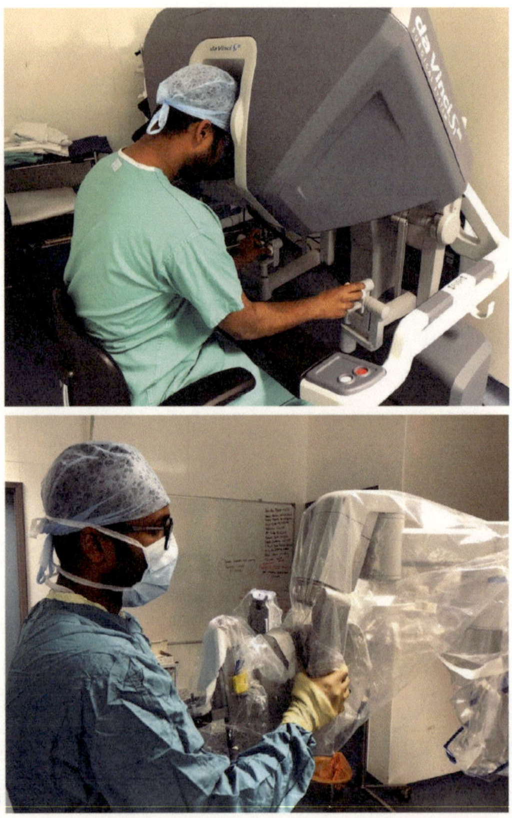

a

b

Figure 3. Resident training. (a) Console training for the robot; (b) Patient-side robotic raining.

Trainee surgeons believe that robotic training is necessary to their future [17], although we know that all will not be robotic surgeons in the current climate. Interesting issues are raised when these trainees only work in robotic centres, where they are only exposed to robotic surgery, effectively missing the opportunities to undertake open surgery.

The robot is a relatively easy tool to use, but the resident will still need the trainer and operating room team to support training, particularly with time pressures in a busy operating room. Incorporating training within the training programme is a significant challenge. The aim should be to train the doctor without lowering the standard of patient outcome. Robotics lends itself to this objective, with stepwise training and short learning curves. Currently, surgical training simulators are being used for teaching, but they only allow initial training [18, 19]. Newer, dual-console robots (dual control) allow the teacher a level of comfort while teaching, but without this there are a number of important teaching processes to assure safety, including combining virtual, augmented training with modular training. It is therefore essential that robotic surgical educators have a comfort level both with performing the surgical procedure and communicating with the assistant to teach the procedure [12, 20] (see **Figure 4**).

Sachdeva et al. [21] summarized three steps involved in trying to train with novel technologies: (i) perceptual awareness, incorporating cognitive understanding of the surgery and visualizing the surgery; (ii) guided learning, in a modular fashion, with immediate mentor feedback, in order to learn correctly; and (iii) autonomous refinement of learning, in which

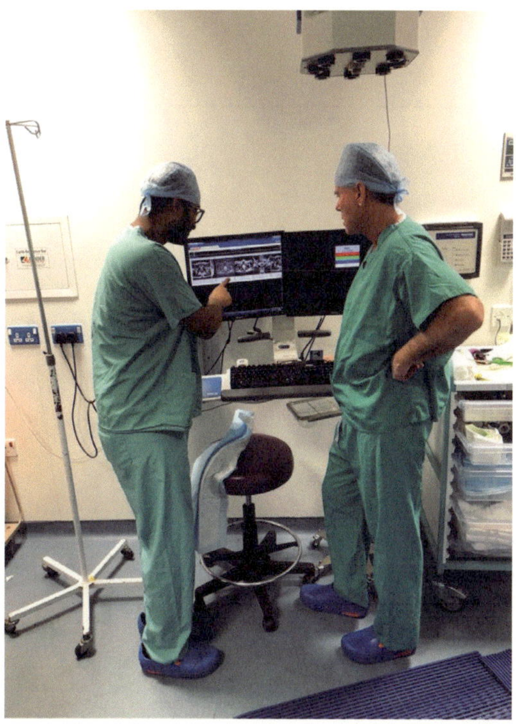

Figure 4. Planning and training presurgery.

No. of		Module				
step	Description of surgical procedure	1	2	3	4	5
1	Placing trocar and dissecting the preperitoneal space	X				
2	Pelvic lymphadenectomy		X			
3	Incising the endopelvic fascia and dissecting the puboprostatic ligaments	X				
4	Ligating Santorini's plexus			X		
5	Bladder neck dissection					
	Anterior and lateral bladder neck		X			
	Dorsal bladder neck			X		
6	Identifying and dissecting the vasa deferentia			X		
7	Dissecting the seminal vesicles			X		
8	Incising posterior Denonvilliers' fascia and mobilizing the dorsal surface of the prostate from the rectum			X		
9	Dissecting the prostatic pedicles			X		
10	Nerve-sparing					X
11	Apical dissection				X	
12	Urethro-vesical anastomosis					
	Dorsal circumference (4, 5, 6, 7, 8 o'clock sutures)				X	
	3 and 9 o'clock sutures		X			
	Bladder neck closure and 11 and 1 o'clock sutures			X		

Modified from Ref. [22].

Table 1. Modular steps for RARP.

precision and efficiency are improved. These steps are logical to any expert trainer, and they are incorporated in the ERUS host robotic training centre curriculum, which are based on modular training [22] (**Tables 1** and **2**).

At present, laboratory-based experience is available for training with the da Vinci Surgical System's inanimate, cadaveric, or animate models [23]. Beyond the point of training laboratories, residents are able to be fellowship train, under supervision by experts within real operating rooms, with the consent of the patients.

The ongoing issue about where robotic surgical training should be deployed (e.g. post-basic training or postgraduate training) continues among robotic trainers around the world. However, surgery in general is becoming more subspecialist, and therefore not all trainee doctors need robotic training.

In our opinion, placing robot-assisted surgery as a category like its predecessor, laparoscopy, is not appropriate. The robot is a facilitating tool, for treating a disease. It would be sensible to train surgeons in robotics as part of specializing in a disease process. The difficulty arises when surgery is superseded by the next iteration of treatments.

http://dx.doi.org/10.5772/intechopen.86026

Step	Module	Description	Competency	Sign off
1a	I	Transperitoneal access—trocar placement, incision of ventral peritoneum, and dissection of Retzius space	Level Date	
1b	II	Extraperitoneal access—trocar placement and dissection of preperitoneal space	Level Date	
2	I	Set-up of da Vinci robot	Level Date	
3	III	Pelvic lymphadenectomy	Level Date	
4	I	Incision of endopelvic fascia and dissection of puboprostatic ligaments	Level Date	
5	II	Anterior and lateral bladder neck dissection	Level Date	
6	III	Posterior bladder neck dissection	Level Date	
7	I	Dissection and division of vas deferens	Level Date	
8	III	Dissection of seminal vesicles	Level Date	
9	III	Incision/dissection of posterior Denonvillier's fascia and mobilization of prostate from the rectum	Level Date	
10a	III	Dissection of prostatic pedicles (non-nerve spare)	Level Date	
10b	V	Dissection of prostatic pedicles (nerve spare)	Level Date	
11	II	DVC ligation	Level Date	
12	IV	Apical dissection	Level Date	
13a	III	Rocco stitch	Level Date	

Step	Module	Description	Competency	Sign off
13b	III	Posterior vesico-urethral anastomosis	Level Date	
13c	II	Lateral and anterior vesico-urethral anastomosis	Level Date	
13d	II	Bladder neck closure	Level Date	

Table 2. Resident diary.

8. Conclusion

Robotic Renal Surgery can be safely adopted and implemented in modern day clinical practice using a team based approach.

Author details

Christopher J. Anderson[1*] and Hiten R.H. Patel[2]

*Address all correspondence to: cja@doctors.org.uk

1 Department of Urology, St Georges University Hospital, ERUS-EAU Host Robotic Training Centre, Accredited Royal College of Surgeons Senior Clinical Robotic Fellowship Centre, London, UK

2 Department of Urology, University Hospital North Norway, Tromso, Norway

References

[1] Joseph JV, Vicente I, Madeb R, Erturk E, Patel HR. Robot-assisted vs pure laparoscopic radical prostatectomy: Are there any differences? BJU International. 2005;**96**(1):39-42

[2] Patel HR, Linares A, Joseph JV. Robotic and laparoscopic surgery: Cost and training. Surgical Oncology. 2009;**18**(3):242-246

[3] Patel HR, Mould T, Joseph JV, Delaney C. Pelvic Cancer Surgery. London: Springer-Verlag; 2005

[4] Ellison JS, Lendvay TS. Robot-assisted ureteroureterostomy in paediatric patients: Current perspectives. Robotic Surgery. 2017;**4**:45-55

[5] Link RE, Bhayani SB, Kavoussi LR. A prospective comparison of robotic and laparoscopic pyeloplasty. Annals of Surgery. 2006;**243**(4):486-491

[6] Scales CD Jr, Jones PJ, Eisenstein EL, Preminger GM, Albala DM. Local cost structures and the economics of robot assisted radical prostatectomy. Journal of Urology. 2005;**174**(6):2323-2329

[7] https://uroweb.org/section/erus/robotic-curriculum/

[8] Ahlering TE, Skarecky D, Lee D, Clayman RV. Successful transfer of open surgical skills to a laparoscopic environment using a robotic interface: Initial experience with laparoscopic radical prostatectomy. The Journal of Urology. 2003;**170**(5):1738-1741

[9] GT S, Gill IS, Hsu TH. Robotic-assisted laparoscopic pyeloplasty: A pilot study. Urology. 1999;**53**(6):1099-1103

[10] Prasad SM, Maniar HS, Soper NJ, Damiano RJ Jr, Klingensmith ME. The effect of robotic assistance on learning curves for basic laparoscopic skills. American Journal of Surgery. 2002;**183**(6):702-707

[11] Hanly EJ, Marohn MR, Bachman SL, Talamini MA, Hacker SO, Howard RS, et al. Multiservice laparoscopic surgical training using the daVinci surgical system. American Journal of Surgery. 2004;**187**(2):309-315

[12] Erridge S, Yeung DKT, Patel HRH, Purkayastha S. Telementoring of surgeons: A systematic review. Surgical Innovation. 2018;**22**:1553350618813250. DOI: 10.1177/1553350618813250. [Epub ahead of print]

[13] https://www.sages.org/publications/guidelines/consensus-document-robotic-surgery/

[14] www.baus.org.uk/_userfiles/pages/files/Publications/Robotic%20Surgery%20 Curriculum.pdf

[15] Patel HRH, Joseph JV, editors. Simulation Training in Laparoscopy and Robotic Surgery. London: Springer-Verlag; 2012

[16] Sood A, Jeong W, Ahlawat R, et al. Robotic surgical skill acquisition: What one needs to know? Journal of Minimal Access Surgery. 2015;**11**(1):10-15

[17] Farivar BS, Flannagan M, Leitman IM. General surgery residents' perception of robot-assisted procedures during surgical training. Journal of Surgical Education. 2015;**72**(2):235-242

[18] Lerner MA, Ayalew M, Peine WJ, Sundaram CP. Does Training on a Virtual Reality Robotic Simulator Improve Performance on the da Vinci Surgical System? Journal of Endourology. 2010;**24**(3):467-472

[19] Patel HR, Patel BP. Virtual reality surgical simulation in training. Expert Review of Anticancer Therapy. 2012;**12**(4):417-420

[20] Budrionis A, Augestad KM, Patel HR, Bellika JG. An evaluation framework for defining the contributions of telestration in surgical telementoring. Interactive Journal of Medical Research. 2013;**2**(2):e14

[21] Sachdeva AK, Buyske J, Dunnington GL, Sanfey HA, Mellinger JD, Scott DJ, et al. A new paradigm for surgical procedural training. Current Problems in Surgery. 2011 Dec;**48**(12):854-968

[22] JU S, Schwaibold H, Bhanot SM, Rabenalt R, Do M, Truss M, et al. Modular surgical training for endoscopic extraperitoneal radical prostatectomy. BJU International. 2005;**96**(7):1022-1027

[23] Schreuder H, Wolswijk R, Zweemer R, Schijven M, Verheijen R. Training and learning robotic surgery, time for a more structured approach: A systematic review. BJOG. 2012;**119**:137-149

Chapter 14

Robot-Assisted Partial Nephrectomy: Evolving Techniques

Mohammed Kamil Quraishi, Edward Ramez Latif, Milan Thomas, Ben Eddy, Elio Mazzone and Alexandre Mottrie

Additional information is available at the end of the chapter

http://dx.doi.org/10.5772/intechopen.89712

Abstract

Robotic-assisted partial nephrectomy is now embraced in urology as a recommended treatment option for small localised renal tumours. There is an increasing trend towards setting up robotic-assisted services in urological centres across the world. Our aim is to review the available published common robotic-assisted partial nephrectomy techniques. We present our institutions' established step-by-step technique for performing robotic-assisted partial nephrectomy, in order to guide aspiring urologists interested in performing robotic-assisted partial nephrectomies. The importance of pre-operative review of imaging in a multi-disciplinary approach is critical. We emphasise certain tips inperforming a safer procedure.

Keywords: robotic, partial, nephrectomy, technique, procedure

1. Anatomy

Specific anatomical consideration needs to be given to the hilar and tumour anatomy. In particular this includes reviewing the size, location within the kidney, and the degree of the exophytic nature of the tumour, in robotic-assisted partial nephrectomy. A thorough pre-operative review of the cross-sectional imaging and patient factors needs to be considered in a multi-disciplinary setting. Each hospital uses their own CT protocol, however we perform a pre-contrast and post contrast nephrogenic phase to assess renal mass enhancement. An arterial and delayed excretory phase may also be added for surgical planning. These phases clarify the presence of variant anatomy including feeding vessels to the tumour or accessory renal veins. It also helps demarcate the distance of the tumour from the renal hilum and the collecting system [1]. The anatomical relations play an important role, particularly in hilar dissection, including the presence of the head of the pancreas and part of the duodenum overlying the right renal hilum. The left hilum is in close proximity to the body and tail of the pancreas, with the left colonic flexure bordering the left kidney anteriorly. In nearly 30% of cases more than one renal artery is identified supplying a kidney, often on the right side [2]. The renal arteries run posteriorly from the aorta to the kidneys, due to the orientation of the renal hilum. The arteries split into four anterior and one posterior segmental branches at the renal hilum [3]. The renal arteries sit in the middle at the hilum, with the renal veins anteriorly and the ureters/collecting systems posterior to the artery [4]. Multiple variants in renal artery anatomy have been reported in the literature, thereby highlighting the close attention warranted during the review of preoperative imaging [3, 5].

2. Introduction

We use a standardised four robotic arm technique using the for renal surgery the Da Vinci Si Surgical system (Intuitive Surgical Inc., Sunnyvale, CA, USA). Suitable training must be achieved to acquire appropriate robotic skills before performing complex renal surgery. We recommend a modular training programme in keeping with European and British board standards [6, 7].

Ensuring that the early stages of the learning curve are supervised with a mentor is essential to reduce errors and aid development of confidence in robotic skills. Evidence on learning curves vary in robotic-assisted partial nephrectomy (RAPN), with a study reporting 44 case requirement by a laparoscopically trained surgeon, to achieve a warm ischaemia time (WIT) of less than 20 min and an operative time of less than 120 min [8]. An alternative report by another centre identified needing to perform 61–90 cases to reach a trifecta of no significant complications, negative surgical margins and WIT of less than 25 min [9]. Needless to say learning curves can be improved with better training techniques, volume and exposure [10]. WIT was found to decrease to 13 from 20 min, following performing 150 RAPN cases compared to the first 10 cases [11]. Robotic trainees under expert supervision were found to have longer operating and warm ischaemia time, but otherwise no worse outcomes than experts performing robotic partial nephrectomies [12]. In addition the patient-side assistant should be appropriately skilled in handling instruments safely and deploying ligature clips. All cases should be subjected to nephrometry scoring (PADUA and RENAL) and a thorough imaging review preoperatively to predict operative complexities and postoperative complications [13–16]. We incorporate the PADUA score due to its standardised use across the national nephrectomy register, collected by the British Association of Urological Surgeons.

3. Patient positioning

The authors recommend this operative approach, based on the available disseminated techniques and preference in their experience and training [17–24]. In order to perform a robotic-assisted partial nephrectomy, the patient is positioned in a lateral decubitus/flank position (**Figure 1**) on the operative table to aid bowel mobilisation [24]. The operative table

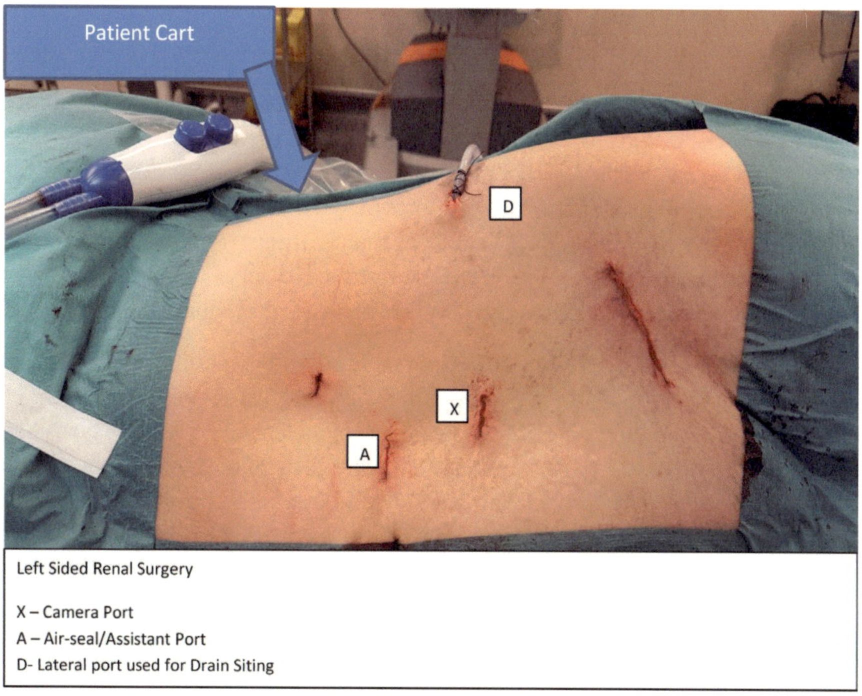

Figure 1. Full flank patient positioning for left RAPN. Note port site marking made prior to knife to skin.

is subsequently broken/flexed. This opens the flank, between the costal margin and the iliac crest. A reported variation may include a slight Trendelenburg position and a flat table [23]. The anterior abdomen lies on the edge of the operative table. The upper arm is flexed at the elbow and kept adjacent to the face [21]. We prefer adhesive tape to secure the patient to the bed, at the level of the iliac crest [23]. Additional adhesive tape used at the level of the mid thoracic cavity should be applied with caution to avoid reduced chest expansion, in the context of ventilation. The back can be stabilised using an additional back support attachment with gel pads. The bottom leg in the lateral position is flexed to 90° at the knee, and is separated from the extended top leg using pillows. All pressure points are padded [23]. A nasogastric tube (NGT) is placed in left sided tumours and a urinary catheter is inserted following anaesthetic induction for all cases, and prior to patient positioning [21]. The NGT is removed in recovery.

3.1. Tips and tricks

- A consistent surgical team who develop skills progressively with the surgeon, specifically for renal surgery is essential for optimal outcomes. Robotic renal surgery is approached differently from pelvic surgery and cannot instantly be translated.
- It is vital that your anaesthetic staff is experienced with patient positioning and moving for robotic renal surgery.

A uniform anaesthetic team will also lead to better pain control in the post-operative phase and consistently enhanced results particularly during the critical on-clamp (WIT) period of partial nephrectomy.

4. Port placement

Precise port placement and patient cart position are important for successful outcomes in robotic renal surgery. Unlike in pelvic surgery, the operative field is wider increasing the potential for robot arms to clash. With some basic principles, success can be replicated case after case. As with radical prostatectomy, the ports must be placed with a minimum 8 cm distance apart. However, with different laterality of renal surgery, an additional consideration is placing arm 3 of the patient cart. In the case of right sided renal tumours, arm 3 should be positioned on the left of the cart stem. The reverse is true for left renal surgery.

We recommend marking the skin to plan port positioning. Formation of a skewed cross or upside-down kite shape should be made with the camera port forming the apex. However the reference point should be the subcostal port, as it offers least flexibility in positioning. The camera port, target organ and patient cart should form a straight line, thereby creating adequate triangulation for safe operating. The contralateral operating port will form a horizontal line to the subcostal port, with the camera port bisecting this line in the middle (**Figure 2**).

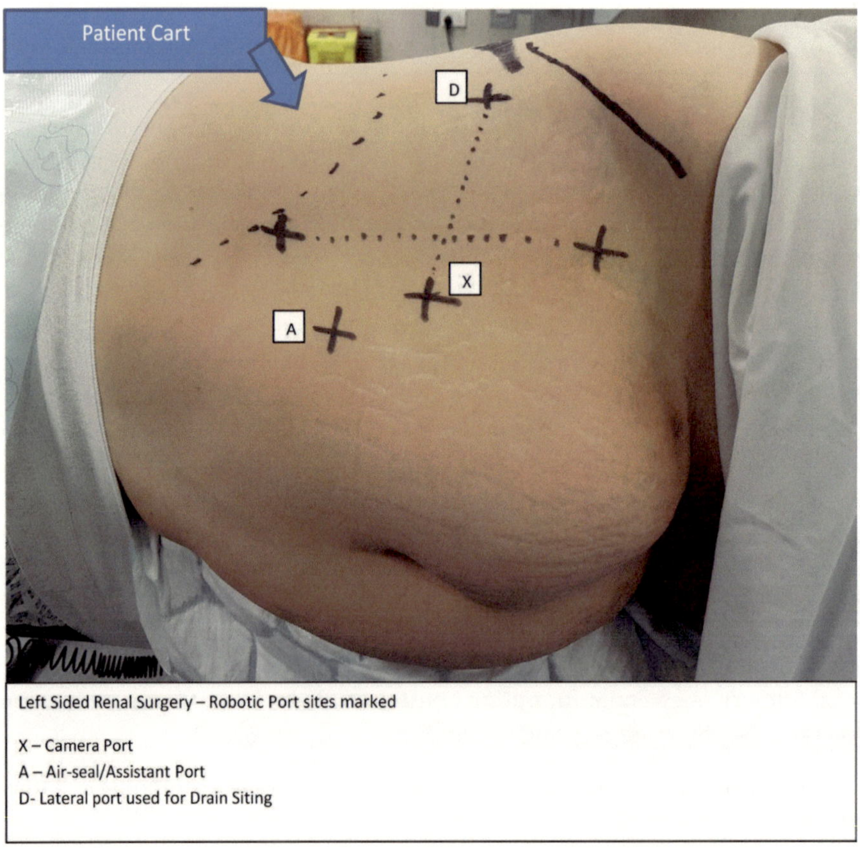

Figure 2. Port site marking for a right RAPN.

This should give adequate room for the 4th robotic arm port, which will then complete the kite or cross shape, placed laterally roughly in the anterior axillary line. It is possible that arm 1 (when operating on the right kidney) can hold the ProGrasp™ forceps, rather than arm 3. The robot is then manipulated to dock over the patient's upper shoulder at an angle of 45 degrees to the kidney.

4.1. Tips and tricks

- Use of the bariatric ports can be beneficial to achieve greater distance between the robot arms, particularly in smaller patients. This will reduce the potential for robot arm clashing.
- Should the arms clash, then 'burping' the ports away from each other can create additional room and potentially avoid restricted movement of the instruments, which can severely limit surgical progress. The ports placed under traction, tents the abdominal wall externally, increasing intra-abdominal space to work in [25].

5. Surgical technique

Evidence from a meta-analysis reveals similar surgical outcomes and complications between transperitoneal and retroperitoneal robot-assisted partial nephrectomies. The retroperitoneal approach may have a specific role in selected cases including posterior tumours and in patients with pervious significant transperitoneal surgery. Absence of the need to mobilise bowel and easy access to the hilar vessels, leads to a shorter operative time [26]. However, the choice between retroperitoneal or transperitoneal approach lies based on surgeon's expertise and patient factors [17].

We recommend a trans-peritoneal approach, particularly in the early phase of the learning curve. This will ensure that adjacent structures can be adequately mobilised away from the kidney. In addition, operative space is optimised when within the peritoneum. This will avoid injury to sensitive structures such as the duodenum on the right and the spleen; tail of the pancreas and duodeno-jejunal junction on the left. The authors recommend using a 0° camera lens in the early learning curve period, unless experienced in 30° downward scope lens from laparoscopic surgery [23]. Use of 30° downward lens has a role in the later stages of dissecting posterior tumours [24]. A pneumoperitoneum of 10–12 mmHg is established. In almost all cases the kidney can be adequately mobilised to expose renal masses to perform a partial nephrectomy successfully in the trans-peritoneal approach. However, some surgeons transferring from retroperitoneal laparoscopic surgery may feel suitably experienced in translating skills to perform retroperitoneal robotic surgery. Guides are available on performing retroperitoneal RAPN [27, 28].

A wide array of instruments and preferences exist in performing a RAPN. The authors perform the procedure with the surgeon holding the EndoWrist® Fenestrated Bipolar Forceps and the EndoWrist® Hot Shears™ monopolar curved scissors in the non-dominant and dominant hand robotic ports respectively. Sharp dissection is performed along the white line of Toldt.

Sharp and blunt dissection is used to reflect the large bowel off the anterior surface of Gerota' fascia [24]. Dissection is directed to the inferior border of Gerota's fascia in order to locate the ureter. Release of attachments from adjacent structures including liver or spleen may be performed to characterise the planes clearly. The psoas major muscle is used as a landmark to help identify the ureter, similar to a laparoscopic approach. The ureter is then dissected cranially to identify the renal hilum [23]. Specific care should be taken to control, or avoid injury to the gonadal vessels. The additional robotic arm, holding the ProGrasp™ forceps can now be deployed to retract the kidney laterally, thereby creating space to dissect the hilum safely away from sensitive medial structures (such as the duodenum or inferior vena cava). The Force Bipolar™ is a new instrument which combines the ProGrasp™ grasping qualities with bipolar diathermy and may be incorporated instead for efficiency. In right sided tumours, the hilum can be approached from a cranial to caudal direction, enabling earlier access to the renal artery. The Inferior Vena Cava just below the liver can be easily identified and followed caudally to reach the renal pedicle in right sided tumours.

Hilar dissection requires sensitive movements to adequately expose all renal vessels (one at a time) to allow for application of clamps later in the operation. This enables precise control in case of unexpected haemorrhage. We recommend clamping the main renal artery early in the learning curve, rather than attempting to selectively clamp more distal segmental branches. Near-infrared fluorescence imaging system with indocyanine green is an available technology allowing identification of intraoperative parenchymal perfusion, thereby enabling selective vessel clamping for limiting ischaemia to the tumour alone. It has been shown to improve early functional outcomes, with better preservation of glomerular filtration rate of the resected kidney on renal scan with Tc 99 m-DTPA [29]. Once the main artery is exposed, a short sling can be placed and held in place by a suitable arterial clip (to the rubber sling ends alone), we use a Weck® Hem-o-lok® ligating clip.

At this stage exposure of the renal tumour proceeds by incising Gerota's fascia and 'defatting' the kidney adequately, preferably along the renal capsular plane. This will enable adequate exposure of the renal tumour and mobilise the kidney to achieve a wide surgical field to perform the excision. The drop-in ultrasound probe is introduced and manipulated by the surgeon using the ProGrasp™ forceps to distinguish tumour margins [17]. The tumour is marked superficially on the renal capsule with the Hot Shears™ curved monopolar diathermy scissors, leaving a 5 mm margin for oncological outcomes.

All accessory equipment is introduced through the assistant port, including the arterial clamps. Two absorbable monofilament sutures such as Poliglecaprone, e.g. Monocryl® 3–0 and two absorbable braided sutures such as Polyglactin, e.g. 0-Vicryl®, cut to size are strategically positioned in the abdomen for easy access during renorrhaphy.

At this stage a brief 'time-out' ensures that the surgeon and the surgical team are aware of the ensuing critical element of the operation—sometimes known as 'on-clamp time'. This provides ample opportunity to ensure that there is adequate insufflation gas in the tanks, that additional sutures are readily available and that the anaesthetist is prepared for potential haemorrhage. At this stage it is recommended to re-review the CT images to ensure that the shape of the renal mass can be translated to the operative field. The authors do not recommend the usage of Mannitol in view of its limited evidence in minimising loss of renal function post operatively in humans [30].

To minimise the dangers associated with, the next step is performed after unanimous readiness of the theatre staff. A Scanlan® Reliance Bulldog Clamp (Scanlan® International, St. Paul, MN, USA) is applied to the renal artery, in selected cases this is followed by another on the renal vein [23]. Satinsky clamp is an option in the rare difficult dissections when bleeding from the renal pedicle impairs ability to clamp the vessels with a bulldog clamp [31]. The clamping marks the triggering of a stopwatch, to measure warm ischaemic time.

The tumour is excised with consideration of surgical margins, with the assistant surgeon ensuring the field is adequately exposed by suctioning away blood. The sliding-clip renorrhaphy principle is applied to close the renal defect, in multiple layers. The deep layer of the renorrhaphy is performed with the poliglecaprone 3–0 suture, with a Weck® Hem-o-lok® ligating clip already attached at one end. A continuous suture runs through the base of the defect closing any open collecting system and small vessels. If arterial bleeds are detected these can be closed individually with additional monofilament sutures to ensure meticulous haemostasis. Once the continuous running poliglecaprone suture is applied, a Hem-o-lok® clip is applied to the needle end. Traction is applied to the needle end to snug the clip down against the renal capsule, bringing the renal defect together. Larger defects will require multiple sutures. We use an early 'off-clamp' technique after the deep sliding-clip renorraphy is complete, in the order of release of renal vein, followed by the artery, where the vein has been clamped. This reduces the warm ischaemic time. We do not use a bolster. At this stage haemostasis is adequate to complete the superficial sliding-clip renorrhaphy suture with a large polyglactin suture. In this layer, clips are applied at every throw through the renal capsule to further close the defect. A second locking clip can be applied above every previous clip on the sliding suture to prevent slipping. Use of adjuncts to haemostasis is not essential but may provide added security and further minimise blood loss. This may be in the form of Floseal®, Surgicel® or Evicel®. The hilum and excision site are carefully inspected following this step, to ensure haemostasis is achieved. We recommend closing Gerota's fascia, which may minimise difficulty in future renal surgery from scarring [24]. An intra-abdominal drain is inserted through the lateral port. The specimen is removed using an endocatch pouch, inserted through the assistant's port.

5.1. Tips and tricks

- A 'time-out' is taken to assess the tumour excision, the associated renal defect and the plan for renorraphy prior to the on-clamp time, will in our experience lead to better planning and a potentially safer procedure.
- Use of intraoperative doppler ultrasound is widely recommended for use in partial nephrectomy.
- Plan your incision on the Gerota's fascia carefully will help with closure after. Practice often on simulators to ensure that your suturing skills are adequate to perform renorrhaphy under the pressure of limited time, whilst the clamp clock is ticking.

- An apron of Perinephric fat can be placed behind the posterior surface of the kidney, to anteriorly displace the kidney. This improves access to posterior and lateral tumours. If there is inadequate Perinephric fat, tonsil swabs can be placed instead.

This is our summarised technique that is performed in our practice, which can be adopted by departments interested in developing a robotic partial nephrectomy service.

6. Indication and guidelines

Both EAU and AUA guidelines advise minimally invasive surgery if possible, however advise caution if perioperative, oncological or functional outcomes are at risk of compromise [32, 33]. In fact, EAU recommend partial nephrectomy over radical in patients with T1 tumours, even if an open approach is warranted. Any approach for PN is valid based on the surgeons skill and preference.

The EAU advise that despite the similar cancer specific survival and recurrence free survival for pT1 tumours in the comparison of partial versus radical nephrectomy; partial nephrectomy is still the ideal treatment in view of minimising impairment to renal function and preventing metabolic and cardiovascular disorders in the long term. Retrospective studies have revealed no difference in long term overall and cancer specific survival between laparoscopic and open partial nephrectomies [34, 35].

Prospective comparison of robotic-assisted versus open partial nephrectomy found significant improvement in estimated blood loss and length of stay in the cohort undergoing RAPN. Early and short term complications, operative time and warm ischaemia time were similar between both approaches [36]. Robotic-assisted surgery was found be superior to laparoscopic PN with regards to conversion to open, conversion to radical nephrectomy, warm ischaemia time and length of stay. This meta-analysis of 23 studies also concluded no difference in short term postoperative complications, operative time, estimated blood loss and positive margins [37].

7. Future developments

We describe a few developing technologies which may be of interest to urologists.

Reconstruction and navigation technology appears to have an emerging role in both preoperative and intraoperative planning and operative assistance. A diverse group of 108 urologists of various training experience changed their views to feel an RAPN over a radical nephrectomy was indicated from 47–75% of the 20 complex cases reviewed following a re-review of the CT scan with three dimensional reconstruction of the renal units [38].

Hyperaccuracy three dimensional (HA3D) is an emerging technology allowing three dimensional reconstructions, enabling virtual mapping of the in-vivo structures with the reconstructed model during the partial nephrectomy. A small sample sized study in complex renal tumours (PADUA >10), using this HA3D technology enabled intraoperative management of the pedicle as preoperatively planned in 90% of the cases [39]. The accuracy of the arterial reconstruction enabled preoperative simulation of vascular ischaemia by selective clamping. This enabled reduction of global ischaemia from 81–24% with the use of the HA3D technology [39].

Near-infrared fluorescence (NIRF) technology using an intravenous contrast medium (e.g. Indocyanine green) enables identification of the segmental vessels perfusing the renal tumour, by switching between white light and fluorescence enhanced views intraoperatively [40]. NIRF RAPN has been found to have a lower loss in renal scan confirmed renal function in the operated unit and a lower reduction in Glomerular Filtration Rate (GFR of 8%)compared to standard RAPN without selective vessel clamping. In three of the 15 NIRF RAPN cases, selective clamping was converted to standard clamping as incomplete ischaemia of the tumour was identified. This demonstrates NIFRs growing benefit over non-NIFR selective clamping.

Urologists participating in a study on 3D (Three Dimensional) printed models of the kidney, favoured its use in preoperative planning, patient counselling and surgical training [41]. The authors report maximal benefit of these models in patients with complex renal vasculature [42].

8. Conclusion

Our technique offers a standardised approach to aspiring urologists in performing robotic-assisted partial nephrectomies. We expect urologists to have the appropriate level of training and supervision prior to performing this procedure. We highlight a variety of tips and tricks that have benefitted our team in performing safer and easier surgery. We describe the stance of guidelines of robotic surgery in partial nephrectomies. We highlight emerging technologies which may become incorporated into the future practice of robotic surgery.

Author details

Mohammed Kamil Quraishi[1]*, Edward Ramez Latif[1], Milan Thomas[1], Ben Eddy[1], Elio Mazzone[2] and Alexandre Mottrie[2]

*Address all correspondence to: mkquraishi@doctors.org.uk

1 Kent and Canterbury Hospital, Canterbury, UK

2 O.L.V. Hospital, Aalst, Belgium

References

[1] Kang SK, Kim D, Chandarana H. Contemporary imaging of the renal mass. Current Urology Reports. 2011;**12**:11. DOI: 10.1007/s11934-010-0148-y

[2] Leung DA, Hagspiel KD, Angle JF, et al. MR angiography of the renal arteries. Radiologic Clinics of North America. 2002;**40**:847-865

[3] Hazırolan T, Öz M, Türkbey B, et al. Diagnostic and Interventional Radiology. 2011;**17**: 67-73

[4] Rocco F, Cozzi G. Renal anatomy, physiology and its clinical relevance to partial nephrectomy. In: Patel V, editor. Robotic Urologic Surgery. London: Springer; 2012

[5] Sampaio FJB, Passos M. Renal arteries: Anatomic study for surgical and radiological practice. Surgical and Radiologic Anatomy. 1992;**14**:113-117

[6] British Association of Urological Surgeons (BAUS) Robotic Surgery Curriculum – Guidelines for Training. Available from: https://www.baus.org.uk/_userfiles/pages/files/Publications/Robotic%20Surgery%20Curriculum.pdf. [Accessed: Sep 2018]

[7] Sridhar A, Briggs T, Kelly J, Nathan S. Training in robotic surgery—An overview. Current Urology Reports. 2017;**18**:58

[8] Dias BH, Ali MS, Dubey S, Krishnaswamy SA, Rao AR, Dubey D. Impact of learning curve on the perioperative outcomes following robotic-assisted partial nephrectomy for renal tumours. Indian Journal of Urology. 2018;**34**:62-67

[9] Omidele OO, Davoudzadeh N, Palese M. Trifecta outcomes to assess learning curve of robotic partial nephrectomy. JSLS. 2018;**22**: pii e2017.00064

[10] Peyronnet B, Tondut L, Bernhard JC, et al. Impact of hospital volume and surgeon volume on robot-assisted partial nephrectomy outcomes: A multicentre study. BJU International. 2018;**121**(6):916-922. DOI: 10.1111/bju.14175

[11] Larcher A et al. The learning curve for robot-assisted partial nephrectomy: Impact of surgical experience on perioperative outcomes. European Urology. 2018;**75**:253-256. DOI: 10.1016/j.eururo.2018.08.042

[12] Khene ZE, Peyronnet B, Bosquet E. Does training of fellows affect peri-operative outcomes of robot-assisted partial nephrectomy? BJU International. 2017;**120**(4):591-599. DOI: 10.1111/bju.13901

[13] Garisto et al. Precise clamping of renal artery with endovascular stents during robotic partial nephrectomy: Technical hints to optimize outcomes. Urology. 2018;**118**:239-240

[14] Corradi RB, Vertosick EA, Nguyen DP, et al. Nephrometry scores and perioperative outcomes following robotic partial nephrectomy. International Brazilian Journal of Urology: Official Journal of the Brazilian Society of Urology. 2017;**43**(6):1075-1083. DOI: 10.1590/S1677-5538.IBJU.2016.0571

[15] Kutikov A, Uzzo RG. The R.E.N.A.L. nephrometry score: A comprehensive standardized system for quantitating renal tumor size, location and depth. The Journal of Urology. 2009;**182**:844-853

[16] Ficarra V, Novara G, Secco S, Macchi V, Porzionato A, De Caro R, et al. Preoperative aspects and dimensions used for an anatomical (PADUA) classification of renal tumours in patients who are candidates for nephron-sparing surgery. European Urology. 2009;**56**:786-793

[17] Novara G, Falce SL, Kungulli A, et al. Robot-assisted partial nephrectomy. International Journal of Surgery. 2016;**36**:554-559

[18] Shwartz MJ, Rais-Bahrami S, Kavoussi LR. Laparoscopic and robotic surgery of the kidney. In: Wein AJ, Kavoussi LR, Partin AW, Peters CA, editors. Campbell-Walsh Urology. 11th ed. Philadelphia, PA: Elsevier; 2016. chap 61

[19] Walsh AJ, Kavoussi LR, Partin AW, et al. editors. Campbell-Walsh Urology; 11th Edition. 2016

[20] Benjamin Pradere B, Peyronnet B, Khene Z, et al. Simplified robot-assisted partial nephrectomy: Step-by-step technique and perioperative outcomes. Journal of Robotic Surgery. 2018;**13**:245-251. DOI: 10.1007/s11701-018-0845-y

[21] Kallingal GJS, Swain S, Darwiche F. Robotic partial nephrectomy with the Da Vinci Xi. Advances in Urology. 2016;**2016**:9675095. DOI:10.1155/2016/9675095

[22] Kaouk JH, Khalifeh A, Hillyer S, et al. Robot-assisted laparoscopic partial nephrectomy: step-by-step contemporary technique and surgical outcomes at a single high-volume institution. European Urology. 2012;**62**:553-561

[23] Kaouk JH, Khalifeh A, Hillyer S, et al. Robot-assisted laparoscopic partial nephrectomy: Step-by-step contemporary technique and surgical outcomes at a single high-volume institution. European Urology. 2012;**62**:553-561

[24] Rogers CG, Singh A, Blatt A, et al. Robotic partial nephrectomy for complex renal tumors: Surgical technique. Urology. 2008;**53**(3):514-521. DOI: 10.1016/j.eururo.2007.09.047

[25] Chang C, Steinberg Z, Shah A, Gundeti MS. Patient positioning and port placement for robot-assisted surgery. Journal of Endourology. 2014;**28**(6):631-638. DOI: 10.1089/end.2013.0733

[26] Xia L, Zhang X, Wang X. Transperitoneal versus retroperitoneal robot-assisted partial nephrectomy: A systematic review and meta-analysis. International Journal of Surgery. 2016;**30**:109-115

[27] Porreca A, D'Agostino D, Dente D, et al. Retroperitoneal approach for robot-assisted partial nephrectomy: Technique and early outcomes. International Braz J Urol. 2018;**44**:63-68

[28] Ghani KR, Porter J, Mennon M, et al. Robotic retroperitoneal partial nephrectomy: A step-by-step guide. BJU International. 2014;**114**:311-313

[29] Mattevi D, Luciani LG, Mantovani W, et al. Fluorescence-guided selective arterial clamping during RAPN provides better early functional outcomes based on renal scan

compared to standard clamping. Journal of Robotic Surgery. 2018;**13**:391-396. DOI: 10.1007/s11701-018-0862-x

[30] Power NE, Maschino AC, Savage C, et al. Intraoperative mannitol use does not improve long-term renal function outcomes after minimally invasive partial nephrectomy. Urology. 2012;**79**(4):821-825. DOI: 10.1016/j.urology.2011.11.064

[31] Abdullah N, Rahbar H, Barod R. Use of the Satinsky clamp for hilar clamping during robotic partial nephrectomy: Indications, technique, and multi-center outcomes. Journal of Robotic Surgery. 2017;**11**:47-51. DOI: 10.1007/s11701-016-0611-y

[32] Ljunberg B, Albiges L, et al. EAU Guidelines on Renal Cell Carcinoma. Renal Cell Carcinoma - Limited Update March 2018. European Association of Urology 2018. Edn. Presented at the EAU Annual Congress Copenhagen 2018. ISBN: 978-94-92671-01-1

[33] Campbell S, Uzzo RG, et al. Renal Mass and Localized Renal Cancer: Aua Guideline. American Urological Association Education and Research, Inc®; 2017

[34] Lane BR et al. 7-year oncological outcomes after laparoscopic and open partial nephrectomy. The Journal of Urology. 2010;**183**:473

[35] Marszalek M et al. Laparoscopic and open partial nephrectomy: A matched-pair comparison of 200 patients. European Urology. 2009;**55**:1171

[36] Masson-Lecomte A et al. A prospective comparison of the pathologic and surgical outcomes obtained after elective treatment of renal cell carcinoma by open or robot-assisted partial nephrectomy. Urologic Oncology. 2013;**31**:924

[37] Choi JE et al. Comparison of perioperative outcomes between robotic and laparoscopic partial nephrectomy: A systematic review and meta-analysis. European Urology. 2015;**67**:891

[38] Bertolo R, Autorino R, Fiori C, et al. Expanding the indications of robotic partial nephrectomy for highly complex Renal tumors: Urologists' perception of the impact of Hyperaccuracy three-dimensional reconstruction. Journal of Laparoendoscopic & Advanced Surgical Techniques. Part A. 2019;**29**(2):233-239. DOI: 10.1089/lap.2018.0486

[39] Porpiglia F, Fiori C, Checcucci E, Amparore D, Bertolo R. Hyperaccuracy three-dimensional reconstruction is able to maximize the efficacy of selective clamping during robot-assisted partial nephrectomy for complex renal masses. European Urology. 2018;**74**(5):651-660

[40] Mattevi D, Luciani LG, Mantovani W, et al. Fluorescence-guided selective arterial clamping during RAPN provides better early functional outcomes based on renal scan compared to standard clamping. Journal of Robotic Surgery. 2018;**13**:391-396. DOI: 10.1007/s11701-018-0862-x

[41] Porpiglia F, Fiori C, Checcucci E, Amparore D, Bertolo R. Ther hyper- accuracy 3D reconstruction is able to maximize the efficacy of selective clamping during robot-assisted

partial nephrectomy for complex renal masses. European Urology. 2018;**74**:651-660. DOI: 10.1016/j.eururo.2017.12.027

[42] Wake N, Bjurlin MA, Rostami P, Chandarana H, Hua WC. Three-dimensional printing and augmented reality: Enhanced precision for robotic assisted partial nephrectomy. Urology. 2018;**116**:227-228